ENDOSCOPIC SURGERY
IN
OPHTHALMOLOGY

MARTIN URAM, M.D., M.P.H.

Retina Consultants
Little Silver, New Jersey

Illustrated by Tommy Graef

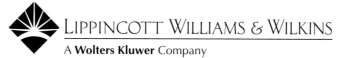 LIPPINCOTT WILLIAMS & WILKINS

A **Wolters Kluwer** Company

Philadelphia • Baltimore • New York • London
Buenos Aires • Hong Kong • Sydney • Tokyo

Acquisitions Editor: Jonathan Pine
Developmental Editor: Grace R. Caputo
Production Editor: Erica Woods Tucker
Manufacturing Manager: Colin Warnock
Cover Designer: Tommy Graef
Compositor: Lippincott Williams & Wilkins Desktop Division
Printer: Walsworth Publishing

Library of Congress Cataloging-in-Publication Data

Uram, Martin.
  Endoscopic surgery in ophthalmology / Martin Uram ; illustrated by Tommy Graef.
    p. ; cm.
  Includes bibliographical references and index.
  ISBN 0-7817-3651-X
  1. Eye—Endoscopic surgery. I. Title.
  [DNLM: 1. Endoscopy. 2. Ophthalmologic Surgical Procedures—methods. 3. Eye Diseases—surgery. WW 168 U72e 2003]
  RE80.U73 2003
  617.7′1—dc21
                                                                                                    2003045799

Care has been taken to confirm the accuracy of the information presented and to describe generally accepted practices. However, the author and publisher are not responsible for errors or omissions or for any consequences from application of the information in this book and make no warranty, expressed or implied, with respect to the currency, completeness, or accuracy of the contents of the publication. Application of this information in a particular situation remains the professional responsibility of the practitioner.

The author and publisher have exerted every effort to ensure that drug selection and dosage set forth in this text are in accordance with current recommendations and practice at the time of publication. However, in view of ongoing research, changes in government regulations, and the constant flow of information relating to drug therapy and drug reactions, the reader is urged to check the package insert for each drug for any change in indications and dosage and for added warnings and precautions. This is particularly important when the recommended agent is a new or infrequently employed drug.

Some drugs and medical devices presented in this publication have Food and Drug Administration (FDA) clearance for limited use in restricted research settings. It is the responsibility of the health care provider to ascertain the FDA status of each drug or device planned for use in their clinical practice.

10 9 8 7 6 5 4 3 2 1

ENDOSCOPIC SURGERY
IN
OPHTHALMOLOGY

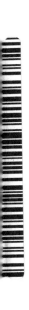

To my brilliant and beautiful wife, Susan Greenberg, M.D.

And to
Catie and Jesse Uram

CONTENTS

PREFACE

I was frustrated. Miffed. Personally, I hadn't had much luck with cyclocryotherapy for managing neovascular glaucoma. Then in 1986, I read an article by Ron Michel's group at the Wilmer Eye Institute. They described their technique for pars plana vitrectomy, lensectomy, scleral depression of the ciliary processes into the view of the operating microscope, and argon laser cyclophotocoagulation. This approach resulted in a high degree of success with little downside.

Later that evening, at a party attended mostly by ophthalmologists, I risked the derision of a few colleagues by expressing my genuine interest in that journal article. I clearly remember expounding on my enthusiasm for this approach although I recognized its severely limited applicability. If the laser could be combined with an endoscope, then surely we would be able to manage almost any form of glaucoma! *Incredulous* would best describe my audience's response.

After several years of letting the notion of a combined laser and endoscope smolder in my mental recycle bin, I found someone who could fabricate such a device, although a stretch in technology would be required. At the time, the smallest commercially available endoscope was 1.70 mm in outer diameter, and my requirement was for one that was 0.89 mm, including a laser fiber that would use 0.20 mm of the total size. All endoscopes had an eyepiece for the surgeon to look through. This arrangement would be too large, clumsy, and impractical for ophthalmic use, however.

The first laser endoscope was designed purely for video imaging, its size streamlined to match the typical endoilluminator or endophotocoagulation probe used in vitrectomy. Of course, this instrument couldn't work until, by trial and error, it was matched with a satisfactory video camera, light source, and video monitor. Ultimately, it proved to function well, and the first human endoscopic cyclophotocoagulation achieved an outstanding result. (Some video footage of this initial procedure can be seen on the accompanying DVDs.)

Over the years, I have gained quite a bit of experience combining endoscopy with anterior and posterior segment procedures. In no way, however, do I present myself as an authority on glaucoma, retinal, or oculoplastic surgery. On these topics, there are experts to whom I defer because of their profound knowledge, experience, and honesty. Rather, the purpose of *Endoscopic Surgery in Ophthalmology* is to share this alternative approach with anyone who might be interested, since I firmly believe that this technique represents a new level of patient care, from both a diagnostic and a therapeutic perspective.

If you are new to endoscopic eye surgery, you may well be dazzled by the photos and illustrations contained within. Most of the endoscopic images in this book and on the DVDs are unique. We believe that combining them with Tommy Graefe's minutely detailed illustrations, so that techniques are portrayed both endoscopically and graphically, increase their instructive value. To augment the text, the DVDs contains video clips of surgical procedures, complete with voiceover narration.

I hope that you will be as excited by this technology as I have always been. I am confident that this book and the DVDs will expand your understanding and skills in ophthalmic surgery.

Martin Uram, M.D., M.P.H.

ACKNOWLEDGMENTS

The initial development and subsequent proliferation of this technology and its associated treatment methodologies have been arduous and would not have materialized without the efforts of many people. I would like to acknowledge some of them here.

Edward Jaeger, M.D., and Thomas Duane, M.D., Ph.D., were instrumental in my education as an ophthalmologist. Vitaliano B. Bernardino, Jr., M.D., was mentor, friend, and iconoclast, who, by example, cultivated my need not only to acquire the classical information and skills in ophthalmology but also to perceive the difference between fact and mythology. Lawrence Yannuzzi, M.D., literally changed the course of my life. His generosity as a person, and especially as a teacher, is unparalleled.

One bizarre twist that ophthalmic endoscopy has made in my life was to force me to initiate, understand, and maintain the design, manufacturing, and regulatory processes associated with this technology—an eye-opening adventure, to be sure. While it might seem superfluous to this book, I can assure you that without the assistance of some key people there would be no ophthalmic endoscopy. Paula Ender has managed the proliferation of this technology with wisdom, grace, and humor. Gene Boccia and Tim Boyce are known to most of the ophthalmic endoscopists in the world for their patience and expertise. Jeff Damanti has become one of the most effective and prolific microendoscope craftsmen in the world. Art McKinley clearly reigns as the king of design optics, as well as a teacher and problem solver.

New technology cannot exist in a vacuum for long. Its survival becomes inextricably tied to commerce. Without establishment and maintenance of this relationship, the most profound development will disappear. Steve Kohn, first as my friend then as president and chief executive officer of Endo Optiks, has guided the steady course of this technology, at great personal expense, since its inception. Rich Camarra and Rob Travis have been instrumental in the proliferation of ophthalmic endoscopy outside of the United States. Mike Furgal, Kevin Burke, Mike Crocetta, Bob Blankemeyer, and Mike Nicoletta of Medtronic Ophthalmics have done a fantastic job in spreading laser endoscopy to a large and diverse audience of ophthalmologists.

Lloyd MacCauley, Esq., has not only been the keeper of intellectual property but also a key advisor in the development and progression of this technology. I doubt that the entire effort would have been initiated without his counsel.

Bill Pulford and Harry Betzel have been the design and manufacturing engineers for this complicated equipment for years. Their intellect, energy, and indulgence not only have made this approach to ophthalmic surgery possible but have seen it through multiple iterations and refinements. I will always be indebted to them.

Richard Ansell, Esq., has been a selfless advisor and great friend in this effort, helping me traverse what at times are some muddy waters, amusement being his only compensation.

There are many others who have helped ophthalmic endoscopy proliferate, too many to acknowledge them all here. Still, I want to thank Fred Blades, M.D., Lawrence Frieman, M.D., Harjit and Barinder Athwal, M.D., Fred Jackson, Ph.D., Dr.Sci., Ralph Del Negro, D.O., Anthony Micale, M.D., Johnny Gayton M.D., Stan Berke, M.D., I. Howard Fine, M.D., Marc Packer, M.D., Mike MacFarland, M.D., Philip Bloom, M.D., John Haley, M.D., and John Hunkeler, M.D.

Special thanks go to a few ophthalmologists who truly staked their reputations on this technology. Michael Lichtig, M.D., inadvertently guided me to a career in ophthalmology, only to become my great friend and unwavering supporter throughout the years. He was also the first ophthalmologist on earth to dare perform a combined phaco-ECP. Norman Medow, M.D., a Surgeon Director of the Manhattan Eye, Ear, and Throat Hospital, has been confidant, advisor, and psychiatrist for years and was first to consider ECP in the management of pediatric glaucoma. Francisco Lima, M.D., and Durval Cavalho, M.D., enthusiastically embraced this technology from its inception and have become perhaps the most experienced ophthalmic endoscopists in the world. Jorge Alvarado, M.D., Ph.D., at the University of California at San Francisco, has been an unwavering judge and proponent of this technology in its application to glaucoma treatment from the beginning, providing unparalleled insight and knowledge. Dave Plager,

M.D., of Indiana University, tremendously extended our understanding and experience using ECP in the treatment of pediatric glaucomas.

Finally, Richard Makool, M.D., who certainly had plenty of other things to do with his time, encouraged the development of this technology and its application in ophthalmology, from the beginning up to the present and that's a long haul. His towering intelligence and skill, combined with his plainspoken manner, have been an inspiration to me.

I would like to express my deep gratitude to the editors at Lippincott Williams & Wilkins, Grace Caputo and Jonathan Pine, for their editorial and counseling skills. For me, having this forum has been the most important aspect of my professional life, and it would not have been possible without them.

1

INTRODUCTION TO OPHTHALMIC ENDOSCOPIC SURGERY

The technique of endoscopy is foreign to most ophthalmologists, for whom the viewing of ocular structures has generally been defined by the slit lamp, indirect ophthalmoscope, and operating microscope. In fact, these devices often enable us to visualize most aspects of the eye in a fashion superior to that afforded by endoscopy. Thus, one might reasonably ask, why is endoscopy or endoscopic laser delivery of much value if we can already view the interior of the eye by other, optically better, means?

The short answer is that certain intraocular areas are difficult or impossible to image by conventional means. Endoscopy allows visualization of the interior of the eye when it cannot be viewed otherwise, such as when anterior segment conditions preclude a posterior view. Corneal opacification, miotic pupil, and lens abnormality—to name a few situations ophthalmologists encounter—would render the operating microscope useless for viewing the ocular interior. Endoscopy circumvents these difficulties with relative ease.

Viewing of the far retinal periphery, pars plana, ciliary processes, and posterior iris region can be difficult or even impossible in a given eye by conventional means. However, the endoscope can easily image and assist laser delivery to these regions.

Some intraocular surgical techniques can be simplified under endoscopic control even if viewing through an operating microscope is possible. For example, it is technically easier to perform intraoperative panretinal photocoagulation with a laser endoscope than to apply photocoagulation while looking through an operating microscope.

Moreover, advances in optical systems development have overcome problems with regard to endoscope size, so that excellent image quality can be obtained with endoscopes smaller than 1 mm in diameter. Simultaneous laser delivery greatly enhances the utility of these instruments, creating the opportunity for novel, effective, and safe endoscopic procedures through the limbus or pars plana.

Finally, new imaging techniques such as intraoperative endoscopic fluorescein angiography are possible.

Simply put, the great advantage of ophthalmic endoscopy is in its capability for letting us "see" (and photocoagulate, aspirate, incise, etc.) when conventional imaging has failed (Table 1-1).

The instrumentation, its application, and the difficulties that one may encounter are described in the following pages. Technical adaptation is mandatory, but the learning curve seems small, and perhaps new opportunities for diagnosis and management of ophthalmic disease will become possible for us all.

TECHNOLOGY

Unfortunately, any new technology necessitates it own terminology. This situation cannot be avoided with endoscopy. On the other hand, only a small number of features need be known to proceed with the technical adaptation that is required for endoscopic surgery by the ophthalmologist.

Technical descriptions tend to be mind numbing. To avoid such overload, the following is not meant to be an

TABLE 1-1. ADVANTAGES OF ENDOSCOPY IN OPHTHALMIC SURGERY

Visualization of inaccessible regions of the eye:
- Behind iris
- Ciliary body
- Pars plana
- Peripheral retina

Internal view despite anterior segment opacities:
- Cornea
- Anterior chamber
- Iris
- Lens

exhaustive analysis of endoscopic optical and video systems. Rather, it is intended to provide an overview of available technology and an understanding of why ophthalmic endoscopes have evolved into their current form.

It is important to appreciate that for a technology to be truly useful it must not only function properly and provide a surgical advantage but also respect cost constraints. Most significantly, the value of any new technology may be severely limited by its complexity of setup, intraoperative use, postoperative maintenance, fragility, and remuneration.

Endoscopic Imaging and Laser Componentry

Two sets of componentry are required in endoscopy. The first is the endoscopes themselves; the second is the video, illumination, and laser sources.

Although there are several types of endoscopes and their hybrid combinations, they share the same basic characteristics. As far as the ophthalmic applications are concerned, the distal end is composed of a small metal tube typically about 30 mm in length and in the range of 1 mm in outer diameter. This represents the intraocular portion of the probe. This segment is connected to a handpiece (Fig. 1-1). From there, depending on the type of endoscope, there are lenses for magnification, focus, and perhaps filtration of particular light wavelengths.

In their most basic form, video endoscopy systems consist of a video camera, a light source, and a video monitor. Video technology has been exploding for some time and will likely continue on this trajectory well into the future, but basically, the images from the endoscope are transmitted to the charge-coupled device (CCD) chips of the video camera and then to the video monitor (Fig. 1-2). These cameras can have one or three chips and are analog or digital. The information can then be passed on to image capture devices, such as videocassette recorders, video printers, and computers.

As far as light sources are concerned, xenon is typically used in nonophthalmic applications and, in general, has also been most useful in ophthalmology. A close second as an illumination source is metal halide. Perhaps the least useful are the halogen sources typically employed in vitrectomy. Although they might seem to be quite bright to the human eye and when viewed through the operating microscope, the CCD chips of most video cameras do not respond as well to them.

Any fiber-delivered laser source used in ophthalmology can be combined with endoscopy for intraocular treatment, including visible and infrared wavelengths. As a practical matter, argon or frequency-doubled neodymium: yttrium-aluminum-garnet (Nd:YAG) lasers that produce the green wavelengths and semiconductor diode lasers that emit the invisible near-infrared (810 nm) wavelengths are the standard.

Most endoscopy systems are essentially a stack of these separate components. However, technology is available with integrated image and illumination, as well as image, illumination, and laser capabilities (Fig. 1-3).

It is important to understand that the surgeon monitors the course of the procedure on the video monitor rather than through the operating microscope. Most surgeons adapt readily to this change, although it can be a significant hurdle for some.

Laser Safety Filter

It is imperative to protect the surgeon and assistants from the potentially damaging effects of laser radiation, and this can be accomplished by introducing a filter for the

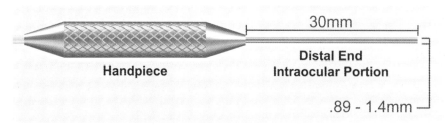

FIGURE 1-1. Ophthalmic endoscope design.

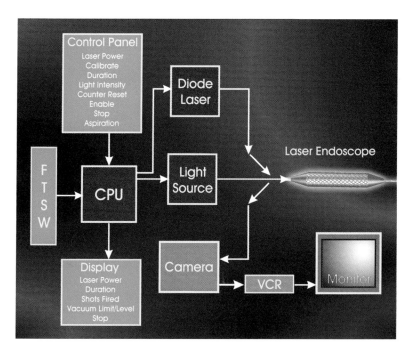

FIGURE 1-2. Schematic depiction of ophthalmic endoscopy componentry.

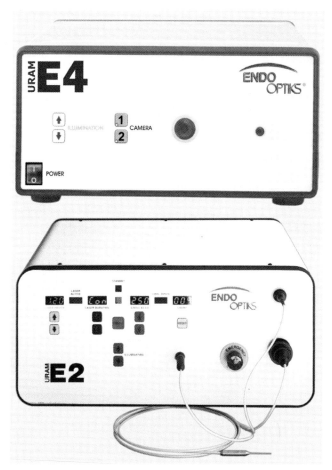

FIGURE 1-3. Integrated ophthalmic endoscopy systems. **Top:** Image and light system. **Bottom:** Image, light, and laser system.

specific laser wavelength along the optical pathway. However, this is necessary only when viewing laser delivery through the operating microscope. This filter is specific for the particular wavelength in use: a 532-nm laser requires a different safety filter than an 810-nm laser. If both green and near-infrared lasers are used, they can be "stacked" together on the operating microscope. The filter of the green laser has an orange appearance, whereas the 810-nm laser is "clear."

Importantly, the major manufacturers of operating microscopes have different fittings for placement of these filters. For example, one cannot use a filter made to fit a Zeiss microscope in a Wilde operating microscope.

It may seem obvious, but it bears mentioning that if laser delivery is observed only on the screen of the video monitor and not through the microscope, strictly speaking, a laser filter is not necessary (Fig. 1-4).

ENDOSCOPE TYPES

Rigid Endoscopes

The typical rigid endoscope employed in nonophthalmologic surgical areas is currently the world standard. It consists of a series of objective lenses in a metal tube with an eyepiece on the proximal end. Illumination is required and is usually accomplished with a right-angle connection to the shaft of the endoscope near the eyepiece (Fig. 1-5). The surgeon looks through this eyepiece directly at the target tissue. Optionally, the eyepiece can be connected to a video cam-

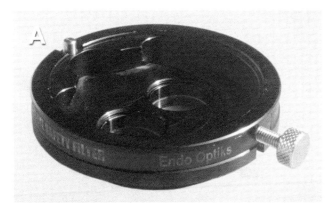

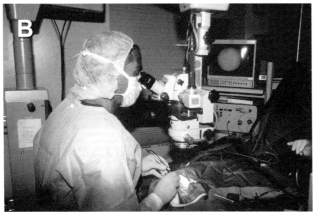

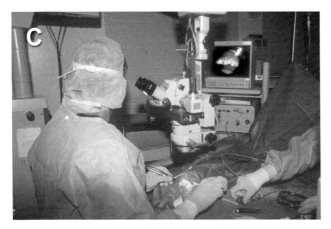

FIGURE 1-4. Laser safety filter. **A:** Filter for operating microscope. **B:** Surgeon viewing laser delivery through the operating microscope. This requires a laser safety filter. **C:** Surgeon viewing laser delivery on the video monitor of the endoscopy system. The safety filter is not important here because the progress of laser application is being followed on the video monitor, where back reflection of the laser cannot occur.

era that is connected to a video monitor, which allows the surgeon to indirectly image the target. This type of endoscope has superior image quality but unfortunately is associated with a number of disadvantages that currently render it impractical. In the ophthalmic application, size is important. Typically, 20-gauge (0.89-mm-diameter) instruments can be used in both the anterior and posterior segments.

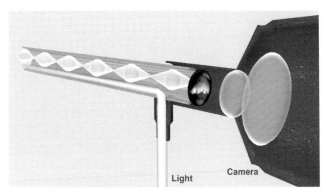

FIGURE 1-5. Rigid endoscope design.

Unfortunately, it is difficult to make such a device in the 1-mm-diameter range. Furthermore, the surgeon cannot look through an eyepiece that is close to the sterile field. To move the eyepiece image away would require an articulated arm of similarly designed lenses attached to the proximal end of the rigid scope or a video interface of some sort. This arrangement would be cumbersome, expensive to manufacture, and time consuming for the operating room staff to sterilize, set up, and maintain. In addition, and depending on the design, it could require an assistant to operate. All in all, not very practical.

Gradient Index Lens Endoscopes

In the gradient index (GRIN) lens format, an objective lens is placed on the distal end of a glass rod. The proximal end is coupled to a set of lenses that determine the ultimate image size and focusing characteristics. This system is then placed in proximity to a video camera that relays the image to a video monitor (Fig. 1-6). Essentially, then, what is required is the placement of a video camera at the end of the endoscope. This necessitates that the surgeon hold the video camera in hand with the endoscope connected to it. The advantages of this type of imaging system are that high-resolution images can be obtained

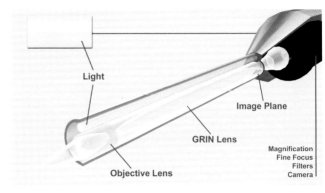

FIGURE 1-6. Gradient index (GRIN) lens endoscope design.

and that the endoscope's outer diameter is in the appropriate range for intraocular use. Such devices are not more costly to produce than other types of commonly used endoscopes. However, their fragility compared with that of fiberoptic endoscopes represents a significant disadvantage. They are also more cumbersome to use because the bulkier camera/endoscope unit must be held together in the surgeon's hand.

Fiberoptic Endoscopes

The fiberoptic type of endoscope is certainly the most commonly used form in ophthalmology. The image guide is composed of a collection of thousands of quartz fibers bundled together. Each individual fiber provides a tiny part of the overall picture. This is called a *pixel*, or picture element. Although the first commercially available ophthalmic endoscope employed a 3,000-pixel image guide, the current standard is the 10,000-pixel iteration. Theoretically, the more pixels, the better the image. However, this assumes that the image size remains the same. Under these circumstances, the apparent resolution improves. There are higher count image guides, such as 15,000- and 30,000-pixel bundles, but increasing the number of pixels also increases the outer diameter of the instrument. Indeed, the challenge in manufacturing fiberoptic image guides is to increase the number of pixels without increasing the diameter.

The pixel count is not the only determinant of image quality in these types of endoscopes. There are several types of fiberoptic image bundles, and 10,000 pixels of one type is not the equivalent of the second type. As the number of pixels increases so does the cost, fragility, imperfections, and outer diameter. Furthermore, there are other imaging characteristics that need to be considered with these fiberscopes.

The first is the field of view. The standard endoscope that was previously discussed has a 30- to 40-degree field of view in water and a slightly larger field in air. Most fiberoptic endoscopes have a 50- to 70-degree field of view in water. The most commonly used ophthalmic fiberoptic endoscope has a 110-degree field of view. This effect is created by the objective lens system on the distal tip of the image guide. Because there is a single imaging system, there is no stereopsis. It is possible to attain stereopsis by various means, and the larger the diameter of the endoscope, the more easily this is achieved. Nevertheless, as a practical matter, stereo endoscopes are not commonly employed in any surgical specialty. Wide-field ophthalmic endoscopes compensate for this, at least partially, by trading stereopsis for panorama. With a wide-field imaging system of 110 degrees, the surgeon can gain visual cues about the location of instruments within the space of the eye as well as assess the effect of these instruments on adjacent ocular tissue, shortening the technical learning curve. This would be more difficult if using an endoscope with a standard field of view or an operating microscope.

There is also the issue of depth of field, which establishes the range in which the image is in focus. One can choose the near and distal focal points, and, again, this is determined by the objective lens system on the distal tip of the fiberoptic image guide. The most commonly used ophthalmic endoscope has a depth of field from 0.75 to 40 mm, meaning that the image first appears clearly when the tip of the endoscope is approximately 0.75 mm from the target tissue and will remain "clear" until the endoscope tip is about 40 mm from the target tissue.

Because the image "begins" at the distal end of the endoscope and is "transmitted" throughout the length of the fiberoptic, these endoscopes are typically several meters in length before they interface with the video unit. Therefore, the surgeon does not hold the video camera in hand, making the instrument far less bulky and cumbersome.

Typically, just before the interface between the fiberoptic image guide and the CCD chips of the video camera is made, there exists another set of lenses that are used for "fine" image focus and for magnification. A "perfectly" focused imaging system will produce a honeycomb effect on the monitor. Many surgeons find this annoying even though it indicates maximal resolution. Depending on elements in the objective lens system distally, and lensing, magnification, and focusing proximally, this effect can be minimized or eliminated (Fig. 1-7).

Next, the endoscopic image is transmitted to the CCD chips of the camera. Here it is possible to dramatically alter color, sharpness, contrast, brightness, and other features before transmission to the video monitor. Similar adjustments can be made on the video monitor as well.

It is important to realize that many factors contribute to the surgeon's overall impression of image "quality" besides the raw numeric value of pixel number in the image guide. All 10K instruments are not created equally!

Fiberoptic endoscopes also require illumination and this may be provided by one or more light fibers adjacent to the image guide. When a standard 30- to 50-degree field-of-view endoscope is made, a single light fiber that would typically be used as an endoilluminator during vitrectomy is

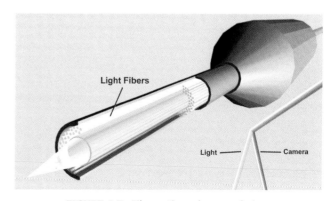

FIGURE 1-7. Fiberoptic endoscope design.

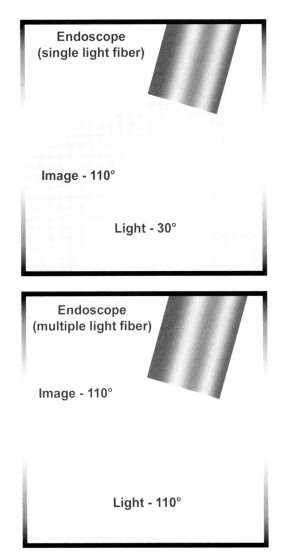

FIGURE 1-8. Comparison of narrow versus wide cone of illumination. A wide field requires a wide illumination cone. If a narrow illumination cone is used, much of the image field will be dark. It is significantly more expensive and technically difficult to fabricate an endoscope with a wide light cone.

adequate to "fill" the image with light. When a wide-field imaging endoscope is constructed, this single illumination fiber that creates a 30-degree cone of light is inadequate. Even though the human eye would perceive light emanating from such a scope to be very bright, endoscopically it would appear like the light of a flashlight in a large room. Multiple fibers (about 35 to 80) would create a 110-degree cone of light, matching the field of view created by the image guide and its objective lens system, filling the field with light (Fig. 1-8).

Curved and Bent Endoscope Configurations

Unlike standard and GRIN lens endoscopes, the fiberoptic variety is innately flexible (unless put into a rigid tube) and can be bent or curved into a variety of shapes. Theoretically,

this feature might be valuable when attempting to image or laser "around a corner" or when the particular anatomic situation in the eye presents an impediment to a straight endoscope. A number of these iterations have been created (Fig. 1-9) to address some of these issues. For example, the distal 3 or 4 mm may be bent at a 35-degree angle, a typical design for endophotocoagulation probes. This permits the surgeon to view and to laser the contralateral portion of the eye in an upward direction. A short intraocular portion that is twisted and is directed upward characterizes another shape. This configuration enables the surgeon to view the ciliary processes from the pars plana on the ipsilateral side. An extremely curved, almost sickle-shaped version can be inserted through the pars plana in a phakic eye to access the contralateral ciliary processes.

While these various iterations seem like they might be helpful, they are, perhaps surprisingly, difficult to use. Recall that when using an intraocular endoscope, the image is derived from the *tip* of the endoscope, so that the surgeon cannot see the instrument in the eye. When using a straight endoscope, the surgeon can readily learn where it is located within the eye. Visual cues, such as image magnification,

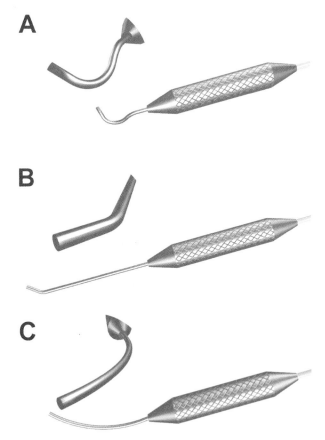

FIGURE 1-9. Various iterations of fiberoptic endoscope design. **A:** "Twisted" laser endoscope for imaging ipsilateral to incision site. **B:** Bent tip for imaging and laser application contralateral to incision site. **C:** Gently curved endoscope.

anatomic structures being viewed, other instruments placed in the eye, and so forth, let the surgeon understand the localization of the probe at any given moment. Although there is a learning curve to acquiring these skills, once they are attained, imaging with the endoscope becomes second nature. By changing the geometry of the instrument, the surgeon's "feel" must readapt. These endoscopes are therefore more difficult and hazardous to use.

Laser Endoscopes

Much of the utility of ophthalmic endoscopes is derived from their ability to deliver laser energy as well as to provide image and illumination. The price paid for this feature is a slight increase in the outer diameter of the endoscope. Fortunately, most of the laser fibers used in ophthalmology are 100 to 200 μm in diameter and so do not significantly change the dimensions of the intraocular portion of the endoscope.

There are two ways to incorporate laser fiber into an endoscope. The first of these is also the typical form used with standard nonophthalmic endoscopes, namely, to construct a channel within the shaft of the endoscope and, when the need arises, pass a laser fiber through it. Here, too, creation of this channel increases the outer diameter of the endoscope slightly and also creates some sterilization issues. Other drawbacks include a bit more setup, cleaning time, and effort required of the operating room staff as well as the

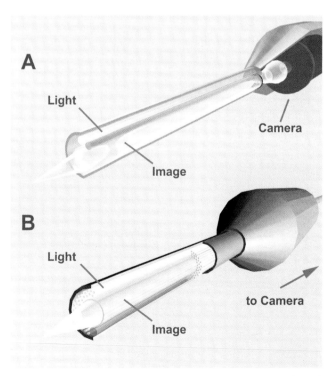

FIGURE 1-10. Laser endoscope design: Gradient index (GRIN) lens **A:** and fiberoptic **B:** laser endoscopes.

expense of the laser fibers, which are typically for single use (disposable). The second approach to this problem is to "build" the laser fiber into the endoscope so that there are no channels or disposable components. This arrangement of intrinsic image, light, and laser can be fashioned with fiberoptic or GRIN-type endoscopes. The most commonly used form of this technology in ophthalmology is the fiberoptic laser endoscope (Fig. 1-10).

HISTORY OF ENDOSCOPY

Mercifully, the history of ophthalmic endoscopy is brief. Most of the ophthalmic uses reported for endoscopy have not been strictly diagnostic in nature but rather have been directed to specific surgical applications. In 1934, Thorpe (1) combined an inverted Galilean telescope with attached intraocular foreign body forceps, with a total outer diameter of 6 mm. The next reported use of ophthalmic endoscopy did not appear until 1981, when Norris and Cleaseby (2–5) employed a 1.7-mm glass rod endoscope for vitrectomy, removal of intraocular foreign bodies, and biopsy. Following interest in the new age of transscleral laser cyclophotocoagulation, in 1985 Shields (6) cleverly attached an argon laser endophotocoagulation fiber to a 1.7-mm-diameter glass rod orthopedic endoscope for the purpose of intraocular cyclophotocoagulation in primate eyes. Variations and improvements on ophthalmic flexible and rigid endoscope design and uses evolved over the next 6 years (7–16). In 1990, the Drs. Leon published an outstanding atlas describing their combined endoscopic and operating microscope technology as well as its application in anterior and posterior segment disease (17).

The next transition occurred in 1991 with the development of a 20-gauge (0.89 mm in outer diameter) ophthalmic laser endoscope using a 3,000-pixel fiberoptic imaging bundle and intrinsic laser fiber. The design of this instrument represented a significant departure from all previous technology in that it was not a derivative of preexisting endoscopes but rather was tailored specifically for intraocular use and video interface. The first human endoscopic cyclophotocoagulation outcomes were reported in a group of patients with neovascular glaucoma (18). Endoscopic photocoagulation of the retina was also reported at that time (19). The instrumentation used in these studies involved, significantly, the first commercially available endoscopes and laser endoscopy system designed specifically for intraocular applications.

Interest in combining endoscopic surgery with various laser delivery systems evolved in oculoplastics and was characterized by novel variations of dacryocystorhinostomy. Reports appeared using the transnasal approach for both imaging and laser application, transnasal imaging with intracanalicular laser delivery, and endocanalicular imaging and laser application (20–23).

Studies detailing technique, results, and complications of endoscopic cyclophotocoagulation in adult and pediatric glaucoma, endoscopic vitreoretinal surgery, and endoscopic goniotomy have expanded the indications for this surgical approach and will be discussed in greater detail later.

REFERENCES

1. Thorpe HE. Ocular endoscope. *Trans Am Acad Ophthalmol Otolaryngol* 1934;39:422–424.
2. Norris JL, Cleasby GW. An endoscope for ophthalmology. *Am J Ophthalmol* 1978;85:420–422.
3. Norris JL, Cleasby GW, Nakanishi AS, Martin LJ. Intraocular endoscopic surgery. *Am J Ophthalmol* 1981;91:603–606.
4. Norris JL. Vitreous surgery viewed through an endoscope. *Dev Ophthalmol* 1981;2:15–16.
5. Norris JL, Cleasby GW. Intraocular foreign body removal by endoscopy. *Ann Ophthalmol* 1982;14:371–372.
6. Shields MB, Chandler DB, Hickingbotham D, Klintworth GK. Intraocular cyclophotocoagulation: histopathologic evaluation in primates. *Arch Ophthalmol* 1985;103:1731–1735.
7. Shields MB. Intraocular cyclophotocoagulation. *Trans Ophthalmol Soc UK* 1986;105:237–241.
8. Lecoq PJ, Billotte C, Combe JC. Interet de la videoendoscopie vitreo-retinienne [Value of vitreoretinal video-endoscopy]. *J Fr Ophthalmol* 1986;9:427–429.
9. Furia M, Hamard H, Puech M. Endoscopie oculaire. I. Modele experimental d'etude de l'implantation en chambre posterieure apres extraction extra-capsulaire du cristallin [Ocular endoscopy. I. Experimental model for studying implantation into the posterior chamber after extracapsular extraction of the crystalline lens]. *Bull Soc Ophthalmol Fr* 1987;87:759–760.
10. Furia M, Hamard H, Puech M, et al. Cloutage retinien avec film video-endoscopique U-MATIC ["Retinal nailing" with U-MATIC video-endoscopy film]. *Bull Soc Ophthalmol Fr* 1987;87:1395–1403.
11. Lecoq PJ, Billotte C, Combe JC, Hamel C. Plaidoyer en favour de l'endoscopie pour certaines interventions retinovitreennes [A plea for endoscopy in various retino-vitreous operations]. *Bull Soc Ophthalmol Fr* 1987;87:575–576.
12. Kora Y, Yaguchi S. Sutured secondary posterior chamber lens with endoscopic control. *Ocular Surg News* 1990.
13. Volkov VV, Danilov AV, Vassin LN, Frolov YA. Flexible endoscope for intraocular surgery. *Arch Ophthalmol* 1990;108:1037–1038.
14. Volkov VV, Danilov AV, Vassin LN, Frolov YA. Flexible endoscopes: ophthalmoendoscopic techniques and case reports. *Arch Ophthalmol* 1990;108:956–957.
15. Eguchi S, Araie M. A new ophthalmic electronic video endoscope system for intraocular surgery. *Arch Ophthalmol* 1990;108:1778–1781.
16. Leon CS, Leon JA. Microendoscopic ocular surgery. Part II. Preliminary results from the study of glaucomatous eyes. *J Cataract Refract Surg* 1991;5:573–576.
17. Leon CS, Leon JA. *Endoscopie chirurgicale oculaire*. Paris: Medsi/McGraw-Hill, 1990.
18. Uram M. Ophthalmic laser microendoscopy ciliary process ablation in the management of neovascular glaucoma. *Ophthalmology* 1992;99:1823–1828.
19. Uram M. Ophthalmic laser microendoscope endophotocoagulation. *Ophthalmology* 1992;99:1829–1832.
20. Levin PS, StormoGipson J. Endocanalicular laser-assisted dacryocystorhinostomy: an anatomic study. *Arch Ophthalmol* 1992;110:1488–1490.
21. Singh AD, Singh A, Whitmore I, Taylor E. Endoscopic visualization of the human nasolacrimal system: an experimental study. *Br J Ophthalmol* 1992;76:663–667.
22. Kong YT, Kim TI, Kong BW. A report of 131 cases of endoscopic laser lacrimal surgery. *Ophthalmology* 1994;101:1793-1800.
23. Uram M. Transcanalicular diode laser dacryocystorhinostomy. Presented at the meeting of the American Society of Cataract and Refractive Surgery, Seattle, WA, June 1–4, 1996.

2

TECHNICAL FEATURES OF OPHTHALMIC ENDOSCOPY

TECHNICAL ASPECTS

Much of ophthalmic endoscopic imaging is self-evident and does not require explanation. Nevertheless, knowing a few technical details can be of great assistance. To be successful with this methodology, the surgeon must gain facility in maneuvering the endoscope, acquiring an adequate image, adjusting illumination, and controlling laser delivery. A review of some of these issues follows.

Image Rotation

The image guide occupies a specific position within the structure of the endoscope. Image orientation is derived from both the proximal and distal ends of the image guide. The visual effect of this is that the image can appear to be rotated obliquely or even upside down. Strictly speaking, it is not important to have proper image orientation because the intraocular target tissue can be viewed or lasered no matter what the rotation. However, as a practical matter, having the image orientation correspond to the anatomy simplifies surgical maneuvers. That is, intraocular endoscopic surgery can be assisted by maintenance of the correct "top" and "bottom" of the image. For example, when one is approaching the ciliary processes from the limbus in an eye with a posterior chamber intraocular lens, the top of the video image should be the posterior iris and the bottom should be the intraocular lens. Changing image orientation is simple: the surgeon merely rolls the endoscope handpiece between the fingers (Fig. 2-1). This rotation can be performed before insertion of the endoscope into the eye or after its introduction into the surgical space. With curved or bent endoscopes, of course, this rotational maneuver becomes more difficult, so the

instrument must be constructed with proper image guide orientation in mind. In straight endoscopes this consideration need not be addressed.

Image Artifacts

If one considers all of the optical interfaces that exist in the video microendoscope, it becomes apparent that there are many opportunities to degrade the image with which the surgeon must ultimately work. Starting distally, debris accumulating on the endoscope tip can create a generally hazy view or black spots of varying size. Because the image guides are of small diameter, typically 300 to 500 μm, it takes very little blood or debris to substantially compromise the view. Wiping the tip of the instrument with a dry sponge or cotton-tipped applicator is usually sufficient to resolve this problem. The proximal end of the endoscope can be similarly affected, with debris accumulation producing a general haze or black spots of varying size. (Powder from the operating room assistant's glove is the most common source of this problem.) The remedy is the same. Less commonly, dust or other debris on the distal or proximal end of the magnifying/focusing/filtering apparatus (connecting the endoscope to the CCD chips of the camera) can also result in a degraded image. This problem can be corrected by cleaning with lens solution or a blast of compressed air (Fig. 2-2).

Fiberoptic endoscopes contain bundles upward of 10,000 small tubes of glass, usually several meters in length. Any physical damage to their integrity along that length will result in broken pixels, typically a large irregular but sharply defined area of blacked-out image. This artifact cannot be corrected without rebuilding the imaging system

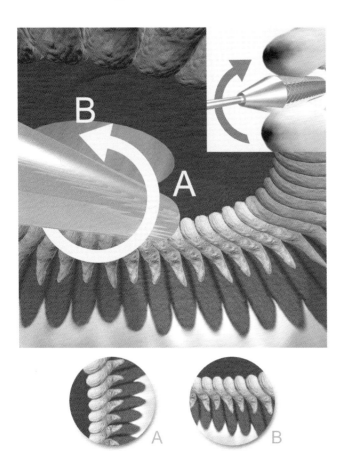

FIGURE 2-1. Image rotation. **A:** By rolling the endoscope handle in one's hand, the image is rotated so that proper orientation can be achieved. **B:** Appearance of the intraocular portion of the endoscope during viewing of the ciliary processes and the effect that physical rotation of the handpiece has on the image as viewed on the video monitor.

of the endoscope. As a practical matter, it is less expensive to buy a new endoscope. If the "scotoma" created by the broken pixels does not hamper the surgeon's overall imaging ability, the scope can still be used (Fig. 2-2).

Illumination Artifacts

The same artifacts that affect the image guides can degrade the light guides. The diameter of this portion of the endoscope is quite small, and light delivery is easily attenuated by debris or inadequate cleaning. Wiping the distal and proximal portions of the light guide will maximize the illumination function of the endoscope.

There are several other sources of apparently degraded illumination. The most common of these reflects not a problem with the endoscope itself but the fact that the brightness setting on the video monitor is too low. By increasing this setting, one should see a dramatic increase in illumination in the endoscopic view. It is also important, when using a nonintegrated endoscopy system, to ensure that the video camera has been maximally adjusted for the light source being used. Specifically, some cameras allow electronic adjustments to the ultimate image that is produced depending on whether the illumination source is halogen, metal halide, xenon, or other.

The surgeon must control the intensity of illumination for optimal imaging. This is because the closer the tip of the endoscope to the tissue, the less light that is needed, whereas the more panoramic the view, the greater the illumination required. If the intensity of light is too high, the video image becomes washed out and white. If illumination

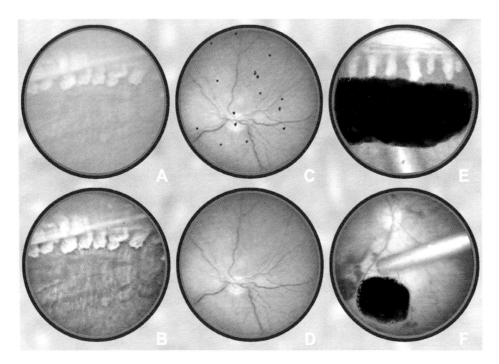

FIGURE 2-2. Image artifacts. **A:** Hazy view of ciliary processes due to blood and debris on the distal tip of the endoscope. **B:** Clear view of gauze after the tip of the endoscope has been wiped. **C:** "Spots" on image from dust on the connection of the proximal end of the image guide as it connects with the video monitor. **D:** Clear image after dust has been removed. **E:** Fiberoptic image with broken pixels, showing a streak of dense, blacked-out image. **F:** Another example of the effect created by broken image guide pixels.

is insufficient, the image is too dark. The most commonly used ophthalmic endoscopy system permits the surgeon to control the level of illumination with a foot switch, circumventing this problem. It is also possible to have an operating room assistant adjust the level of illumination at the light source, although this approach can become tedious if frequent changes are required.

GETTING STARTED: TECHNICAL ADAPTATIONS

Endoscopy is a foreign experience for most ophthalmologists, and to become facile in its use technical adaptation is mandatory. Perhaps this is because endoscopy seems to violate a basic tenet of ophthalmic surgery—specifically, that the surgeon is not to manipulate an instrument within the eye when it cannot be seen. With the operating microscope, there is simultaneous viewing of the instrument tip and its proximity to other ocular structures. Manipulation can then be visually judged. This control limits inadvertent contact with and damage to intraocular structures. This precept is usually set aside in endoscopy, primarily because the endoscope allows viewing, laser delivery, and surgical manipulation to areas that are not visually accessible by the operating microscope. Because the image originates at the distal tip of the instrument, the endoscope itself cannot be seen. It must be advanced within the eye according to what it "sees." The surgeon must learn to recognize the "endoscopic" features of the eye that may differ from its familiar appearance when viewed by conventional means. Visual cues must be taken from the surrounding anatomy to ultimately enable manipulation of the endoscope and other instruments in the eye.

This brings us to the second technical adaptation that must be made: viewing the progress of surgery on the video monitor rather than the operating microscope. For some this can be a difficult transition. Typically, the endoscopy componentry and video monitor are placed on either side of the surgeon but within arm's reach. This instrumentation is placed on the opposite side of the patient from the other surgical consoles, such as phacoemulsification or vitrectomy machines. Certainly, numerous variations of this arrangement can be made to accommodate a particular surgeon's preference or the physical requirement of the operating room.

Before surgery, pupillary dilation is helpful. As the surgeon gains experience with endoscopy, this feature becomes less important; however, use of familiar visual cues imaged through the operating microscope can simplify and accelerate the learning process.

Interestingly, the endoscopic image on the video monitor changes little with pupillary dilation, when the room lights are off or on, or when there is operating microscope illumination. For example, this feature can allow the operating room staff to function with the room lights on (rather than working in the dark) without disturbing the surgeon's progress.

When anterior segment conditions preclude a more posterior view or when otherwise inaccessible anatomy is being approached, the ability to endoscopically image, surgically manipulate, or deliver laser energy to ocular structures is not diminished, but a higher degree of skill is required on the part of the surgeon. All visual location cues must be taken from the video monitor. At first, it can be disorienting to realize that virtually an entire intraocular procedure can be performed without a microscope. However, it is not necessary to be a purist but rather to use whatever works best in a given situation. For example, if the posterior view through the operating microscope during vitrectomy is good, then endoscopic imaging will not be especially helpful. However, if pupillary miosis impedes the surgeon's progress later in the procedure, merely shifting to the endoscopic view will enable expeditious continuation.

RETINAL PHOTOTOXICITY

One might be concerned that light sources other than halogen may produce retinal damage, but scientific evidence supporting this fear is scant. Only a handful of publications have reported this problem, and the cases are about equally distributed between halogen and others. The commonality appears to be that most of these reports are generated around lesions created during extended macular surgery. It has been conjectured that holding the tip of the endoilluminator close to the retina creates a thermal effect. Often, however, the endoscope is placed at a distance from the target tissue to take advantage of its panoramic viewing capabilities, so there is actually less light on the retinal surface. Furthermore, most of the light emanating from the light source is "lost" at its connection with the light guide. Only a small percentage of light delivered to the endoscope is actually transmitted to the eye; the rest is "thrown away."

With use of a combined imaging and illumination system or an integrated imaging, illumination, and laser console, one of the critical engineering tasks is to adequately dissipate the heat. Aside from a burn risk to the surgeon or assistants, video cameras do not function well when they are hot. Xenon light sources, in particular, are notorious for creating this problem. Semiconductor diode lasers are also a source of unwanted heat, although they malfunction when overheated. However, all of these problems occur before or at the connection of the endoscopy componentry with the endoscope and must be resolved simply to permit functioning of the system. In more anterior applications of endoscopy, such as cyclophotocoagulation, illuminator phototoxicity is a nonissue because of the large distance between the tip of the endoscope and the macula or optic nerve. There has never been a reported incident of retinal phototoxicity created by an endoscope.

3

ENDOSCOPIC ANATOMY

One of the unique aspects of ophthalmology, in comparison with other fields of medicine, is the practitioner's strong reliance on visual inspection for diagnostic and therapeutic decision making. Experience can be a powerful teacher, especially when a single pathologic entity may present itself in many different forms. Through years of training and practice, ophthalmologists have gained intimate knowledge of anterior segment microscopic anatomy as well as that of the posterior pole. Viewing of the more peripheral aspects of the retina by routine methods is somewhat more difficult, and its variations in normal and pathologic states are less well recognized. The appearance of the pars plana, ciliary body, and posterior aspects of the iris are not well known in vivo to most ophthalmologists.

When first using the endoscope to view the interior of the eye, the surgeon may experience disorientation. The more anterior structures are less familiar when approached from their posterior aspect, and the nonstereoscopic view adds to a sense of disorientation. If the endoscope alone is introduced into the eye, the absence of a second imaging instrument also contributes to the confusion. A bit of practice on animal or cadaver eyes can easily overcome these obstacles, and the learning curve typically is short.

A brief review of normal anatomy as imaged through the endoscope might be helpful. Pathologic states that alter the anatomic appearance will follow. This is not meant to be an exhaustive review of ocular anatomy and its many nuances, but rather is intended to orient the novice endoscopist to what may be an alternative and novel view of intraocular structures.

POSTERIOR SEGMENT

Perhaps the most familiar region, when viewed endoscopically, is the posterior pole. The disc, vessels, and macula appear much as they do when viewed by conventional means (Fig. 3-1). Advancing the endoscope closer to these structures will magnify the image but reduce the field of view. Depending on the type and quality of endoscope and viewing system used, high-resolution images can be obtained that are comparable or superior to those created by the operating microscope. When working in the posterior segment, the surgeon can easily achieve orientation by starting at the posterior pole and then following the course of one of the major vascular arcades to a more peripheral area of interest.

If the vitreous is intact, the endoscopic image has a slightly hazy or weblike appearance because the eye is being illuminated from within (Fig. 3-2). One must recall that, typically, ophthalmic diagnostic and surgical instruments follow a format of external to internal lighting. As an example, it is interesting to observe a "bright spot" on the surface on the retina that is produced by the illumination source of the operating microscope (Fig. 3-3). One might conjecture about the relationship between this observation and the development of postoperative cystoid macular edema or macular "burn."

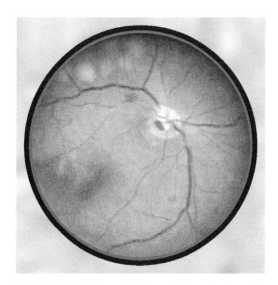

FIGURE 3-1. Endoscopic view of the posterior pole.

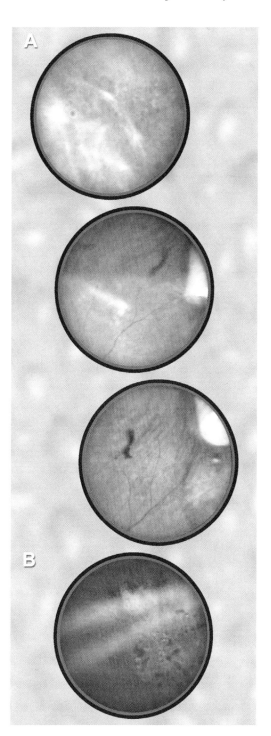

FIGURE 3-2. Endoscopic appearance of the vitreous. **A:** The weblike structure stands out because of internal illumination and imaging, rather than the more conventional method of illuminating and viewing from the outside to the inside of the eye. **B:** Appearance of the vitreous base.

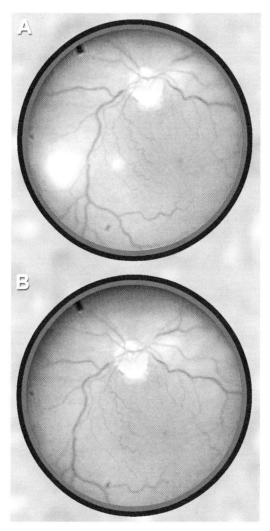

FIGURE 3-3. Endoscopic views of the posterior pole. **A:** Operating microscope light creates a spot of illumination on the macula. **B:** The spot disappears after the microscope light is extinguished.

PERIPHERAL RETINA

Progressing more anteriorly, the endoscope allows an easily accessible view of the peripheral retina (Fig. 3-4). There is some variability in the retinal pigment epithelial coloration. Several types of peripheral retinal pigment epithelial degenerations easily observed by this methodology, such as "cobblestone" degeneration, are of little clinical significance but have striking appearance. There is also substantial variability to the appearance of the retinal insertion at the pars plana. The ora serrata is often more pronounced nasally with distinct "bays" and "teeth," while the retinal insertion is less distinct temporally. The oral teeth may extend for a short distance anteriorly or may be quite long, actually contacting the ciliary processes.

A whispy white appearance is often present endoscopically in the region of the peripheral retina, which results from internal illumination of the vitreous base.

PARS PLANA

Moving more anteriorly, the pars plana region is encountered. This zone is the continuation of the choroid anteri-

orly without overlying retina. It is usually mottled and dark brown and may be observed to have fine black pigmentation oriented in a radial fashion (Fig. 3-5). The external surface of the globe that extends from approximately 3.0 to 5.5 mm from the limbus correlates with this region internally. An incision in this area may avoid damaging the lens anteriorly or the retina posteriorly.

CILIARY PROCESSES

As the view continues in an anterior direction, the ciliary processes are encountered. There are approximately 70 to 80 of these structures arranged in a ring fashion. Color varies from white to orange to dark brown, and their appearance can range from a translucent fluffy texture to a compact and stiff form. The anterior "head" of each process is often wider and thicker than the narrower and flat posterior potion, or "tail," that arises from the pars plana. There is also some variability in their grouping, with some eyes revealing tightly packed and wedged-together processes, whereas others have narrow processes with wide gaps or "valleys" between them (Fig. 3-6). Mostly, the processes are all aligned in a vertical

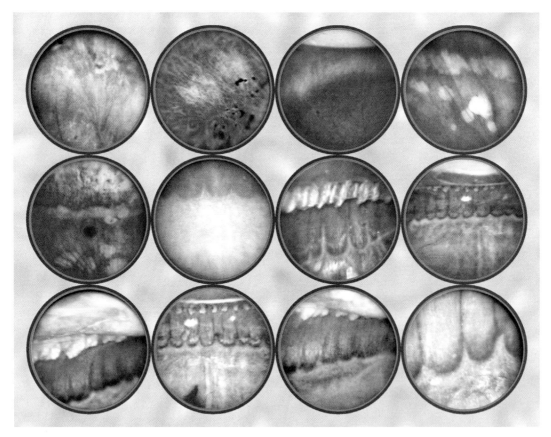

FIGURE 3-4. Endoscopic views of the peripheral retina, showing variability in pigmentation and vasculature. This is also a variability in the appearance of oral bays and teeth. The vitreous base often appears to be a diffusely white band straddling the peripheral retina.

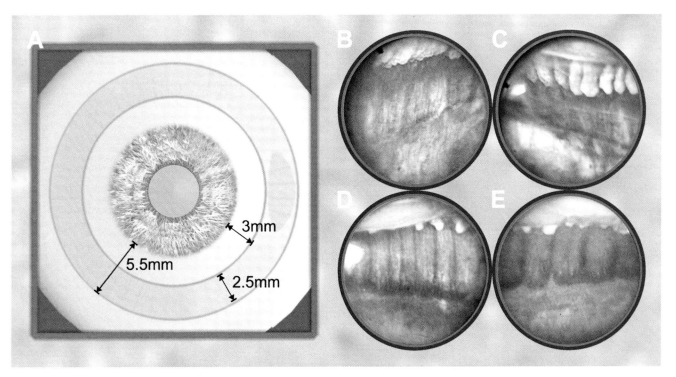

FIGURE 3-5. A: Diagram of the internal pars planan location on the external surface of the eye. As measured there, the pars plana "begins" 3.0 mm from the limbus and extends 5.5 mm from it. It is 2.0 to 2.5 mm wide. **B–E:** Various images of the pars plana viewed endoscopically.

fashion, but occasionally they may be twisted, overlapping, bifurcating at the head or tail, or slanted obliquely. None of these physical characteristics seems to have much pathologic significance. It should be noted, however, that anterior retraction and distortion of the processes are frequently observed in eyes with previous anterior segment surgery. Juvenile glaucoma patients typically exhibit distorted and anomalously positioned ciliary processes. These matters will be examined in greater detail later.

LENS AND ZONULES

In the phakic eye, the lens is positioned centrally and, even when not opacified, appears to be translucent to white when viewed through the endoscope. Again, this phenomenon seems to arise from internal illumination of the structure. It also appears to be more globular and spherical in nature than one might expect. Sometimes an instrument may be introduced through the pars plana and advanced across the eye to the opposing peripheral retina without traumatizing the posterior capsule because the lens is relatively flat. At other times it may be extremely spherical, to the degree that a surgeon might not permit the pars plana instrument to approach the midline for fear of abrading the posterior capsule.

The zonules are fine white whispy structures that arise from the tails and areas between the ciliary processes and are attached to the lens posterior to the equator and onto the peripheral edge of the posterior lens surface (Fig. 3-7). Various postsurgical and pathologic states can alter this appearance, and these changes will be discussed in greater detail.

POSTERIOR CHAMBER INTRAOCULAR LENSES

Posterior chamber intraocular lenses may also have a white appearance when they are enveloped by capsular material, again as a consequence of internal illumination (Fig. 3-8). Whatever portion of the optic that is not covered by capsular material will appear clear.

The haptics, especially blue or brown ones, are quite distinct and easily seen whether they are within or outside of the capsular bag. Their malpositioning (e.g., extruding through the capsule, piercing a ciliary process, penetrating the iris) can be easily detected. On the other hand, if the haptics are clear, they are more difficult to detect, especially if they are within the capsular bag.

CILIARY SULCUS

Just anterior to the "heads" of the ciliary processes is an indentation surrounding the eye, which is the ciliary sul-

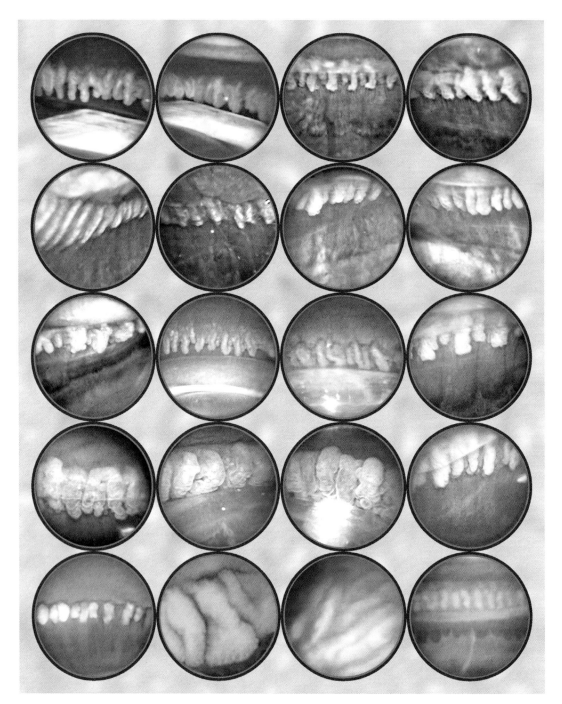

FIGURE 3-6. Endoscopic views of the ciliary processes. While most eyes appear to be similar in this effect, there are variations in width, length, number, and interprocess spacing.

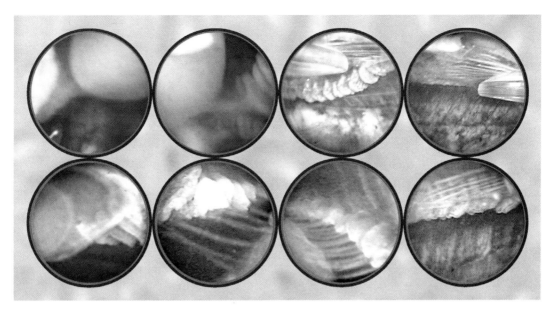

FIGURE 3-7. Endoscopic appearance of the zonules. These attachments to the lens capsule can have a variable appearance depending on a number of factors, including the type of endoscope used to view them, their thickness, variability in illumination, and the angle at which they are approached.

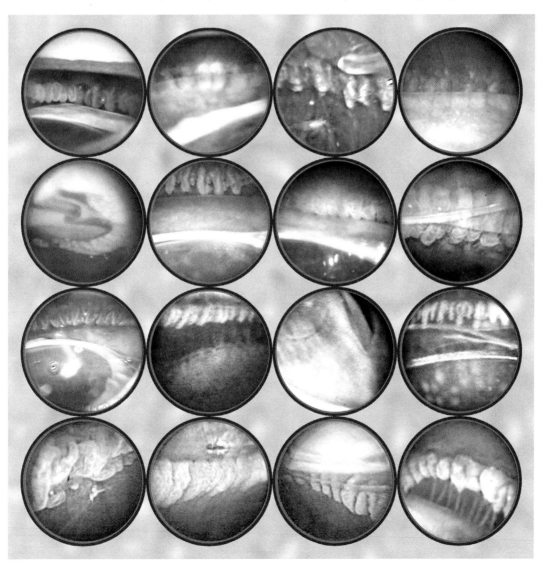

FIGURE 3-8. Endoscopic appearance of the posterior chamber intraocular lenses and their haptics. There is variability in capsular fibrosis, and the haptics can be seen both within and externalized from the bag. These issues are important for endoscopic cyclophotocoagulation.

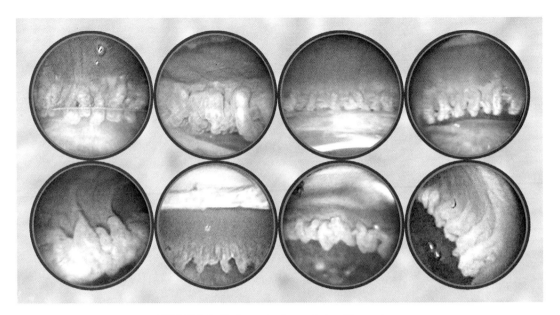

FIGURE 3-9. Endoscopic views of the ciliary sulcus.

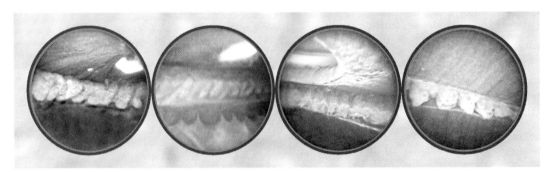

FIGURE 3-10. Endoscopic views of the posterior aspect of the iris.

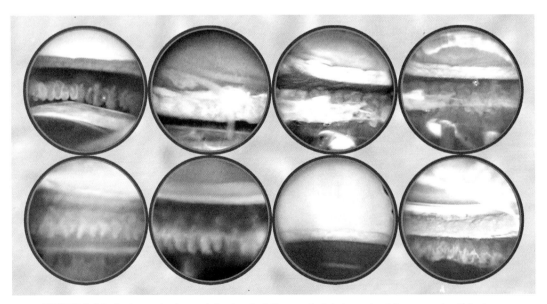

FIGURE 3-11. Endoscopic views at the level of the pupil. It is important to recognize this structure for proper orientation during surgical maneuvers.

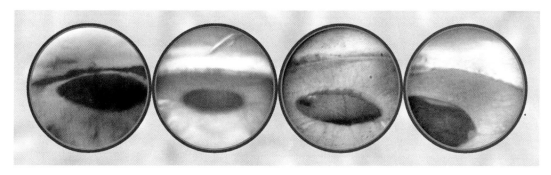

FIGURE 3-12. Endoscopic views of the anterior chamber.

cus. This region is affected by a number of pathologic entities and surgical misadventures. It is easily accessible from the anterior or posterior segment endoscopically, although it is generally impossible to reach for diagnostic evaluation or surgical manipulation through the operating microscope. The sulcus typically has a dark brown appearance regardless of other ocular pigmentation (Fig. 3-9).

IRIS

The posterior aspect of the iris is typically uniformly dark brown no matter the patient's anterior iris or fundus coloration (Fig. 3-10). There may be several concentric fine white rings as a normal variant. Iridotomy, iridectomy, and trabeculectomy sites can be viewed from this posterior aspect. Interestingly, iris neovascularization rarely seems to involve the posterior iris, even in highly ischemic florid examples of this problem.

In the aphakic or anterior chamber pseudophakic eye, a view can be obtained in the plane of the pupil. The edge of the iris in the pupillary space often droops posteriorly for a short distance when not supported by a lens.

ANTERIOR CHAMBER

Imaging in the anterior chamber can be accomplished from a posterior approach, through the pupillary space; or through a limbal incision. When viewed endoscopically, the aqueous appears slightly translucent. If the anterior chamber is filled with a viscoelastic or with a gas such as room air, the image becomes crystal clear. The cornea is moderately translucent when viewed posteriorly. If an object, such as a forceps, is held over the eye, it has a hazy appearance even though the ocular media and cornea seem to be transparent. Anterior chamber lens implants appear pretty much as one would expect when viewed through the endoscope (Fig. 3-11).

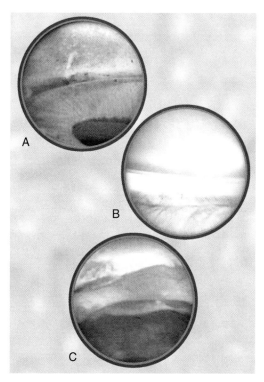

FIGURE 3-13. Endoscopic views of the angle structures. **A:** Post-cyclocryotherapy eye with pigment splattering on the corneal epithelium. **B:** Anterior chamber intraocular lens and open angle. **C:** Fine vessels and blood in the angle of a patient with neovascular glaucoma.

ANTERIOR CHAMBER ANGLE

The anterior chamber angle appears endoscopically as it would by gonioscopy. In the aphakic or anterior chamber pseudophakic eye, this region can be accessed anteriorly from not only a limbal approach but also posteriorly from the pars plana (Fig. 3-12). If the angle is open, trabecular meshwork can be observed; if the angle is closed, the iris can easily be seen in contact with the endothelium (Fig. 3-13). This view will be familiar to most ophthalmologists, but having an appreciation for the endoscopic approach enables goniotomy and angle dissection by viscoelastic.

CORNEA

The cornea can be approached through a limbal incision or from the pars plana in the aphakic and anterior chamber pseudophakic eye. Even though the cornea may be clear, internal illumination makes it appear to be translucent. Interestingly, if the cornea is opaque, its appearance is not significantly different, again being characterized by translucence.

4

SURGICAL MANAGEMENT OF GLAUCOMA

PHYSIOLOGIC BASIS OF GLAUCOMA

All ophthalmologists know that intraocular pressure (IOP) represents the balance between aqueous production, or inflow, and its drainage, or outflow. When this relationship experiences a pathologic imbalance, the IOP rises. Damage to the ganglion cells and, ultimately, to the optic nerve produces visual field defects that establish the diagnosis of glaucoma. This inflow/outflow imbalance can arise from a number of pathophysiologic mechanisms, each of which has its own particular set of clinical peculiarities. Most patients with glaucoma respond to topical and systemic medications or noninvasive laser treatment, but when these measures prove to be inadequate, more aggressive intervention is required. From a pathophysiologic viewpoint, one can make the following assumptions:

1. Virtually all cases of glaucoma result from obstruction to outflow.
2. Glaucoma is never the result of aqueous "overproduction."
3. Aside from neovascular glaucoma arising from ischemic diabetic ophthalmopathy or from ischemic central retinal vein occlusion, glaucoma is not associated with diminished inflow.

The physical goal of surgery is to manipulate either side of the inflow/outflow equation, although, strictly speaking, there is no reason that both sides cannot be addressed simultaneously. As a disclaimer, one should recall that the mechanism of cell death, optic nerve damage, and visual field loss is obscure and perhaps not entirely related to the IOP. However, as a practical matter, the only way to manage a glaucomatous eye is to somehow lower the IOP.

ALTERATION OF OUTFLOW

Filtration Surgery

It would be fair to say that most surgical glaucoma patients today are treated by increasing aqueous outflow. Essentially, two procedures, and their seemingly infinite variants, are in use. The first of these is filtration surgery, typically trabeculectomy; and the second is tube implantation with drainage reservoir. The success and complications experienced with these methods depend, at least in part, on such factors as patient race, age, mechanism of glaucoma, lens status, previous intraocular surgery, previous glaucoma surgery, ability to comply with postoperative management, and the skill and experience level of the surgeon.

Trabeculectomy was first described by Koryllos in 1967 (1) and then by Cairns in 1968 (2). Simplistically, a full-thickness opening is created in the eye wall with an overlying flap of sclera and conjunctiva, permitting drainage of fluid from the ocular interior. There are many variations of this technique, and a considerable body of literature addresses the other details, such as results and complications of surgery, mechanisms of action, and failure. These issues have been elucidated by hundreds of others and so do not require attention here except in the context of endoscopic applications. Concisely, though, it should be recalled that the ultimate purpose of filtration surgery is to control IOP and prevent vision loss.

Nevertheless, even with best efforts, one third to one half of patients with open-angle glaucoma (presumably the least difficult mechanism of glaucoma to manage surgically) experience progressive visual loss despite "successful" control of IOP when followed up for the very long term.

Trabeculectomy shares many complications associated with essentially any type of intraocular surgery. Typically, a small percentage of patients develop what is euphemistically referred to as minor complications, including anterior or posterior segment hemorrhage, inflammation, accelerated cataract formation, cystoid macular edema, and transiently elevated IOP or hypotony. These problems are typically self-limited and often do not require intervention.

Then there is a set of problems peculiar to filtration surgery patients. These are often the consequence of altered intraocular fluid dynamics, created by the sclerostomy. If too much fluid drains from the eye, the anterior chamber can flatten, which might result in the formation of peripheral anterior synechiae (PAS) and the ultimate development of a second and more ominous mechanism of glaucoma than that with which the patient started. If the eye continues to overfilter, hypotony evolves with its attendant complications, including maculopathy and visual loss. Conjunctival holes leak aqueous, and scleral flaps that are too loose can permit overfiltration, both of which require intensive postoperative care or reoperation and add to the misery of the patient and surgeon.

If, on the other hand, underdrainage of fluid from the eye may cause failure to control IOP and its implications for progressive visual loss. Furthermore, if insufficient drainage occurs, the conjunctival bleb overlying the trabeculectomy site has an enhanced opportunity to close and to scar, resulting in permanent failure of the procedure. If the scleral flap is too tight, drainage cannot occur, leading to bleb failure. Other bleb problems can plague the postoperative course, such as inflammation (blebitis), development of an overly large bleb that obscures vision by several possible mechanisms, or the evolution of a thin-walled bleb.

This leads us to what is perhaps the most threatening bleb problem of all: the development of infectious endophthalmitis. Two statistics are of importance here. The first is the risk of endophthalmitis as a direct consequence of intraocular surgery, which is 0.1%. The second is peculiar to this type of surgery. Specifically, the cumulative risk for the development of endophthalmitis after trabeculectomy is 1% per year. There are a number of risk factors that can potentiate this problem. Although most of the studies concerning this issue are small, recurring themes are apparent. Inferior bleb location, high bleb configuration in association with blepharitis, bleb leak, use of mitomycin or 5-flu-

orouracil, full-thickness procedures, early postoperative flat chamber, wound leak, suprachoroidal hemorrhage, intermittent or chronic use of postoperative antibiotics have all been considered significant risk factors for the development of this problem.

Devastating complications can also arise from trabeculectomy, including massive intraocular hemorrhage, choroidal effusion (serous and hemorrhagic), retinal detachment, lens dislocation, permanent hypotony, and phthisis. Many of these difficulties require surgical intervention, and the outcomes are often discouraging for patient and ophthalmologist.

Reoperations are common after any type of glaucoma surgery, and in the case of trabeculectomy, the risk that further intervention would be required can be affected by a host of factors, including mechanism of glaucoma, previous glaucoma surgery, previous eye surgery, patient age, patient race, lens status, complications of the first surgery, and use of antimetabolites. Needless to say, reoperations have a dramatically smaller chance of being successful than the initial procedure.

Another issue related to filtration surgery is the long-term performance of an initially "successful" procedure. Typically, at about the 2-year postoperative mark, the late failure rate of trabeculectomy begins to increase and continues on this course for years. This is the so-called decremental response.

Ultimately, the trabeculectomy patient with the best long-term prognosis is a Caucasian individual with uncontrolled open-angle glaucoma in an eye without previous glaucoma surgery that is phakic. Any alteration to these variables can dramatically reduce the long-term outlook for successful management.

In the "best" prognostic patient populations (open-angle glaucoma), trabeculectomy is only moderately effective in the long term and is not applicable in many glaucoma patients at all. Still, it is unequivocally true that trabeculectomy is the singular choice for invasive glaucoma treatment by most ophthalmologists today despite its limitations. Perhaps this is the case not because it best addresses the underlying pathogenesis of the disease and is therefore the most efficacious approach, but rather because it has been historically the least offensive of all glaucoma surgical procedures.

Finally, it should be recalled that many trabeculectomy patients require intensive postoperative follow-up and a high level of skill on the part of the surgeon to maximize the potential for a successful outcome. This feature alone can discourage many ophthalmologists from treating surgical glaucoma patients.

Tube Implantation Surgery

In refractory glaucoma or in eyes with glaucoma mechanisms that are poorly responsive to filtration, aqueous shunting procedures are used. First introduced by Molteno in 1969 (3), this approach can be highly successful. The technique is demanding and relatively unforgiving. Postoperative care is typically intensive. Often the eye is hypotonous during the first few weeks, and shallow anterior chamber, choroidal effusion, and visual loss may ensue. Then, as fibrous encapsulation develops around the plate, IOP can rise to unacceptable levels. Complications peculiar to this approach also include migration or frank expulsion of the tube or the plate, corneal edema, ocular motility disturbance, conjunctival melting, and loss of visual acuity. Numerous preventive and treatment measures can be used to address these problems. Successful long-term control of IOP is typically in the 50% to 70% range. Because of the demanding nature of this approach to glaucoma treatment, it is typically the province of subspecialists in glaucoma rather than a tool for most practicing ophthalmologists.

It would be fair to say that most practicing ophthalmologists today rarely perform trabeculectomy and never undertake tube implantation or cyclodestructive procedures. That is hardly a ringing endorsement for the state of the art.

ALTERATION OF INFLOW

Transscleral Cyclodestruction

Consider the alternative approach to glaucoma treatment: diminishing the inflow side of the equation. Diathermy, cryotherapy, and various laser wavelengths have been applied to the external surface of the eye for the purpose of destroying the ciliary body and "turning off" aqueous production. Less aqueous presumably means lower IOP.

All of these modalities were applied transsclerally. In this approach, the location of the ciliary body is estimated on the outside surface of the globe, largely by our historical knowledge of where this structure is assumed to be located inside the eye. Then, one of these "destructive" sources is applied to this area, theoretically destroying the underlying portion of ciliary body yet hopefully sparing adjacent tissue. It is not possible to directly view the target tissue by these methods.

Weve (4) first described this inflow-reducing approach by using penetrating diathermy in 1933, and other reports followed some time later (5,6). Because of its brutality, low success rate, and high incidence of complications, cyclodiathermy was abandoned.

Cyclocryotherapy

An alternative inflow procedure did not present itself until 1950, when a freezing probe was placed on the outside surface of the eye and repeated freeze–thaw cycles were applied from 90 degrees to 360 degrees around the globe, over one or multiple sessions. Other reports established the value of this surgical option, cyclocryotherapy (CCT), in the management of intractable forms of glaucoma. This technique was noninvasive, simple to perform, and repeatable, while

requiring a minimum of instrumentation that was not particularly expensive, comparatively little skill on the surgeon's part, and no surgical assistant or operating room. Postoperative care was minimal. On the negative side, CCT was brutish and painful, and was associated with a significant failure rate as far as controlling IOP was concerned. CCT resulted in a host of minor and devastating complications, including a 10% to 20% incidence of phthisis and a 70% incidence of visual loss. Nevertheless, considering the practice patterns of all ophthalmologists worldwide, this more than 50-year-old approach is the standard inflow procedure today.

Laser Transscleral Cyclophotocoagulation

With the availability of lasers in ophthalmology, Beckman and colleagues (7–9) were the first to report laser transscleral cyclophotocoagulation (TSCPC), initially with the ruby laser and shortly thereafter with the neodymium:yttrium-argon-garnet (Nd:YAG) laser. His landmark 10-year follow-up study included a very large population of ruby laser–treated patients and established without doubt the moderate efficacy and safety of the transscleral approach in patients with refractory forms of glaucoma as well as the superiority of this "destructive" force to CCT (Fig. 4-1).

Most studies of laser TSCPC involved the Nd:YAG laser. Comparisons between the contact and noncontact application of laser indicate that the noncontact method has a greater incidence of postoperative pain, inflammation, and other complications. This approach has largely been abandoned in favor of the contact technique.

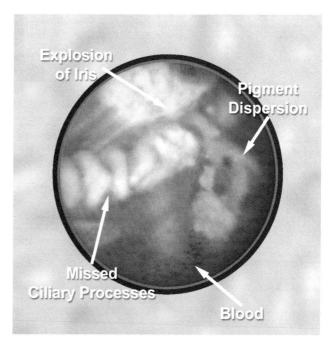

FIGURE 4-1. Effect of transscleral cyclophotocoagulation on the ciliary processes and adjacent tissue in vitro.

Typically, successful IOP control with TSCP has been reported in the 50% to 70% range, representing a considerable improvement over the outcomes experienced with CCT. On the other hand, a significant incidence of serious complications still plagues this approach.

TSCPC, then, shares many of the advantages of CCT. Specifically, it is noninvasive and simple to perform, needs a minimum of instrumentation, does not require a surgical assistant or operating room, and can be repeated. Disadvantages of this approach are similar to those of CCT in that it is painful for the patient and is associated with an array of minor and severe complications. A significant incidence of hypotony and phthisis is associated with certain glaucoma mechanisms, and this technique bears a 40% to 50% risk for visual loss. In addition, Nd:YAG lasers are expensive, placing this technique beyond the reach of most ophthalmologists, hospitals, and patients. However, the proliferation of less expensive, compact semiconductor diode lasers has expanded interest in TSCPC.

A number of factors can control the outcome of TSCPC in a given eye. As far as laser wavelength is concerned, it seems that it is virtually irrelevant whether the lesion is created by a red (640 nm) ruby or krypton source, the near-infrared (810 nm) of the semiconductor diode laser, or a somewhat longer infrared (1064 nm) source of Nd:YAG laser.

The pressure applied to the eye wall with the contact TSCPC laser probe can dramatically increase the laser delivery to the tissue. This factor can potentiate the risk of "overtreatment" or perforation. Energy delivery to tissue can also be affected by such seemingly minor variations such as tilt of the transscleral laser probe as it contacts the eye.

It has also been demonstrated that laser energy delivered transsclerally to the ciliary body region in the pseudophakic eye can damage IOL haptics that are incorporated into the treatment zone, resulting in an inflammatory response.

However, the "blind" approach of laser delivery to the ciliary processes is by far the major determinant of treatment success or failure. Transscleral probe placement, tilt, and pressure can alter laser transmission to the target tissue, resulting in overtreatment or undertreatment or partially or completely missed processes. Inadequate power delivery results in an inadequate IOP response. Overly intensive treatment, on the other hand, is responsible for many of the complications experienced by those who use this technique. Pain, inflammation, hemorrhage, choroidal effusion, diminished vision as a consequence of cystoid macular edema, hypotony, and phthisis are the eye's response to overtreatment of the ciliary processes or "missing" of the target tissue altogether, as well as damage to adjacent structures such as the iris, pars plana, and retina. "Pops" are an example of this in that they indicate explosion of the tissue at the laser delivery site, presumably by overheating and gas bubble formation. Some take comfort in hearing this reaction because they assume that this indicates that the target (the ciliary process) has been appropriately localized and that it has been successfully ablated. This conclusion is erroneous. Any ocular tissue treated in an overly intense manner will explode. One can easily demonstrate that the retina, pars plana, or iris can be popped by delivering a higher power laser application to these structures through the laser endoscope (where this reaction can be visualized) in a practice animal eye (Fig. 4-2).

Because of its limitations, TSCPC is applicable primarily in (a) patients with refractory forms of glaucoma, (b) those who are likely to fail filtration, (c) those with a high risk for filtration complications, and (d) those who already have poor central vision.

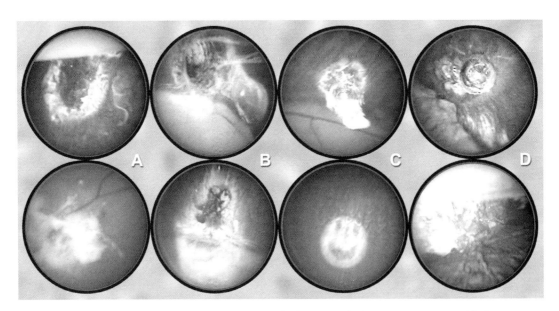

FIGURE 4-2. A: Appearance of transscleral cyclophotocoagulation overtreatment with "popping" (explosion) of retina **B:** pars plana **C:** ciliary body **D:** iris.

The most important limitation to this approach is the 40% to 50% incidence of visual loss, being perhaps slightly better than what may be expected with CCT.

ARE INFLOW PROCEDURES INHERENTLY NEGATIVE?

One might conclude that there is no place for an inflow procedure in most ophthalmic practices based on the difficulties encountered with this approach. Poor to moderate success in controlling IOP, limited applicability in most glaucoma mechanisms encountered in the typical ophthalmology practice, and a significant incidence of unhappy or devastating outcomes translate into avoidance.

But is there some ill-defined yet inherently dangerous feature of the ciliary processes that leads to poor results? The short answer is no.

Historical Perspective

A small body of literature specifically addresses laser treatment of the ciliary processes under direct visualization. Early reports were of the transpupillary approach in eyes with large iridectomies or aniridia, which permitted a slit-lamp view of the target. Argon laser applications to these areas resulted in some eyes having improved IOP control, but overall the outcomes were disappointing. Of perhaps greater significance was the absence of serious complications. This approach to the ciliary processes was not a practical solution to the universe of patients with surgical glaucoma problems because, as we all know, a sufficient number of ciliary processes cannot be viewed (or treated) except under extraordinary circumstances.

In 1985, Charles (10) reported on a patient with neovascular glaucoma and vitreoretinal disease. After vitrectomy and lensectomy, the ciliary processes were scleral depressed into the view of the operating microscope and a xenon arc endophotocoagulation probe was inserted through the pars plana. The ciliary processes were viewed through the pupil and, under this direct visualization through the operating microscope, were photocoagulated (Fig. 4-3). The postoperative IOP was lowered but long-term data were not presented, primarily because the neovascular glaucoma treatment was not the point of the study. This, however, was the first report of the transvitreal approach to cyclophotocoagulation.

Patel and colleagues (11) and later Zarbin and associates (12) reported a large series with long-term follow-up of intractable glaucoma patients, mostly neovascular, treated by the transvitreal method using the argon laser. The outcomes were remarkable, with almost 90% success in controlling IOP yet few significant complications. Given the extremely poor prognosis for these patients, the transvitreal approach was an outstanding accomplishment.

One might conjecture that if this most treacherous form of glaucoma could be so effectively managed in this manner, why can't other mechanisms of the disease? The only major disadvantage of this approach was the prerequisite of an aphakic and vitrectomized eye.

Shields (13) recognized this dilemma and reported on the experimental juxtaposition of an endoscope with an argon laser endophotocoagulation fiber. The ciliary processes in cadaver eyes were photocoagulated and then studied.

Putting this into historical perspective, the smallest gauge commercially available endoscope at that time was used in orthopedic surgery and was 1.7 mm in outer diam-

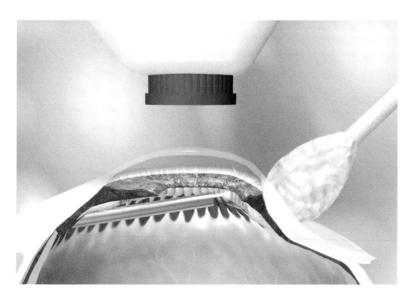

FIGURE 4-3. Transvitreal approach to cyclophotocoagulation. After vitrectomy and lensectomy, the endophotocoagulation probe is inserted through the pars plana while the ciliary processes are scleral depressed in the view of the operating microscope. If the cornea is not clear, if the pupil is mitotic, or if there is a lens implant, it will not be possible to see the target tissue and effect treatment. This technique represented the first surgical approach to photocoagulating an extensive area of the ciliary ring under direct visualization.

eter. Combining with a laser fiber resulted in a diameter of more than 2 mm. Furthermore, the optics of this endoscope would in no way image from within the human eye. The portion of the instrumentation that was in the surgeon's hand was very large, cumbersome, and impractical.

Most endoscopes used in other surgical areas have a characteristic design and—no matter whether rigid or flexible, used in gastrointestinal, pulmonary, general surgical, or gynecologic applications—are physically more or less the same. If endoscopy were to become practical in ophthalmology, a complete departure from the "standard" instrumentation was required.

If one were to imagine what physical changes in this imaging system would be required, perhaps the first item on the list would be elimination of the eyepiece for direct viewing. To simply adapt this component to a lensing and video camera system would only make the already cumbersome endoscope even more awkward and impractical. Second, the outer diameter of the smallest endoscope, even if it had the appropriate optics, was twice as large as would be acceptable and so would require reduction. Finally, to make such an instrument widely useful in ophthalmology, it would be desirable to have it subserve a function beyond mere observation, so that incorporation of a laser fiber into the design would transform a diagnostic into a therapeutic instrument.

In 1991, a laser video endoscope with an outer diameter of 0.89 mm (20 gauge) and a 3,000-pixel image guide was developed and received U.S. and other nationality patents, as well as Food and Drug Administration clearance for use in vitreoretinal surgery and cyclophotocoagulation. The first group of patients with intractable neovascular glaucoma who were treated by endoscopic cyclophotocoagulation (ECP) carried out with a diode laser through a pars plana incision was reported. The outcomes were similar to those experienced with the transvitreal approach, with achievement of IOP control in the 90% range and less than devastating complications. The technique was far simpler than the transvitreal approach.

Shortly after the evolution of this instrument it became apparent that phakic patients could not realistically be treated from the pars plana, even with curved probes. The posterior aspect of the lens was observed to be quite spherical in many eyes, so that the shaft of the endoscope would traumatize the posterior lens surface during ECP, resulting in acute cataract formation. To address this problem, a clear corneal limbal approach was developed. Although it will be discussed in greater detail shortly, the key was to open the potential space that exists between the posterior aspect of the iris and the anterior lens surface and to maintain it throughout the procedure. Ultimately, it was found that a sodium hyaluronate viscoelastic could be used to displace the iris forward and the lens posteriorly, permitting access to the ciliary processes and allowing their controlled, directly visualized, photocoagulation.

Once this limbal approach was refined for phakic eyes, it became clear that it could be applied regardless of the patient's lens status. Furthermore, vitrectomy was not a prerequisite for this approach. The door was opened for management of an array of glaucoma mechanisms with widely variable anatomic and lens conditions, from either the anterior or posterior segment, by ECP. Technically, combining cataract surgery with ECP became feasible, and for the first time an inflow procedure could be mounted concomitantly for management of cataract and glaucoma.

Pediatric glaucomas present another stubborn management problem for the ophthalmologist. Many of these patients can present under desperate circumstances, having failed all treatment modalities even when performed multiple times. The corneal and lens status of these patients, along with surgically or congenitally induced anatomic abnormalities and the presence of prosthetic devices such as drainage tubes or lens implants, confounds therapy. ECP has shown significant efficacy and a minimum of morbidity in this difficult group and will be discussed in further detail in Chapter 13. In addition, many congenital glaucoma patients present with corneal opacification, making goniotomy a problem. Endoscopic visualization of the angle would seem to be a logical solution to this dilemma. Combining endoscopy with goniotomy has indeed been shown to be a technically simple and effective approach.

REFERENCES

1. Koryllos K. Trabeculectomy: a new glaucoma operation. *Bull Soc Hellen Ophthalmol* 1967;35:147–157.
2. Cairns JE. Trabeculectomy: preliminary report of a new method. *Am J Ophthalmol* 1968;66:673–679.
3. Molteno AC. New implant for drainage in glaucoma: clinical trial. *Br J Ophthalmol* 1969;53:606–615.
4. Weve H. Die Zyklodiatermie das Corpus ciliare bei Glaukom. *Zentralbl Ophthalmol* 1933;29:562–569.
5. Stocker FW. Response of chronic simple glaucoma to treatment with cyclodiathermy puncture. *Arch Ophthalmol* 1945;34:181–186.
6. Walton DS, Grant WM. Penetrating cyclodiathermy for filtration. *Arch Ophthalmol* 1970;83:47–48.
7. Beckman H, Kinoshita A, Rota AN, Sugar HS. Transscleral ruby laser irradiation of the ciliary body in the treatment of intractable glaucoma. *Trans Am Acad Ophthalmol Otolaryngol* 1972;76:423–436.
8. Beckman H, Sugar HS. Neodymium laser cyclocoagulation. *Arch Ophthalmol* 1973;90:27–28.
9. Beckman H, Waelterman J. Transscleral ruby laser cyclocoagulation. *Am J Ophthalmol* 1984;98:788–795.
10. Charles S. Endophotocoagulation. *Retina* 1981;1:117–120.
11. Patel A, Thompson JT, Michels RG, Quigley HA. Endolaser treatment of the ciliary body for uncontrolled glaucoma. *Ophthalmology* 1986;93:825–830.
12. Zarbin MA, Michels RG, de Bustros S, et al. Endolaser treatment of the ciliary body for severe glaucoma. *Ophthalmology* 1988;95:1639–1648.
13. Shields MB. Cyclodestructive surgery for glaucoma: past, present, and future. *Trans Am Ophthalmol Soc* 1985;83:285–303.

ENDOSCOPIC CYCLOPHOTOCOAGULATION FOR GLAUCOMA: THE BASICS

SURGICAL CONSIDERATIONS

This above outline has delineated the reality that an inflow procedure exists that is widely applicable across a spectrum of glaucoma mechanisms and anatomic conditions, and that can be safely and efficaciously performed by most ophthalmologists.

Now for the details. Armed with an understanding of the historical precedents of endoscopy and the evolution of inflow and outflow surgical glaucoma procedures, one must next consider how exactly to perform endoscopic cyclophotocoagulation (ECP) under various anatomic scenarios.

It is important to appreciate that a triple-function laser endoscope must be used to perform ECP. A combination of coaxial image, illumination, and laser is the *only* feasible configuration to simultaneously visualize and laser the ciliary processes. Dividing these functions and employing a bimanual approach is difficult to impossible. Essentially, ECP is a one-handed technique. The surgeon's sec-

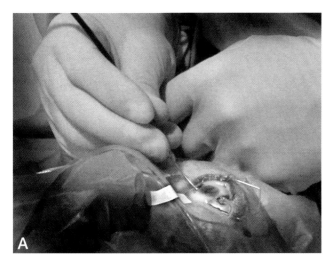

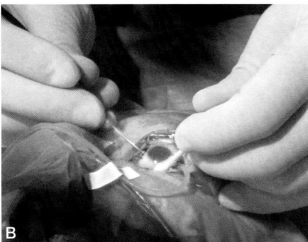

FIGURE 5-1. A: The laser endoscope is held with one hand and supported by the other. **B:** Alternatively, one hand holds the endoscope while the other hand depresses the sclera.

ond hand is used to support the one with the laser endoscope or, occasionally, to perform scleral depression (Fig. 5-1).

Anesthesia

The ciliary processes are very sensitive to contact by instruments, prosthetic devices, and, in particular, the application of any ophthalmic laser wavelength. Happily, it is simple to achieve adequate anesthesia. General anesthesia is effective but rarely necessary. Exceptions to this are in the treatment children or other patients who could not otherwise cooperate with surgery under lesser conditions. Any form of local anesthesia with or without sedation is typically sufficient. Retrobulbar, peribulbar, and intraocular approaches are quite effective. Purely topical anesthesia, however, is insufficient for this purpose. Topical application can be augmented by intraocular anesthesia to obtain the desired

result however. Pretreatment with analgesics is not necessary. Interestingly, postoperative analgesic requirements are usually minimal.

Ciliary Process Access

The surgeon must clearly understand how to access the ciliary processes from the pars plana or the limbus in the phakic, anterior chamber pseudophakic, posterior chamber pseudophakic, or aphakic eye as well as at the time of cataract surgery. It is curious that this is the most significant technical consideration that the surgeon must make. Facility with each approach is essential to maximize the outcomes to ECP. Fortunately, these variations are easily mastered.

Surgeon Placement

The surgeon can sit in any position around the patient's head but usually is situated superiorly or temporally. The operating microscope is placed over the patient's eye and is used primarily for creating and closing incisions and inserting and removing the endoprobe. Once the endoscope has been introduced into the eye, the microscope is no longer needed and the surgeon must direct attention to the video monitor, where the endoscopic image appears. This monitor can be placed in any location that the surgeon finds comfortable. Usually, the endoscopy console is positioned on the opposite side from other major instrumentation, such as the phacoemulsification or vitrectomy unit.

Lighting

After the endoscope is positioned in the eye, the illumination from the operating microscope can be turned off; it usually does not contribute much to the endoscopic image. However, if the endoscope being used has poor illumination characteristics, the microscope's light can be helpful.

The surgeon increases or decreases the endoscope's illumination, depending on the proximity of its tip to the target tissue. The closer the target, the less illumination required for optimal visualization. Too much light "whites out" the view, and too little illumination results in a dark picture with loss of tissue detail, sometimes to a critical degree.

The most widely used laser and endoscopic system permits the surgeon to control the illumination level and laser application with a single footswitch or by an assistant changing these parameters on the system control panel. Others demand that the assistant always manually alter the level of illumination.

Endoscope Removal from the Eye

Before proceeding with the details of each specific approach to the ciliary processes, one must consider how to withdraw the endoscope from the eye. Recall that endoscopy ignores one of the "rules" of operating microscope surgery, that is, to always be able to see the instruments tips within the eye. Because the image is derived from the tip of the endoscope, it cannot be seen unless one is using the operating microscope or some other means of direct visualization. It is important to ensure that the endoscope (or any other instrument, for that matter) is not adherent to any intraocular structures. There has been a single case report of iris avulsion arising as a consequence (1). Gayton (1) has elucidated that careful removal of the endoscope at the completion of surgery under direct visualization will ensure that this problem does not occur.

ANTERIOR SEGMENT APPROACH

General Considerations

Entry Sites

Because the laser endoscope must be of a small outer diameter, an elaborate set of anterior segment incisions is not necessary. Typically, the conjunctiva need not be disturbed. This is helpful because it limits the potential for bleeding and shortens operative time. It is also best not to manipulate the conjunctiva in eyes with filtering blebs, tube implants, corneal sutures, or chronic injection from a variety of causes. A clear corneal flat incision is fashioned near the limbus. Although endoscopes are typically less than 1.0 mm in outer diameter, a generous incision that allows lateral movement is best. It is not important to have a "tight" wound because such a wound can inhibit intraocular manipulation of the endoscope. As you will see, it is often helpful to create a flat anterior chamber during the procedure, so again, there is no advantage to a "watertight" incision. Further, endoscope management in a tight incision seems to promote postoperative corneal edema as a consequence of repeated torsion on the tissue. Any blade that can create a straight flat incision is adequate. Some surgeons prefer a keratome, others an MVR blade, still others a 15-degree blade.

Placement of the incision is usually arbitrary. Some surgeons prefer to sit in a temporal position to the patient's head while others may prefer a superior position. It might be beneficial to avoid functioning and nonfunctional trabeculectomy sites and the areas adjacent to them on the external ocular surface. An inadvertent conjunctival buttonhole, for example, might alter the filtration dynamics of a given eye, creating a host of complications. Even multiple tube implants do not present much of an obstacle for performing ECP, but one must plan entry sites that will not disturb the conjunctiva or scleral patch overlying the tube. Other physical obstacles that are commonly encountered include broad-based areas of iridocapsular adhesions, displaced lens implants, and dense accumulations of cortical

remnants after cataract surgery. Maneuvers to circumvent these obstacles will be reviewed shortly.

It is important to appreciate that ECP is a relatively minimalist procedure when performed from the anterior segment, especially in view of the fact that, at least ideally, the only ocular tissue that the surgeon contacts is the edges of the corneal wound.

External Surface Hemorrhage

Typically, bleeding from incision sites is an issue of minor concern because a clear corneal approach is relatively avascular. Still, even a small amount of blood creates a film on the endoscope tip. Recall that the image is derived from the distal end of the probe, so blood will obscure the view, like ketchup on spectacles. It is important then to irrigate or dry this entry site during endoscope insertion (Fig. 5-2).

Corneal Opacification

Many ocular disorders are associated with corneal opacification. This can be a problem when using the operating microscope for obvious reasons. On the other hand, the endoscopic image is independent of this feature. With very

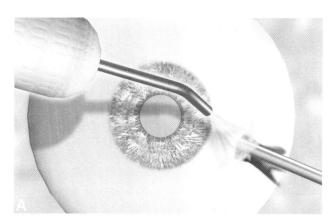
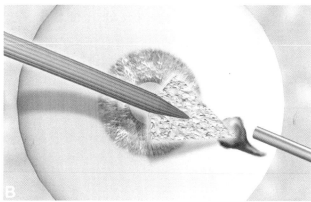

FIGURE 5-2. Insertion of the endoscope into the bleeding limbal incision. **A:** Blood is cleared with irrigation. **B:** Blood is cleared with a sponge.

little experience, the ophthalmologist can attain proficiency in intraocular maneuvers without being able to actually see the instruments in the eye. This attribute is helpful when dealing with eyes for which corneal transplantation is undesirable. Consider an eye with an opaque cornea and suspected advanced glaucoma. By simply visualizing the posterior pole from the anterior segment, the surgeon can assess the general health of the optic nerve and retina to determine whether initiation of a more involved procedure is warranted or whether there is so much preexisting damage that extensive intervention would be fruitless. In vitreoretinal surgery, endoscopic imaging can almost always eliminate the need for additional surgery that involves removal of the opacified cornea, placement of a temporary keratoprosthesis, and subsequent corneal transplantation.

Hyphema

When inserting the endoscope into the anterior segment, clear imaging demands clear media. Ocular trauma, intraocular surgery, iris neovascularization, vitreous hemorrhage with extension into the anterior chamber, intraocular lens (IOL) haptic erosion of ciliary body or iris, and many other problems are frequent sources of anterior segment hemorrhage. To endoscopically image anterior segment or posterior iris structures, blood must be removed from the eye. This is usually a simple task that requires a minimum of instrumentation (Fig. 5-3). One technique is to make a small flat stab incision through the clear cornea near the limbus and a second flat stab incision at the limbus opposite to it. An anterior chamber maintainer with balanced salt solution (BSS) is used to irrigate through one of the incisions while a forceps is used to open the second site. The cannula of the anterior chamber maintainer can be moved horizontally and vertically to irrigate blood from the surface of the iris or corneal endothelium. Switching the anterior chamber maintainer to the second incision site can help to remove blood that did not clear initially. These maneuvers are often successful in removing most or all of the hemorrhage from the anterior and posterior chambers within a few minutes. The incisions do not require sutures, except sometimes in children.

Surgical Planning

Now that we understand the theoretical basis for ECP and its relationship to other glaucoma procedures, have a background in the technology of endoscopic imaging and laser delivery, and possess the tools to access the target tissue and deliver laser energy to it, the next step addresses surgical planning. Unlike other forms of glaucoma surgery, the status of the lens and of the vitreous is the primary consideration, while mechanism of glaucoma, intraocular pressure (IOP), previous surgical interventions, visual acuity, and visual field status are of lesser importance.

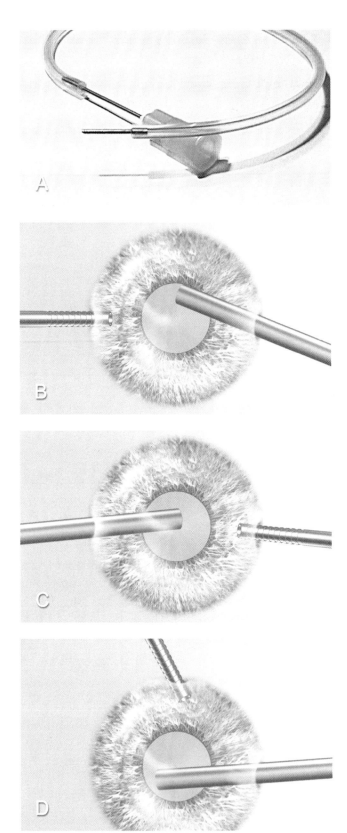

FIGURE 5-3. Removal of blood from the eye. **A:** Anterior chamber maintainer. **B:** Endoscope in one incision and anterior chamber maintainer in another. **C:** Positions switched. **D:** Third incision site.

Viscoelastic Use and Removal

The ciliary processes can be accessed from an anterior segment incision in a phakic, pseudophakic, or aphakic eye, and ECP can be combined with cataract surgery and IOL implantation or corneal transplantation. Incisions can be made in clear cornea, at the limbus, or in the sclera just posterior to the limbus.

The first human ECPs were performed from a pars plana incision in vitrectomized aphakic or pseudophakic eyes. Even though the clinical outcomes were remarkable, it soon became apparent that if this technique were to be generally useful to most surgical glaucoma patients and executed by most ophthalmologists, a less involved technique must evolve. Ideally, this approach would not necessitate lensectomy and vitrectomy as prerequisites but rather would circumvent these anatomic conditions to access the ciliary body. Fortunately, it did not require much of an intellectual leap to solve this problem. Basically, injection of a sodium hyaluronate viscoelastic posterior to the iris displaces the crystalline lens, posterior chamber IOL, or lens remnants posteriorly and flattens the anterior chamber anteriorly, easily permitting access to the ciliary processes. If there is no lens, IOL, or lens material posterior to the iris, then a viscoelastic is not required.

Use of viscoelastics is central to the execution of ECP from the anterior segment. By far, their most significant function is to open the potential space that exists between the iris and lens, IOL, or lens remnant. Furthermore, they must remain in place throughout the surgical procedure, creating adequate exposure for the surgeon. There is some evidence that these substances can exert a hemostatic effect. Finally, they must be easily removed at the completion of surgery

Sodium hyaluronate viscoelastics are the only products appropriate for this task. Viscoelastics not in this group are typically inadequate because they do not open the space behind the iris well, do not remain in this area for long, and typically ooze posteriorly. Once this occurs, these substances cannot be removed from the eye sufficiently to prevent complications, such as elevated postoperative IOP.

It is important to remove as much viscoelastic as possible from the eye at the completion of surgery (Fig. 5-4). Failure to do so will almost assuredly result in an IOP spike during the first postoperative day or two, with the patient experiencing a number of problems, including severe pain, nausea and vomiting, and blurred vision. If the eye is highly threatened because of advanced visual field loss, it is especially important to avoid this situation.

The exception to this is the vitrectomized eye, in which viscoelastic removal is less critical because retention frequently will not result in IOP elevation. It is sometimes difficult to remove viscoelastic from these eyes because it may slip into the posterior segment during the procedure.

Perhaps the best method for removing viscoelastic from the anterior segment is to use the standard irrigation/aspi-

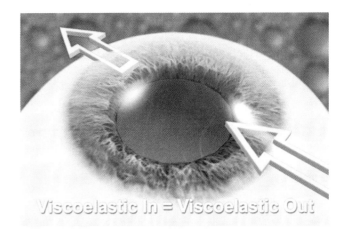

FIGURE 5-4. It is important to remove as much of the inserted viscoelastic from the eye as possible at the end of the procedure.

ration setup employed in cataract surgery. Although some instrumentation and experience is required to effect this technique, most surgeons and operating rooms are familiar with this approach.

Another simple and effective approach is to inject BSS from a 3-mL syringe through a small-gauge needle into the anterior chamber from the limbus at a site opposite the surgical incision. While the solution is being injected, the surgical incision is held open with a forceps or other instrument. Typically, the viscoelastic extrudes from the surgical incision in several globs (Fig. 5-5). This maneuver can be repeated as needed until there seems to be no residual viscoelastic behind the iris.

Viscodissection

Adhesions frequently occur between the posterior aspect of the iris and the lens, IOL, or lens remnants. Some of these are visible preoperatively in the form of posterior synechiae.

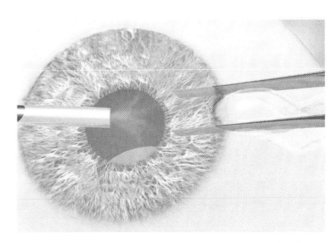

FIGURE 5-5. Viscoelastic globs out when balanced salt solution is injected into the eye.

A more subtle manifestation of this is posterior dimpling of the iris, especially in pseudophakic eyes. When there is a history of anterior segment uveitis or of iris neovascularization, there almost always are areas of iridolenticular or iridocapsular adhesion, even if these problems have become quiescent or regressed.

Previous intraocular surgery, such as phacoemulsification or trabeculectomy, often incites adhesion development. Typically, their presence is of little clinical significance, but their existence impedes the surgeon's access to the ciliary processes during ECP. Viscoelastics are effective at gently dissecting or breaking these adhesions. A word of caution, however: If there is a strong, broad-based pillar of posterior iris connected to anterior lens or capsule surface, or a fragment of lens material that does not easily displace with this maneuver, it is best to *avoid* it and find some other area of the ciliary body to address (Fig. 5-6). In some problem eyes, four or more incisions may be required to access a sufficient number of ciliary processes to effect adequate treatment. This is a relatively simple task. One of the great benefits of ECP is that it can be performed rapidly with minimal disturbance to the intraocular terrain, limiting potential complications. Overzealous manipulation of these difficult adhesions can lead to intraocular hemorrhage, IOL dislocation, vitreous extrusion, posterior or anterior dislocation of old lens fragments, and a host of other problems that defeat the purpose and advantages of this approach.

Unsuspected Pathologic Anatomy and Other States

Endoscopy is an exciting tool if for no other reason than portions of the eye that were previously visually and surgically inaccessible can now be reached. During the course of ECP, the surgeon may encounter pathologic states that were unsuspected preoperatively. This is particularly true in pseudophakic eyes, in which lens remnants, extruding IOL haptics, and other surprises are not uncommon. The temptation to address these situations should be avoided unless they directly contribute to the pathogenesis of the patient's surgical problem. Although this philosophy is not based on a scientific foundation, "gilding the lily" often does not seem to reward the surgeon or the patient. One of the great advantages of ECP is that it can circumvent anatomic and pathologic impediments to accessing and photocoagulating the desired amount of ciliary process tissue. To be diverted from this physical goal can be counterproductive.

Pupillary Dilation

For the experienced anterior segment endoscopic surgeon, pupillary dilation is not very important. Recall that most of the surgery is performed without the benefit of operating microscope, loupe, or direct visualization. Sometimes it is even helpful to have a relatively miotic pupil. When the ciliary processes are imaged from the anterior segment, the posterior aspect of the iris acts endoscopically as the "ceiling," defining the "top" of the surgical space. The greater the pupillary dilation, the less there is of it. Still, for the novice, it is usually easier to have a dilated pupil simply because there is greater opportunity to manipulate the endoscope into its proper position by direct visualization. Under these conditions, if the endoscope is advanced across the anterior chamber to the edge of the pupil, the target tissue is almost in view. Furthermore, less viscoelastic is required because there is less iris to displace. Merely injecting viscoelastic posterior into the iris often results in significant pupillary dilation. Any mydriatic will usually suffice, depending on the surgeon's preference. Cyclopentolate 1% has proven to be adequate for this purpose. Finally, it is important to avoid abrading the posterior aspect of the iris while maneuvering the endoscope behind it. This is facilitated by a well-inflated sulcus.

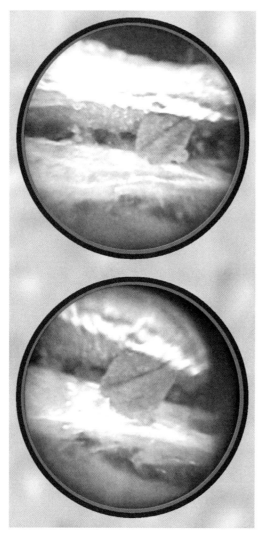

FIGURE 5-6. Endoscopic views of dense iridocapsular adhesion obscuring view of ciliary processes.

Scleral Depression

It is sometimes helpful to combine scleral depression of the ciliary body area with ECP. This maneuver is quite simple. Recall that ECP is typically a one-handed technique, so the surgeon's second hand is available for other tasks. By using a cotton-tipped applicator or some other instrument to depress the opposing sclera just posterior to the limbus, endoscopic access to the ciliary processes can be enhanced. This technique may "splay" open the processes (Fig. 5-7), allowing access to the spaces between them for more complete photocoagulation, or it may simplify the presentation of certain portions of the processes that for technical reasons are difficult to image or laser in the usual manner. This technique can be applied to any of the variations in surgical approach in the performance of ECP from the anterior or posterior segment or when it is combined with cataract surgery. Because the amount of force to the external eye

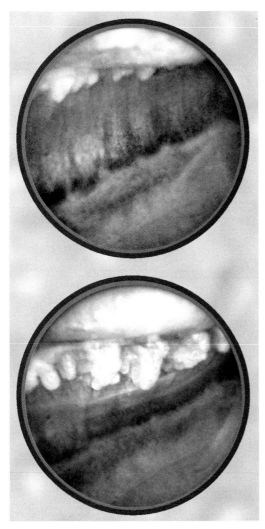

FIGURE 5-7. Endoscopic views of ciliary processes splayed open by scleral depression.

wall is minimal, no complications from this variation of technique have been encountered.

Vitrectomy

A small amount of instrument manipulation in the posterior segment or in the vitreous-filled anterior segment probably would not be harmful. Still, it would be difficult to quantify these parameters. Thus, an accepted precept of intraocular surgery is that vitreous must be removed from the anterior or posterior chamber, or both chambers, before instruments are introduced and maneuvered. While some vitreoretinal techniques are involved and require specialized training and extensive experience (and perhaps even luck), the performance of basic vitrectomy involves little training and just a minimum of practice to achieve facility. Being successful with ECP under a variety of ocular anatomic conditions demands that the surgeon possess some technical versatility. One of the interesting aspects of ECP, and a surprise to many, is that the ciliary processes can be accessed from the anterior segment and that vitreous is usually not found in the working area. However, if vitreous is present in the treatment zone during an anterior segment approach, it must be removed. Going a step further, if the surgeon is to attain maximum flexibility in dealing with the array of anatomic situations that may present themselves, the pars plana approach to the ciliary processes must be learned. Vitrectomy is usually an integral part of this method because most of these eyes have not undergone previous vitreous surgery. The following is a description of some simple vitrectomy techniques for the anterior segment, which can be helpful in achieving surgical goals with a minimum of difficulty.

Maintaining Intraocular Pressure

Because vitrectomy instruments aspirate fluid and other material from the eye, they will, by definition, lower the IOP intraoperatively to the point where the eye would collapse. This situation makes it a little difficult to continue with the procedure (not to mention how it increases the risk of certain complications, such as hemorrhage and choroidal effusion). In standard three-port pars plana vitrectomy, this problem is overcome by placement of an infusion cannula through one of the three sclerotomy sites. It would be fair to say that most anterior segment surgeons do not feel comfortable with this maneuver and would not adopt a technique that requires it. Fortunately, insertion of a pars plana infusion cannula is not necessary in any of the technical variations of ECP. As discussed previously, there are several ways to maintain IOP throughout surgery that are quite simple. If only a small amount of vitreous is to be removed, whether from an anterior or posterior segment approach, infusion may not be necessary at all. But, typically, if a significant anterior vitrectomy is required, having some form of infusion is advisable (Table 5-1).

TABLE 5-1. OPTIONS FOR MAINTAINING INTRAOCULAR PRESSURE DURING VITRECTOMY

- Infusion sleeve around vitrector
- Anterior chamber maintainer
- Pars plana infusion of balanced salt solution

One elementary solution is to place an infusion sleeve around the vitrector (Fig. 5-8B). The incision site must be enlarged to accommodate the larger outer diameter of the instrument, but this technique works well from either the anterior or the posterior segment. Once vitrectomy has been completed and the instrument removed from the eye, the infusion sleeve can be removed from the vitrector and placed on the endoscope if the surgeon desires. In this manner, a single incision is all that is required to achieve vitrectomy and 180 degrees of cyclophotocoagulation.

A second variation would be to insert an anterior chamber maintainer through the limbus (see Fig. 5-8A), permitting a constant infusion of BSS into the eye. This method is useful whether accessing the ciliary processes through the anterior or posterior segment. The fluid delivery through this device is relatively smaller than what may be expected through a 20-gauge infusion cannula, which is typically used in vitrectomy. If the surgeon discovers that the flow is

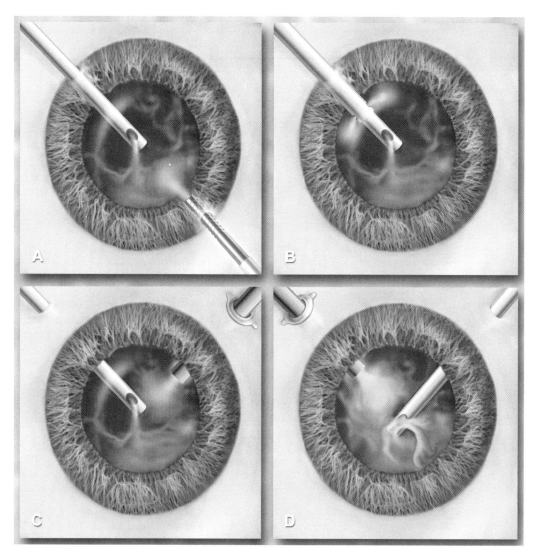

FIGURE 5-8. Methods for maintaining globe formation during vitrectomy for endoscopic cyclophotocoagulation (ECP). **A:** Anterior chamber maintainer inserted through the limbus. **B:** Infusion sleeve placed around the vitrector. **C, D:** Pars plana infusion option involves two incision sites: one for the vitrector and then the endoscope (10-o'clock position) and one for the infusion cannula (2-o'clock position). The instruments are then *switched* in the sites so that ECP can be performed on the opposite side.

insufficient, the height of the BSS bottle can be raised to compensate.

A third approach would be to place a standard pars plana infusion cannula in one sclerotomy site and proceed with vitrectomy and ECP from a second anterior or posterior segment incision site (see Fig. 5-8C, D). This technique has the advantage of allowing the surgeon to switch instruments from one site to the other, so that cyclophotocoagulation to be executed for 360 degrees. As an example, pars plana incisions are made at the 10- and 2-o'clock positions. The infusion cannula is inserted at 10 o'clock and the vitrector followed by the laser endoscope at 2 o'clock. Once adequate vitrectomy and ECP have been performed from this position, the infusion is moved to the 2-o'clock position, and the vitrector and laser endoscope are inserted through the 10-o'clock position to complete treatment on the opposite "side" of the eye. A trocar system for placing the infusion cannula is useful because it is simple to place, does not require sutures, and can be switched to the opposite-side incision in less than a minute.

Vitrector Parameters

Although historically there have been many vitrectomy devices available with variations in their cutting characteristics, most current vitrectomy units function in a similar manner. Although there may be wide variation in what the surgeon can preselect on the vitrectomy control unit, a single set of parameters is typically all that is required to perform most cases. Ultimately, the goal is to remove the vitreous without being so vigorous as to induce tractional forces sufficient to tear the retina.

First, a guillotine cutter is necessary. This instrument has a vertical chopping effect that minimizes the traction between vitreous and retina when in use. Rotary cutters are to be avoided. Their spinning motion can spool strands of vitreous that can ultimately tear the retina.

Second, a balance must be reached between cutting speed and efficacy of removing the vitreous. Slower cut rates can amputate more vitreous and thereby accelerate the course of surgery. On the other hand, aspirating and cutting larger segments of vitreous can increase vitreoretinal traction, with its attendant complications. Alternatively, a very fast cut rate is useful for tissue cutting associated with minimal traction. Removing vitreous from the surface of the retina in traction retinal detachment surgery typically requires a very fast cut rate. Faster cut rates also give the surgeon greater control over the tissue effect during the course of vitrectomy. The disadvantage is that the faster the cut rate, the less vitreous is removed. A good compromise, however, is to set the cut rate at 400 to 600 cuts per minute. This setting typically gives the surgeon good control and minimizes retinal traction.

The final parameter to consider is the level of aspiration. Phacoemulsification and irrigation/aspiration techniques of cataract surgery use variable and relatively high suction lev-

els. This is ill advised and unnecessary in vitrectomy. High suction can markedly increase tractional forces on the retina, whereas levels that are too low do not adequately draw enough vitreous into the vitrector and hold it there for cutting. A preset maximum of 100 mm H_2O is typically sufficient to remove the vitreous without the creation of iatrogenic breaks or detachment.

Anterior Segment Approach to Anterior Vitrectomy

When vitreous is in the anterior or posterior chamber, it can be adequately removed for ECP by approach through the anterior segment. A clear corneal, limbal, or scleral beveled incision is fashioned, usually in a temporal position. The vitrector's cut rate and aspiration levels have been preset, as discussed. The vitrector is inserted with the cutter port facing upward, so that the surgeon can continuously view the aspiration and cutting through the operating microscope (Fig. 5-9). The procedure is continued until no vitreous can be seen in the microscope's field of view. The tip of the vitrector should not venture behind the iris or so far posteriorly that it cannot be well seen and focused by the microscope. If the eye appears to be softening, it should be infused with BSS, as previously discussed. This procedure is all that is required to adequately remove the anterior vitreous for ECP. Often, a good deal of vitreous remains in the eye, but that is acceptable since the purpose of this venture was to remove enough vitreous to enable a safely executed ECP. With a bit of experience, this can be achieved in a few minutes.

The vitrector can then be withdrawn from the eye and the laser endoscope inserted through the same incision site.

Posterior Segment Approach to Anterior Vitrectomy

Although many anterior segment surgeons have some trepidation about using a pars plana approach under any circumstances, it can actually be quite simple and in many

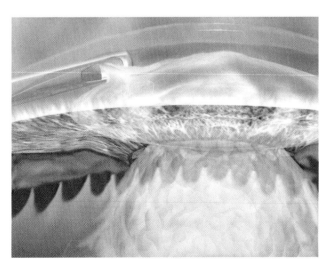

FIGURE 5-9. Anterior segment approach to anterior vitrectomy.

instances is more effective than proceeding through the anterior segment. The same principles of IOP maintenance apply here as in the anterior segment approach. An infusion sleeve can be placed around the vitrector or the endoscope, or an anterior chamber maintainer can be inserted at the limbus while a pars plana access is used for vitrectomy and ECP. Alternatively, a second pars plana incision can be created to permit infusion.

A small conjunctival incision is made beginning a few millimeters posterior to the limbus, usually in a temporal position. Then, with use of a caliper, a stab incision is created with an MVR blade 3.5 to 4.0 mm from the limbus. It is important for the novice pars plana surgeon to direct the blade posteriorly, as if aiming for the optic nerve. The blade need not enter the eye for more than 5 or 6 mm. Care should be taken not to advance the blade further within the eye because this will not make the incision any more useful

but may inadvertently damage some intraocular structure. As the blade is being withdrawn, the sclerotomy is enlarged to facilitate insertion and manipulation of the vitrector and endoscope (Fig. 5-10). While most MVR blades are said to create a 20-gauge incision, this dimension is measured on the external surface of the eye. The internal geometry of the wound is smaller, and so the surgeon often discovers that 20-gauge stab incisions are not large enough to permit insertion of a 20-gauge instrument. If the incision proves to be too small, the best technique for enlarging the wound is to reinsert the blade and enlarge the site as the blade is being withdrawn. A very short MVR-type blade has been

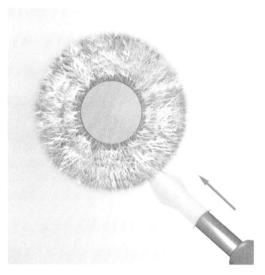

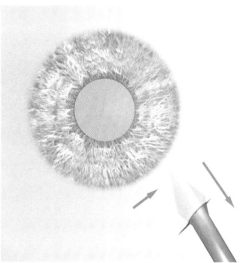

FIGURE 5-10. Creating and enlarging the pars plana incision using an MVR blade.

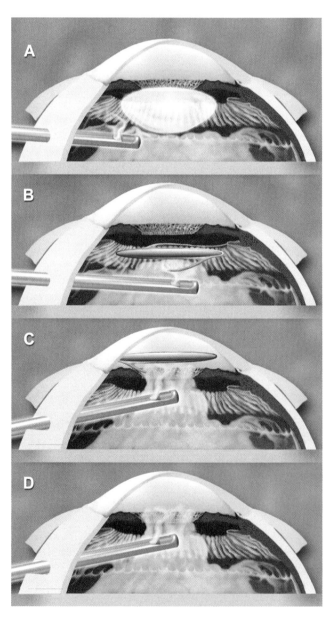

FIGURE 5-11. Anterior vitrectomy approached from the posterior segment. **A:** Phakic eye. **B:** Posterior chamber intraocular lens. **C:** Anterior chamber intraocular lens. **D:** Aphakic eye.

developed expressly for the purpose of pars plana endoscope insertion; it can be advanced up to its hilt, diminishing the possibility of inadvertent intraocular damage, and it is large enough to create the proper size wound with a single pass.

The vitrector is then inserted with the port facing upward, so that the progress of vitrectomy can be monitored through the operating microscope. The cut rate and aspiration parameters have been set, as discussed previously. All vitreous that is visible through the microscope is removed, with care taken not to advance the vitrector behind the iris and out of the microscope's view or so posteriorly that the cutting port cannot be seen clearly. Such care will minimize the likelihood of unwanted contact with intraocular structures.

If the eye is phakic, the surgeon must be careful not to traumatize the posterior lens surface. If a second incision was created, it is best not to cross the midline but rather to switch the vitrector to the opposite entry site. The presence of a posterior chamber IOL is of less concern, especially as regards crossing the midline, but care should still be taken not to traumatize the capsular bag. In the presence of an anterior chamber IOL or in an aphakic eye, the vitrector can be directed in such an anterior direction as to enter the pupillary space from behind and easily remove all of the vitreous in the region (Fig. 5-11). Once completed, the instrument can be removed from the eye and the laser endoscope inserted.

Posterior Segment Approach to Posterior Vitrectomy

Surgical intervention in the posterior vitreous cavity requires a pars plana vitrectomy. When trying to remove lens material from the posterior segment, or extracting a foreign body, or peeling gliotic tissue from the retina, vitrectomy must precede all other maneuvers. Most ophthalmologists are not facile with this aspect of surgery, although the basic technique is not particularly difficult to learn. The same principles that guide the permutations of anterior vitrectomy are unchanged when working posteriorly. The only added dimension is that an additional imaging system is required when using the operating microscope to view more posteriorly into the vitreous cavity.

First, a peritomy must be fashioned nasally and temporally. This is usually begun starting about 1 or 2 mm from the limbus to minimize surface hemorrhage that can occur when a more limbal incision is initiated. After adequate hemostasis is obtained, sclerotomy sites are fashioned 3.5 to 4.5 mm from the limbus. A stab incision is made with the MVR blade just above the horizontal nasally and temporally. If the surgeon elects to perform a two-port procedure, these are the only incisions that are required. The vitrector can be inserted through one site and the laser endoscope through the other. An infusion sleeve must be placed around one or the other of these instruments.

In a three-port procedure, which is more or less the standard in vitreoretinal surgery, a third sclerotomy is made,

usually inferior temporally, and a dedicated infusion line is placed. Depending on surgeon preference and the patient's particular anatomic status, the placement of these sclerotomies can vary (Fig. 5-12); it is not very important. Before infusion is initiated, the surgeon must ascertain that the cannula is in the vitreous cavity and not under the pars plana, choroidal effusion, detached retina, and so forth. Finally a lens must be used to neutralize the optical elements of the eye, allowing a posterior view. Typically, this is accomplished with a handheld or sewn-on contact lens, although wide-field noncontact imaging systems are popular among retinal surgeons. While the surgeon watches through the operating microscope and illuminates the field, most of the vitreous can be removed from the eye. When surgery is completed, the sclerotomy sites must be sutured and the overlying conjunctiva reapproximated.

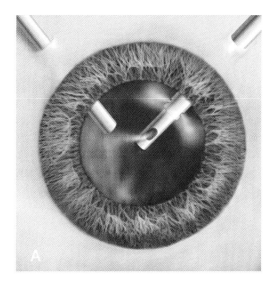

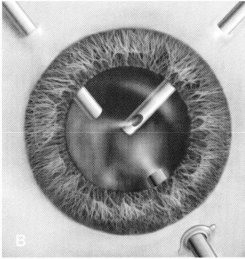

FIGURE 5-12. Posterior vitrectomy approached from the pars plana. **A:** Two-port procedure with infusion sleeve around the infusion cannula. (Sleeve could have been placed around the endoscope instead.) **B:** Three-port procedure.

Lens Status

At this point, let us consider some specific techniques for accessing the ciliary processes from an anterior segment approach. Perhaps the most useful device for classifying these methods is based on the patient's lens status.

Posterior Chamber Pseudophakia

Because the degree of surgical difficulty is typically related to the status of the lens and vitreous rather than the severity of glaucoma, the posterior chamber pseudophakic eye represents one of the less difficult situations for the novice to address. These cases can present ideal conditions for gaining access to the ciliary processes, even when they have failed multiple filtration or cyclodestructive procedures. Once the posterior iris region is filled with viscoelastic, the posterior chamber IOL becomes the "floor" and the posterior iris the "ceiling," and the only other structure in the space is the ciliary body. If this working space is sufficiently expanded, the surgeon can maneuver the endoscope with ease and have little concern for inadvertently bumping in to some other structure that should best be avoided. It is critical to understand that adhesions of varing degree almost always exist between the lens and/or its capsule and the posterior iris. Severing these adhesions, tyically with viscoelastic most often breaks them clearing the way for ECP. These posterior adhesing may not be clinically evident prior to surgery.

Typically, under operating microscope visualization, a flat clear corneal incision 1.5 to 2.0 mm in length is fashioned. A 30-gauge cannula is introduced and passed across the anterior chamber, and a small amount (0.1 to 0.2 mL) of viscoelastic is inserted posterior to the iris. It is important to inject enough so as to open the potential space and permit treatment of each entire process. Care should be taken to place the viscoelastic over the anterior capsule. When this is properly executed, the surgeon will have a clear view of up to 180 degrees of ciliary process tissue from a single incision site and be able to laser this region of the ciliary body. It is the surgeon's choice whether to image and laser from a panoramic viewpoint or to advance the tip of the endoscope closer to the target tissue, which allows higher magnification but a smaller field of view (Fig. 5-13). Depressing the sclera with the surgeon's second hand may enhance the ability to laser between each process or may assist in gaining access to portions of the ciliary body that cannot quite be reached.

As with any surgical procedure, numerous opportunities for misdirection present themselves. One common error in this approach is the injection of viscoelastic into the capsular bag rather than over the anterior capsule. Misplacement in the viscoelastic cannula is typically the cause. When this problem occurs, the capsular bag expands around the lens implant and balloons in front of the ciliary processes (Fig. 5-14). This situation usually does not present a critical impediment because laser energy can be delivered through the capsule and adequate treatment of the ciliary processes can be

effected. The imaging through this structure becomes somewhat hazy, however, and the laser delivery may be attenuated, requiring higher power settings or longer duration of application because the translucent capsule is now insinuated between the tip of the endoscope and the target tissue.

Perhaps of greater importance is the potential for injection of too much viscoelastic over the capsule in the presence of a posterior capsulotomy. Care should be taken to avoid this situation because it may cause extrusion of the vitreous through the capsulotomy or around the zonules and into the anterior chamber. The elegance of the over-the-capsule approach to ECP is that the vitreous need not be manipulated. When this problem arises, however, an anterior vitrectomy often becomes necessary. Careful injection of the viscoelastic, especially in the presence of a large capsulotomy, is usually sufficient to prevent this problem.

One might think that zonular rupture would be a common experience, but it is amazing how resilient these structures are. Even with the insertion of large amounts of viscoelastic, with posterior displacement of the capsular bag and IOL posterior to the ora serrata, zonular rupture is rare, even focally, let alone to the extent that subluxation or dislocation occurs. Diode laser (810 nm) energy applied to the ciliary processes does not cause zonular rupture in and of itself because the zonules do not absorb this wavelength. It is possible to focally rupture the zonules, however, if they are substantially stretched and then the portion of the ciliary process adjacent to their attachment (usually the more posterior "tail") is "overtreated" with the laser. Even when this occurs, it does not create much of a problem but should serve as a warning for the surgeon to make some type of technical alteration (usually decreasing the laser power). Although there has never been a reported case of dislocated IOL as a consequence of ECP, the surgeon should take great care not to disturb the placement of the implant. This is especially true when the IOL is not in the capsular bag but rather is sutured or simply wedged in the sulcus. Posterior displacement with viscoelastic may dislodge the implant, converting a simple procedure for the surgeon and patient into a complicated affair with an uncertain outcome.

Combined Cataract Surgery and Endoscopic Cyclophotocoagulation

Perhaps it may seem that this is an odd juncture to present what appears to be an esoteric application and technique of ECP. After all, how often do most ophthalmologists perform combined procedures? There are two reasons to discuss this situation. First, as it turns out, combining cataract surgery with ECP is the most common use of ophthalmic endoscopy in the world today. Second, there are numerous variations of the surgical technique used in this situation that are an outgrowth of what has already been discussed. Facility with these methods will expand the surgeon's versatility in dealing with each patient's unique anatomic and pathologic status.

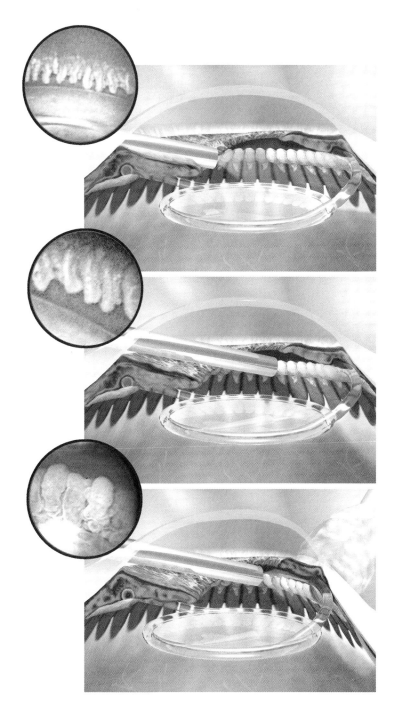

FIGURE 5-13. Posterior chamber approach over the intraocular lens in pseudophakia, showing more distant **(top)** and closer **(center)** position of the endoscope relative to the ciliary processes, as well as use of scleral depression to enhance view of ciliary processes **(bottom)**. The endoscopic views in the insets are pre–endoscopic cyclophotocoagulation.

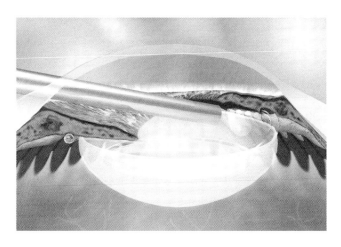

FIGURE 5-14. Pitfall of posterior chamber approach over the intraocular lens in pseudophakia. Viscoelastic has been inadvertently injected into the capsular bag, rather than the anterior capsule, and has ballooned in front of ciliary processes.

There are three approaches from which the surgeon may choose in this situation. The first of these is the *"over-the-bag" technique,* which is theoretically the safest and most useful for the novice endoscopist. In this scenario, phacoemulsification or extracapsular surgery is completed. Then, through the same incision site, viscoelastic is placed between the anterior capsule and posterior to the iris. This maneuver collapses the capsular bag and displaces it posteriorly while creating an iris bombé effect anteriorly. The laser endoscope is inserted through the cataract incision, through the pupillary space, and directed toward the sulcus (Fig. 5-15). The ciliary processes are then easily viewed, and photocoagulation can begin. Usually, at least 180 degrees of ciliary process tissue can be treated through the cataract incision, but if more extensive laser application is planned, one or more of the side ports can be enlarged to accommo-

date the laser endoscope and treatment can continue, or a curved endoscope can be used.

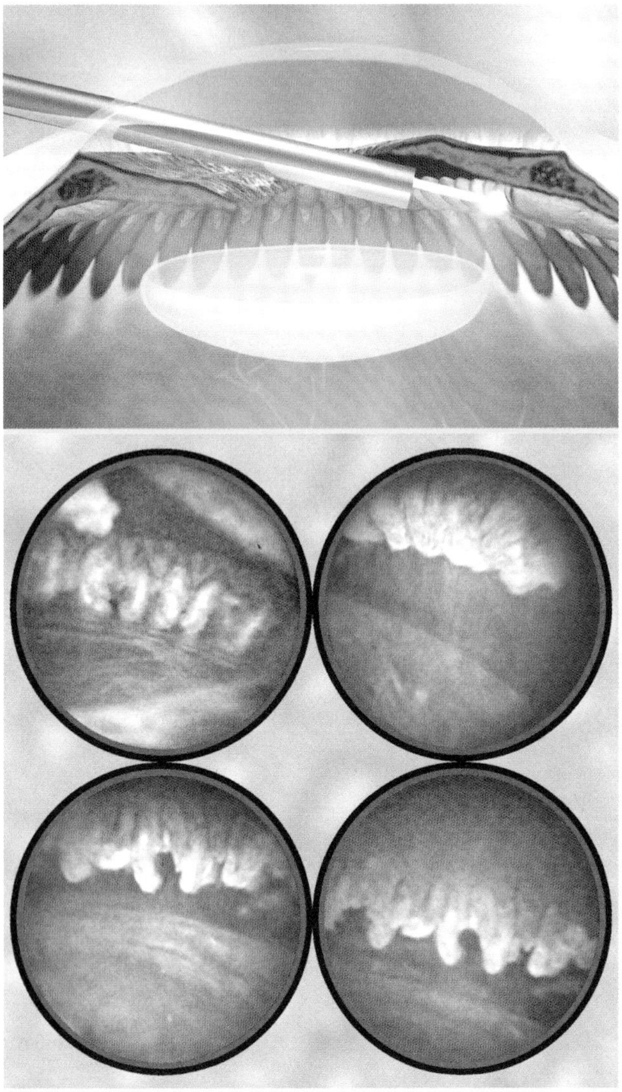

This approach is among the simplest and safest methods for the performance of ECP. The underside of the iris is the "ceiling," the capsular bag is the "floor," and the only other visible structure is the target, the ciliary processes. The vitreous is protected on the posterior side of the capsular bag and should be of no concern. It is difficult for the surgeon to cause a problem with this method because the space between the capsular bag and the iris can be safely expanded to a considerable degree. It would be unlikely for the surgeon to inadvertently damage the bag or the zonules posteriorly or abrade the underside of the iris anteriorly. Because the lens implant has not yet been inserted, displacement or frank dislocation is not a realistic possibility. If there are any cortical or nuclear remnants hidden behind the iris, the surgeon now has an opportunity to remove them. After cyclophotocoagulation is performed, the viscoelastic is removed, usually by the irrigation/aspiration method, and then IOL insertion can proceed in the usual manner.

A second alternative is the *"through-the-bag" technique.* At the completion of cataract surgery, viscoelastic is injected into the capsular bag, ballooning it to its "normal" size. The laser endoscope is insert through the pupillary space, through the anterior capsulotomy, and directed toward the sulcus (Fig. 5-16). Once the processes are viewed, photoco-

FIGURE 5-15. Combined cataract surgery and endoscopic cyclophotocoagulation using the over-the-bag technique.

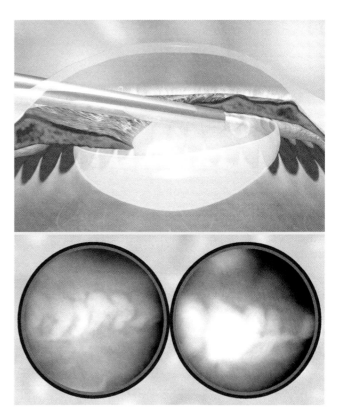

FIGURE 5-16. Combined cataract surgery and endoscopic cyclophotocoagulation using the through-the-bag technique.

agulation through the capsular bag is performed. The image will be slightly hazy using this method because the capsule is somewhat translucent when illuminated from within and it is insinuated between the tip of the endoscope and the target tissue. Laser power may also be mildly attenuated as well, so that a slightly higher power setting or longer duration of laser application is often required. Once treatment has been completed, the endoscope is removed from the eye and the IOL can be inserted in the surgeon's usual fashion. Again, this technique is easily mastered and is quite safe. There is substantial room for manipulation of the endoscope but not much to inadvertently traumatize, the IOL cannot be displaced, and the vitreous is posterior to the surgical field. However, care is required not to damage the capsule.

A variant of this technique has been reported by Cavalho and Lima (personal communication), in which it is combined with scleral depression. This maneuver presents more ciliary process tissue and the valleys between them for laser application (Fig. 5-17). The originators have suggested that this approach may be especially useful in the management of eyes with cataract and more stubborn forms of glaucoma.

Although this through-the-bag approach presents relatively few opportunities for mishaps, it is important that the surgeon take care to avoid tearing the capsule or physically distort the bag in a manner that will rupture the zonules.

In the third approach, the surgeon completes the cataract surgery and lens implantation in their usual manner, and all viscoelastic is removed from the eye. Then viscoelastic is injected between the anterior capsule and posterior iris, inflating the sulcus region. The laser endoscope is inserted through the pupillary space and over the capsule, and directed toward the sulcus. The ciliary processes are easily accessed and photocoagulated by this method (Fig. 5-18). This is the same approach as described for ECP in the

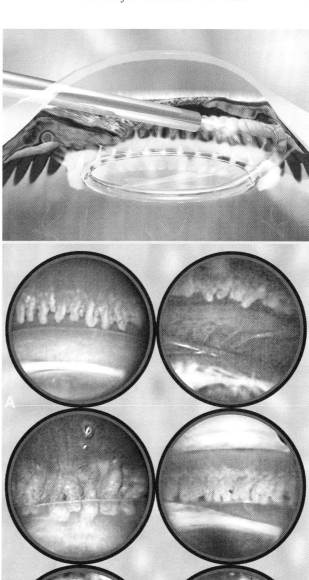

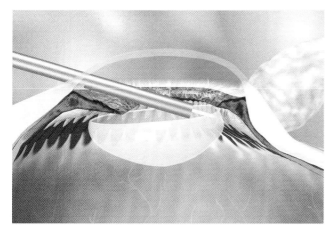

FIGURE 5-17. Combined cataract surgery and endoscopic cyclophotocoagulation using the through-the-bag technique combined with scleral depression

FIGURE 5-18. Combined cataract surgery and endoscopic cyclophotocoagulation (ECP) using the over-the-intraocular lens approach. The cataract surgery and intraocular lens insertion are completed before ECP in this procedure. **A:** Images of ciliary processes when the sulcus is inflated, as viewed from the limbus. **B:** Images of the posterior chamber intraocular lens after sulcus inflation, as viewed from the posterior segment. Note the peripheral cortical remnants in the bag as well as the stretched zonules.

posterior chamber pseudophakic eye and, as it turns out, is the most commonly used method by most surgeons. A theoretical disadvantage would be the possibility that manipulation of the endoscope might displace the lens implant, and so perhaps it would be better to perform ECP first and then follow with IOL implantation. As a practical matter, however, this problem has not been reported.

These combined-procedure approaches are the simplest to learn and execute and should probably be the first carried out by the novice endoscopist.

The Phakic Eye

The phakic eye presents a greater degree of difficulty. An anterior segment approach to the ciliary processes is the only option. A generous beveled incision is fashioned, usually through the clear cornea. Recall that a "tight" wound inhibits manipulation of the endoscope and makes it more difficult to shallow the anterior chamber and posteriorly displace the lens. The space between the lens and iris should be sufficiently expanded with viscoelastic so as not to traumatize the lens during insertion and manipulation of the laser endoscope (Fig. 5-19).

Although this method seems to be straightforward, it is perhaps the most difficult to execute. These cases should not be among the first attempted by the novice. In the posterior chamber pseudophakic eye and in eyes undergoing cataract surgery, the ophthalmologist has quite a bit of latitude with regard to the movement of the endoscope posterior to the iris. The important structures have been "pushed" out of harm's way, and learning to maneuver the instrument is fairly simple, even if the space between iris and capsule has not been ideally expanded. To safely and effectively perform ECP in the phakic eye, however, the surgeon must be adept at maximizing the dimensions of this working space as well as be confident with endoscopic imaging and laser delivery.

There is also another important factor that may confound the best efforts of even the most experienced laser endoscopist. In some eyes, even after the anterior chamber has shallowed or flattened following the incision and aqueous drainage, the injected viscoelastic extrudes from the incision site. The space between iris and lens cannot be opened, and therefore the laser endoscope cannot be introduced and treatment cannot be performed. This event most likely occurs because the IOP remains elevated despite opening the eye. To minimize the potential for this event, it is best to lower the IOP as much as possible preoperatively with topical or systemic agents or by mechanical means, such as digital massage or balloon. However, in many cases this is not possible, inability to lower IOP being the reason for surgery in the first place. In eyes with extensive visual field loss, it is not advisable to raise IOP even transiently, and so mechanical pressure applied to the eye would not be a realistic option.

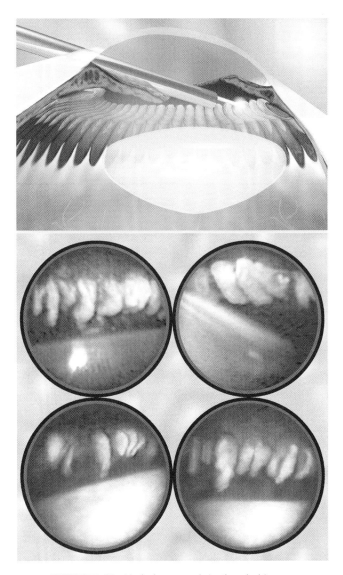

FIGURE 5-19. Limbal approach in the phakic eye.

When confronted with this situation, the surgeon has several alternatives, all of which increase the complexity of the procedure. One choice would be to fashion a pars plana incision and perform an anterior vitrectomy (the variations of this technique for the anterior segment surgeon will be discussed shortly). This approach is quite simple, can be performed in a few minutes, and will not traumatize the crystalline lens. In so doing, the IOP is dramatically lowered, and a space is created for posterior displacement of the lens after injection of viscoelastic posterior to the iris. When properly performed, this technique contributes little to the risks of the procedure. A second, perhaps less tolerable, option would be to remove the lens, converting the surgery to a combined procedure. It is best to prepare the phakic patient undergoing ECP for these potential solutions to the vitreous extrusion problem.

Aside from the basic set of hazards associated with the performance of any intraocular surgery and ECP, a few complications are peculiar to this situation. Certainly, any intraocular procedure, such as trabeculectomy or vitrectomy, increases the phakic eye's risk for the subsequent development of cataract. In most ECP studies, the incidence of this complication is about 30%. This outcome compares favorably with the potential for cataract formation in phakic vitrectomy and phakic trabeculectomy. Still, most ECP-related cataracts develop in the early postoperative period, whereas in the case of vitrectomy and trabeculectomy this problem evolves more slowly. Loss of accommodation is an extremely uncommon ECP-related complication, but it can be quite disturbing to the patient. Typically, resolution does not occur. This untoward event does not seem to be related to overly intensive treatment or zonular rupture.

Anterior Chamber Pseudophakia

The technique of ECP in eyes with pseudophakia of the anterior chamber type is straightforward. Because there is no lens or implant posterior to the iris, viscoelastic is not required (although it may be helpful to place a bit between the IOL and cornea to protect the corneal endothelium). An anterior segment incision is created, the laser endoscope is inserted, and the tip is directed through the pupil and advanced toward the ciliary processes. When it is in the appropriate position, ECP can be initiated (Fig. 5-20).

As mentioned earlier, most patients with anterior chamber IOLs have undergone complicated cataract surgery. While the pupillary space and posterior segment may appear to be clear and free of debris, these eyes often have cortical and capsular remnants overlying the ciliary processes and adherent to the posterior iris surface, making it difficult to access the target. Tissue retraction in an anterior direction from previous surgery can increase the difficulty of maneuvering the laser endoscope into proper position for ECP. Indeed, this might represent one of the situations in which an upwardly curved endoscope may be of value. At any rate, combining this approach with scleral depression is usually effective.

Residual lens material overlying the ciliary processes does not preclude laser delivery. After all, patients with significant cataract formation routinely undergo laser treatment at the slit lamp. Attenuation of laser delivery does occur, so that higher power levels, longer duration, closer placement of the laser endoscope to the target tissue, or a combination of these will successfully circumvent this anatomic problem (Fig. 5-21).

Even these maneuvers sometimes will not surmount the obstruction created by a large, dense piece of residual lens material or fibrotic capsule. The surgeon's choice is to then remove these impediments, manipulate them so that they are temporarily out of the way, or to skip the region alto-

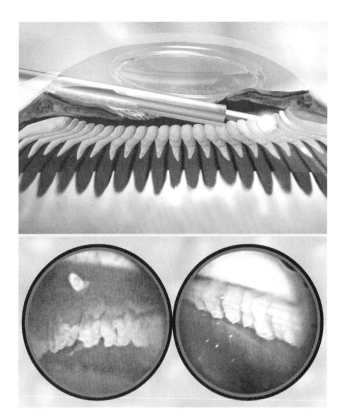

FIGURE 5-20. Anterior segment approach in anterior chamber pseudophakia. The endoscope is positioned under the intraocular lens.

gether, moving to some other portion of the ciliary processes.

Typically, it is best to leave these obstructions in place. They may be strongly adherent to surrounding tissue, creating an inadvertent avulsion when manipulated. There may also be an element of vascularization to these tissues, a disturbance of which may lead to significant intraocular hemorrhage, converting a simple procedure to a drama.

Gentle tissue manipulation with an additional instrument through a second incision (Fig. 5-22) or displacement of the obstruction by injection of viscoelastic sometimes is effective. These are especially helpful maneuvers when a particular region of the ciliary process tissue cannot be left untreated for some reason.

Finally, discretion may be the better part of valor. Changing the area of interest to an adjacent accessible portion of the ciliary body is usually the best choice. The procedure may continue along its expeditious performance and complications arising from surgical misadventures are minimized. In other words, it is best to move on!

A general rule of ophthalmic surgery is not to manipulate any instrument in the presence of vitreous. Tractional forces induced by these movements have the potential to create retinal breaks and detachment. Many anterior chamber pseudophakic eyes, as stated previously, have experienced complicated cataract extraction, and a significant

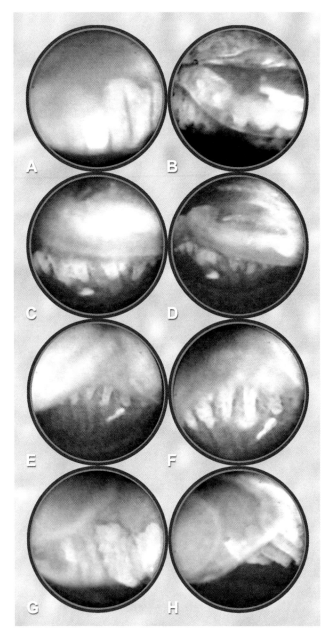

FIGURE 5-21. A-H: Different cases of ciliary processes undergoing endoscopic cyclophotocoagulation through a lens remnant.

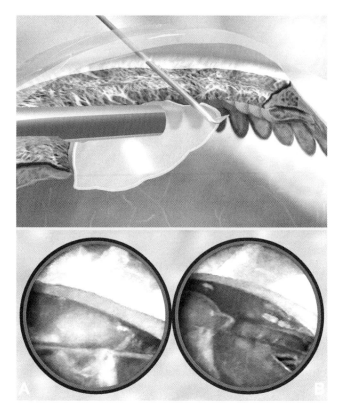

FIGURE 5-22. Use of a second instrument to move lens remnant from the surface of the ciliary processes. **A:** Obstructed ciliary process view. **B:** Same eye after a metal instrument pushes the cortical material posteriorly, permitting a view of the processes.

proportion of them have also undergone anterior vitrectomy. If there is no vitreous just posterior to the iris, the laser endoscope can be manipulated freely without the concern of creating iatrogenic retinal pathology. On the other hand, if vitreous is present, before the endoscope is inserted, an anterior vitrectomy must be performed. This is quite a simple task and can be approached from the anterior segment or from the pars plana. Once completed, the ciliary processes can be addressed with impunity.

Another peculiarity of this set of anatomic conditions is the potential for intraoperative hypotony. Eyes that have

undergone vitrectomy and lensectomy can be considered as single chambered. Aqueous from the anterior and posterior segments easily escapes from the anterior chamber incision site, and these eyes can actually collapse during the course of ECP. Interestingly, if the eye is very soft but not collapsed, it is simple to laser the ciliary processes, sometimes well beyond the maximum of 180 degrees that would be expected through a single incision site. If the eye collapses, however, the door is open for significant complications to evolve, particularly the development of hemorrhagic or serous choroidal detachment.

If a single-chambered eye seems to be collapsing, there are a few alternatives that can remedy the situation (Fig. 5-23). The laser endoscope can be inserted through an infusion sleeve and then replaced in the eye. This will result in immediate reformation and maintenance of the normal globe architecture. Intraocular pressure can then be controlled largely by raising or lowering the BSS infusion bottle. A corollary of this solution would be to place an anterior chamber maintainer through a limbal port. Again, the height of the infusion bottle will determine the IOP. This is also a simple and useful technique that can be rapidly effected if the need arises. Another option is to inject BSS

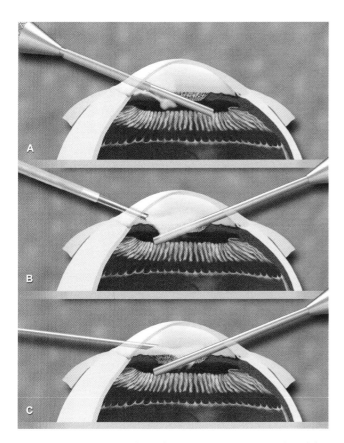

FIGURE 5-23. Methods for reforming or maintaining the globe during the anterior segment approach to endoscopic cyclophotocoagulation. **A:** Infusion sleeve added to the endoscope. **B:** Anterior chamber maintainer placed though a limbal port. **C:** Syringe injection of balanced salt solution into the anterior chamber.

Aphakia

The technique and peculiarities of this approach are similar to those for anterior chamber pseudophakia. A generous flat anterior segment incision, usually in clear cornea, is fashioned. No viscoelastic is required because there is no lens to displace. The laser endoscope is inserted through the pupillary space and is directed toward the sulcus. Once the ciliary processes are adequately imaged, photocoagulation may begin. This might appear to be the most straightforward and simple of procedures yet described, and it often is.

Imagine for a moment a patient with refractory aphakic glaucoma who has not had success with maximal medical therapy and previous filtration surgery. Through one or two sutureless corneal incisions, ECP can be completed in a few minutes with a high potential for success, a minimum of postoperative care, and low risk of significant complications. This scenario is the likely outcome. At times, however, appearances can be deceiving. Just as in cases of anterior chamber pseudophakia, many aphakic patients have had complicated cataract surgery or vitrectomy with lensectomy. Significant anatomic obstacles prohibiting access to the ciliary processes may linger. It is best for the surgeon to anticipate these problems and be prepared to create several incision sites. Vitreous must be removed from the region of the ciliary body. Again, because these eyes are usually single chambered, the possibility of intraoperative hypotony developing through leakage of aqueous from the incision sites demands that the surgeon be prepared to reform the globe with BSS or air inserted through an infusion sleeve, anterior chamber maintainer, or syringe injection. Scleral depression in combination with ECP can be quite helpful in these eyes. A curved endoscope can be of assistance as well.

Curved Laser Endoscopes and Single-Incision Endoscopic Cyclophotocoagulation

Accessing a ciliary process arc of about 180 degrees is what might typically be expected with use of a straight endoscope. With this style of probe, at least two incisions are required for more extensive treatment. If the surgeon prefers to use a single incision, it is possible to access about 300 degrees (ten clock hours) through a single incision using a curved endoscope (fiberoptic only). Once a bit of experience has been gained with the straight endoscope, transition to this method is quite simple. Basically, the endoscope is introduced into the eye as one might a corneoscleral scissors "to the right" and "to the left." There is one other trick, though: Because of the fixed configuration of the image guide in the handpiece and the curve of the tip, the surgeon cannot rotate the endoscope for proper image orientation. However, by simply having an operating room assistant rotate the image guide connector as it interfaces with the video system, proper orientation can be achieved. This must be separately adjusted for introduction

into the anterior chamber through the endoscope insertion site or through a pars plana entry, refilling the eye. A 3- or 5-mL syringe filled with BSS and outfitted with a short, small-gauge needle is sufficient for this purpose. This is a quick and effective solution for the problem of a deflating eye, its only drawback being that this reformation usually does not last long, so that the approach is useful only if the surgeon is willing to repeat it or if the intraoperative hypotony occurs near the end of the procedure. Air can be substituted for BSS injection with the same effect. One benefit is that air generally remains in the eye longer than the more rapidly egressing BSS. On the down side, if the air bubble becomes segmented ("fish eggs"), it is more difficult to image and laser the ciliary processes. It is not necessary to remove it from the eye at completion of surgery because it usually disappears over the course of a few days. However, the patient will notice black circles or a watery-wavy effect in part of his or her visual field and so should be forewarned about what to expect.

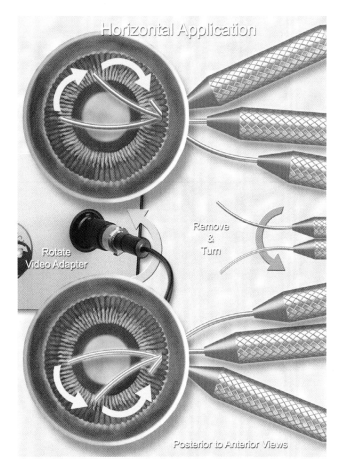

FIGURE 5-24. A curved endoscope used in a horizontal fashion to access a 300-degree view of the ciliary processes. The operating room assistant must rotate the image guide connector at the video adapter *(green arrow)* for proper image orientation.

to the right and to the left. The simplest technique is to insert the endoscope and direct it 180 degrees from the entry site. ECP proceeds laterally so that the tip of the endoscope ultimately is adjacent to the entry site. Then the endoscope is withdrawn and reinserted in the opposite "direction." Again, the processes 180 degrees from the entry site are accessed, and ECP proceeds toward the entry site. In this fashion, about 300 degrees of the arc can be photocoagulated (Fig. 5-24).

Using the curved endoscope in this horizontal manner can be helpful in rapidly treating a large segment of the ciliary processes. If this same instrument is rotated for use in a vertical fashion from an anterior segment approach, the image and laser delivery can be effected in an upward direction (Fig. 5-25). This approach is most useful for photocoagulating the ciliary body from an anterior segment approach in the aphakic eye. In this scenario, the processes often seem to be retracted anteriorly, almost onto the posterior aspect of the iris. The curved endoscope directs the image in an upward direction, improving access and enhancing the potential for more effective treatment.

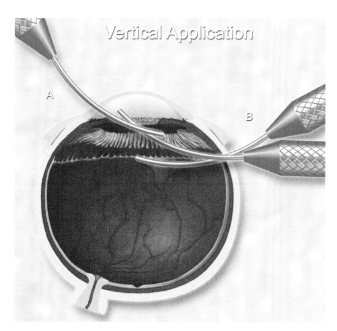

FIGURE 5-25. A curved endoscope used in a vertical fashion to access the ciliary process in an aphakic eye from an anterior segment approach.

POSTERIOR SEGMENT APPROACH

When accessing the ciliary processes through the pars plana, the surgeon must understand that the ciliary processes are actually "above" (superior to) the pars plana incision sites, so the laser endoscope and other instruments must actually be tilted "upward" after insertion into the eye to approach the target tissue. Most of time, intraocular instruments are directed in a "downward" (posterior) direction, and so the feel of this maneuver can seem strange at first. Moreover, the ciliary processes in the phakic eye cannot be accessed by this approach because the posterior aspect of the crystalline lens extends so far posteriorly that the shaft of the endoscope will traumatize it (Fig. 5-26), initiating rapid cataract formation. All phakic eyes must be treated through an anterior segment incision site.

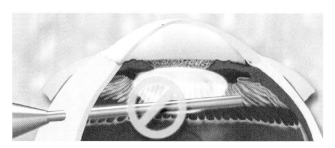

FIGURE 5-26. Pars plana insertion of laser endoscope in phakic eye demonstrating the shaft of the endoscope hitting the lens. To avoid such a complication, phakic eyes *must* be treated by an anterior segment approach.

Anterior Chamber Pseudophakia

Once the anterior vitreous has been removed, it is simple to access the ciliary processes. The laser endoscope is inserted through one of the sclerotomies and tilted upward as it is advanced across the eye (Fig. 5-27). When the tip is 3 to 5

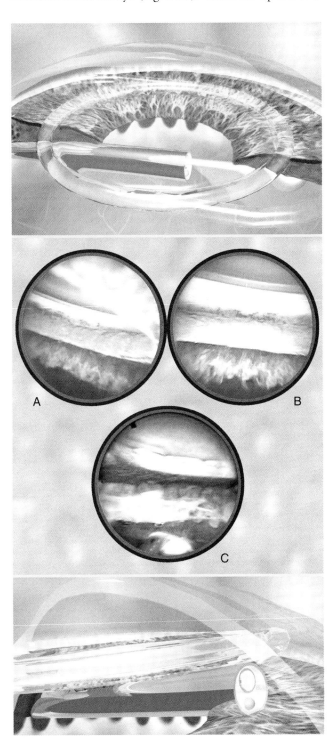

FIGURE 5-27. Pars plana approach in anterior chamber pseudophakia. The endoscope can be advanced through the pupil into the anterior chamber with the anterior chamber intraocular lens in place. **A:** Image through pupil. **B:** Image at level of pupil. **C:** Image posterior to iris.

mm from the processes, cyclophotocoagulation can begin. Access to 180 degrees of ciliary process tissue can typically be achieved through one incision site, and the extent of treatment can be enhanced with scleral depression or by creating temporary hypotony. Aside from the risks associated with intraocular surgery of any type in a single-chambered eye, this approach to ECP is easily effected. It is quite remarkable that some refractory forms of glaucoma can be so simply and effectively managed by this technique. The anterior chamber can also be accessed from this approach by directing the endoscope anteriorly and through the pupil. Of course, care must be taken to avoid displacing the anterior chamber IOL or pushing it into the corneal endothelium.

Posterior Chamber Pseudophakia

In the situation of posterior chamber pseudophakia, the laser endoscope is inserted through one of the pars plana incisions after adequate vitrectomy has been performed. It is then tilted anteriorly and directed across the vitreous cavity toward the contralateral ciliary processes. Once the target is adequately imaged, the aiming beam of the laser is projected onto the processes and ECP can begin. One need not be fearful of crossing the midline in this scenario because there is no crystalline lens to potentially traumatize.

In some eyes, the capsular bag/IOL complex can limit complete visualization and treatment of the ciliary processes. This is especially true when a ring of residual peripheral cortex is present within the bag. While this condition does not affect the patient's vision, the bulging peripheral capsular bag can obstruct the surgeon's view of the ciliary processes. It is interesting to observe how common this situation is. To circumvent this problem, the surgeon has three options: move the treatment area to a different region of the ciliary body, change to an anterior segment approach where viscoelastic is used to posteriorly displace the obstruction, or combine the pars plana approach with scleral depression (Fig. 5-28). This last choice usually proves to be effective in surmounting this obstacle for imaging and laser delivery to the ciliary processes. Finally, it should be clear that the anterior chamber cannot be accessed under this set of conditions.

Aphakia

The approach in an aphakic eye is also straightforward, with insertion of the laser endoscope through one of the sclerotomy sites after vitrectomy has been completed. The probe is directed anteriorly and across the eye to access the processes, and ECP can begin (Fig. 5-29). The surgeon must remember that aphakic eyes usually have undergone complicated cataract surgery or other serious ophthalmic processes, increasing the likelihood that impediments to visualization of the target tissue will be present. The options

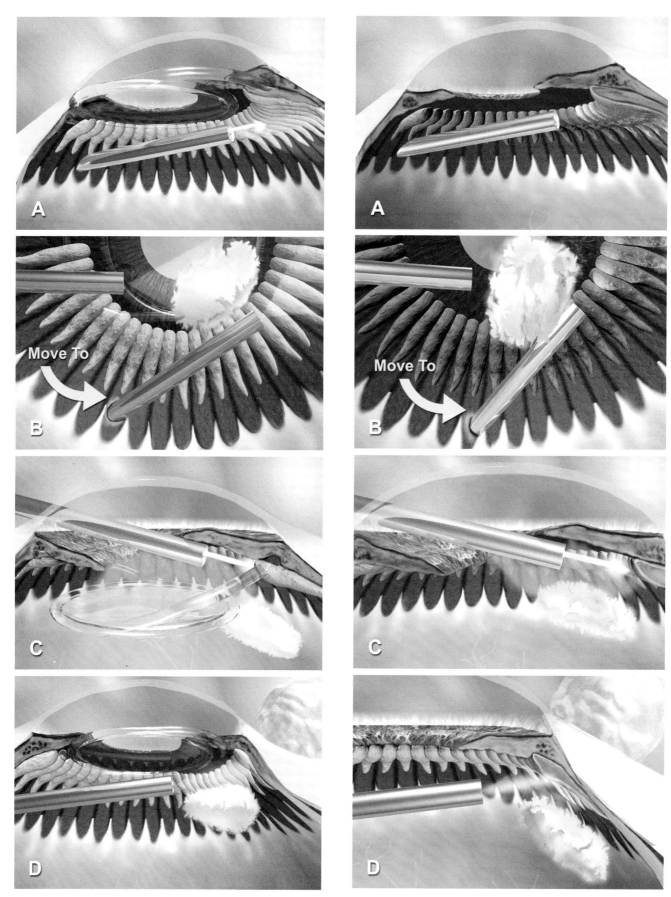

FIGURE 5-28. A: Approach in posterior chamber pseudophakia. **B:** Regular view. If residual cortex is in the way, there are three options: switch incision sites in the pars plana, **C:** switch to an anterior segment approach, **D:** or add scleral depression.

FIGURE 5-29. A: Pars plana approach in aphakia. **B:** Regular view. If residual cortex is in the way, there are three options: move to another incision site, **C:** switch to an anterior segment approach and use viscoelastic or another instrument to move the obstruction, **D:** or add scleral depression.

are to direct attention to another area of the ciliary body, change to an anterior segment approach and use viscoelastic or a second instrument to push the obstruction out of the way, or use scleral depression to move the target into a more beneficial position.

LASER DELIVERY IN ENDOSCOPIC CYCLOPHOTOCOAGULATION

Now that we appreciate the theoretical value of direct visualization and laser application to the ciliary processes, understand the technology required to execute this treatment, and have the technical ability to access the target in a given eye depending on its lens and anatomic status, the next critical step is learning how to attain the desired tissue effect. Specifically, we must delineate the laser treatment end point for each ciliary process and, of perhaps equal importance, establish how much of the ciliary body to incorporate in the treatment zone.

Tissue Effect

Because most of the world literature on inflow procedures has been accumulated using the transscleral approach, little historical assistance existed to help determine the proper method of ciliary process photocoagulation under direct visualization. The first human ECP study (2) indicated that specific treatment parameters using an 810-nm diode laser correlated with the ultimate clinical effect in the management of neovascular glaucoma, a difficult problem that nevertheless tends to respond "well" to inflow procedures. Modifications, mostly to the extent rather than manner of treatment, have subsequently evolved for other mechanisms of glaucoma and surgical conditions. The goals of treatment, as far as tissue effect is concerned, are outlined in Table 5-2.

Laser Power Density

An understanding of the concept of laser power density and of how its components can be used to optimize treatment is crucial. What actually takes place at the tissue level represents the culmination of three factors, which together con-

TABLE 5-2. GOALS OF ENDOSCOPIC CYCLOPHOTOCOAGULATION

- Whiten the ciliary process.
- Photocoagulate the entire surface of the process and as much of the intervening valleys as possible.
- Shrink the tissue.
- Incorporate the appropriate extent of ciliary process tissue in the treatment zone.

stitute laser power density: laser power delivered through the endoscope, duration of laser delivery, and distance of the laser source (the tip of the instrument) from the target (Fig. 5-30A-D). Alteration in any of these variables will modify the tissue response in some way. As an example, consider the desired outcomes of tissue whitening and shrinkage. If the laser power and duration are set but an inadequate response is observed, the surgeon can increase the laser power setting, increase the duration of application, move the tip of the endoscope closer to the process, or any combination of these options. If, on the other hand, the response is too intense, the surgeon can decrease the laser power setting, decrease the duration of application, move the endoscope further away from the target, or some combination of these.

Laser Power Setting

Typically, the initial power setting of the 810-nm diode laser is between 300 and 500 mW. This parameter can be altered as needed. The higher the power, the faster the tissue responds. Lower power levels can achieve the same effect but require the surgeon to use a longer duration, move the endoscope closer, or both. For the novice, the combination of lower power and longer duration provides greater control of the tissue effect. If the laser fiber within the endoscope is degrading, the connector to the laser not properly cleaned, the media hazy, or treatment to the processes made through lens or capsular material, then the laser power will be attenuated and the power density equation must be altered in some way. Increasing laser power, duration, or closeness to the target will overcome these problems. Rarely, however, would as much as 1,000 mW of power be required.

Laser Duration

When using ophthalmic lasers in their typical manner, short bursts of exposure time, usually a small fraction of a second, are the norm. In the case of visible-wavelength laser sources, such as argon or green, the surgeon sees the tissue effect after laser delivery has been completed. Usually this is not a problem, but if this setting were too intense, tissue explosion, hemorrhage, pigment dispersion, and pain might occur.

Endoscopic cyclophotocoagulation incorporates a novel style of laser delivery. The laser duration is set on the continuous-wave (CW) mode. What this means is that as long as the surgeon depresses the footswitch, the laser will fire; when the footswitch is released, laser delivery ceases. This function translates to a significant technical advantage for the surgeon. Consider that the 810-nm laser is invisible when fired, so the tissue effect can be continuously monitored during the course of laser application. Using a long, low-intensity application, the sur-

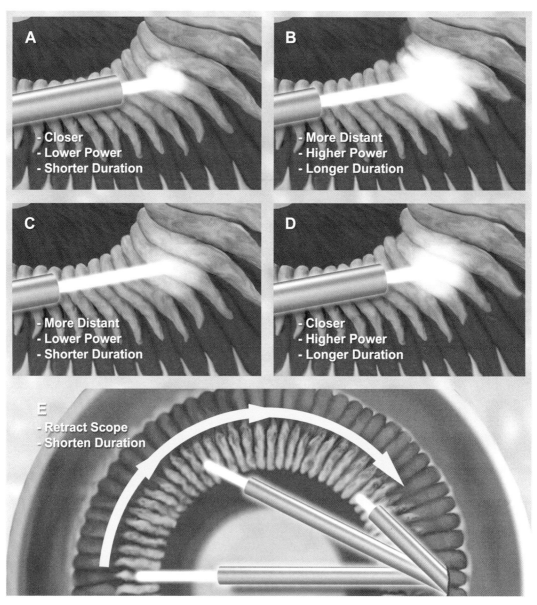

FIGURE 5-30. Laser power density is a function of laser power setting, duration of exposure, and distance of laser endoscope from target. **A:** Smaller spot. **B:** Larger spot. **C:** Less intensity. **D:** More intensity.

geon can substantially control what happens at the tissue level. This is not possible with a visible-wavelength laser fired for a fraction of a second. This characteristic minimizes overtreatment and undertreatment, contributing to the success of the procedure and reducing its complications.

Laser Distance from Ciliary Processes

When the retina, iris, or angle is being photocoagulated through a slit-lamp delivery system, the target tissue is essentially always on the same plane. The distance from the

laser source is more or less constant. When the surgeon is maneuvering the endoscope within the eye, this constant no longer exists. Recall that the ciliary body is a ring-shaped structure, so that when one moves from one process to the next, the distance changes. ECP takes place over an arc, not a straight line. When one views ciliary processes directly across from the entry site, a certain set of laser parameters will achieve the desired effect. But, as the laser endoscope is directed laterally, the processes are actually closer, so that the laser effect occurs more rapidly and intensely. The simplest method for addressing this change in working distance is to simply pull back on the laser endoscope. The next approach would be to shorten the duration of the laser application. If the effect is still too intense, decreasing the laser power should resolve the issue. Although these maneuvers seem to be involved, once the surgeon has gained some experience, they most often are effected subliminally. Through adjustment of any or all of the components that constitute laser power density, a tissue effect that is uniform across the entire treatment zone can be achieved (Fig. 5.30E).

Number of Incisions

Whether using an anterior or posterior segment approach or a combination of both, it now may be evident that multiple incision sites are often necessary to treat glaucoma patients. After all, about 180 degrees of ciliary process tissue is the maximum that can be accessed through a single incision site with a straight endoscope. If a broader treatment zone is needed, a second incision can be created 90 to 180 degrees from the first incision. This usually permits access to the remaining ciliary processes. The precise location of this site depends on a number of factors, among them the particular architecture of the eye in question and the surgeon's comfort. As discussed previously, in some difficult situations, a number of anterior and posterior segment incisions are required to circumvent problem anatomy and access a sufficient number of processes to achieve a good result.

A few maneuvers can increase somewhat the extent of treatment deliverable through a particular incision. One is to rotate the laser endoscope. This will orient the image obliquely while also rotating the laser fiber, which may allow treatment of a few more processes. If this maneuver is performed at both extremes of the treatment zone, a clock hour or two of additional ciliary process tissue may be accessed. Another option is to have the eye become soft. Hypotony will cause collapse of the ciliary ring, bringing a fair amount of additional process tissue into view. Finally, scleral depression of the ciliary body not only increases the treatment field to a small extent but also opens the spaces between the processes, which seems to enhance efficacy per clock hour of ECP.

Single Process Versus Painting

Once the surgeon becomes comfortable with endoscopic imaging and instrument manipulation and laser delivery, two methods can be used to effect treatment. The first of these is to apply the laser to each ciliary process, one at a time. The laser application is made from the superior to inferior portion of the process and, when deemed adequate, the next ciliary process is addressed. The alternative is to "paint" the tissue (Fig. 5-31). In this method, the power is raised a bit to compensate for changing power density. The laser endoscope is fired as it sweeps across the

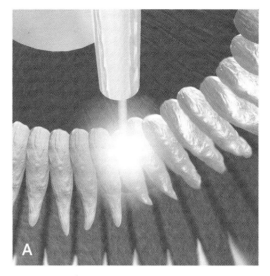

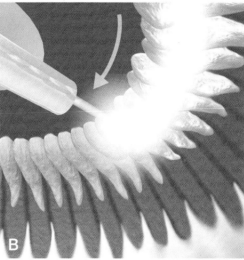

FIGURE 5-31. Two methods of treating the ciliary processes. **A:** The laser is applied to each process completely, one at a time. **B:** The laser is applied to a number of processes at once with the painting technique.

arc of the ciliary ring. In this way, a significant portion of each ciliary process can be photocoagulated for up to 180 degrees in just a few minutes. Typically, several passes are required to treat most of the surface of each process. Although this approach seems to be less controlled than the individual method (which it is), the clinical results cannot be distinguished. Ultimately, it is a matter of personal preference.

Extent of Treatment

How much treatment to deliver is a pivotal question, the answer to which is a powerful determinant of the clinical outcome. Although there is a wealth of literature available regarding the results of transscleral laser cycloablation, it was evident early in the course of ophthalmic endoscopy that this information would lead to an erroneous conclusion if extrapolated to ECP. In one study (3), eyes that had failed transscleral cyclophotocoagulation and were to undergo further treatment by ECP were typically found to have far less actual ciliary process ablation than reported by their surgeons. Although this will be discussed later, of 20 patients with 360 degrees of reported transscleral cyclophotocoagulation and failed outcomes, none had more than 120 degrees of actual ciliary process ablation and most had significantly less. Although it could be argued that these eyes had failed but many others that were not in the study succeeded, it makes one ask how much of the ciliary processes we should treat.

Review of the literature related to the transpupillary approach of slit-lamp-delivered cyclophotocoagulation, which typically incorporated a small amount of ciliary process tissue in the treatment zone, revealed a poor success rate (4–6).

We could conclude from these studies that if less than 120 degrees of ciliary process tissue was actually photocoagulated, the effect would not be particularly efficacious. But how much more cyclophotocoagulation is required to achieve a generally good response? Scientific deduction is not helpful because there is no practical way of measure aqueous inflow in a given eye; we can only measure outflow. The solution was to gradually increase the extent of treatment and monitor the patient's postoperative IOP response and associated complications. Most of the patients treated early on had neovascular glaucoma, and some very good results were obtained with relatively small amounts of ECP, from 90 degrees to 120 degrees (2). However, this was misleading in a way because ischemic eyes respond better to ECP than nonischemic eyes. When "healthier" eyes were treated by this method to the same extent, the results were disappointing. Clearly, more of the ciliary body had to be treated to gain a significant benefit. While each mechanism of glaucoma may have its own peculiarities in this regard, and will be discussed shortly, most eyes require 180 to 360 degrees of ECP to derive a long-term benefit. Generally, less than this amount will have little or no effect.

Completeness of Treatment

Although the goal is to apply the laser to the entirety of each ciliary process in the treatment zone, whiten its surface, and effect shrinkage, the reality is that this may not be possible for a variety of reasons. Rather than be a "purist," if a particular process or region presents problems, it is best to go elsewhere. Treating a larger area, albeit less completely, is better than potentially creating a complication by seeking the ideal. The novice may find this to be particularly true when performing a reoperation. During the course of ECP, one may think that all of the treatment parameters have been met only to discover during the subsequent procedure that portions of many processes were indeed untreated. It is the sum of the adequately photocoagulated tissue that determines, to a large extent, the final IOP. For example,

the same effect can be attained from a meticulous 180-degree treatment as from an incomplete 360-degree ECP. Some surgeons even prefer this latter approach.

Endoscopic Internal Needling of Failed Filtering Blebs

There may come a time during the course of ECP that the surgeon has an opportunity to view and puncture the inter-

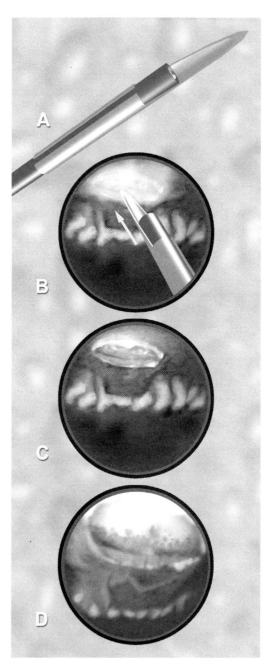

FIGURE 5-32. Endoscopic internal needling of failed blebs. **A:** Endoscope blade. **B:** Opening bleb with blade on endoscope. **C:** View of opened membrane after needling with endoscope blade. **D:** Magnified view of internal aspect of the bleb.

nal aspect of a closed (failed) filtration bleb. This situation may be encountered in the phakic, pseudophakic, or aphakic eye from an anterior segment approach or in the aphakic or anterior chamber pseudophakic eye from a pars plana approach. It is straightforward to push the endoscope tip through the occlusive membrane, reestablishing aqueous access to the subconjunctival space. There is also a blade that can be attached to the shaft of the endoscope that can effectively sever any membranes or adhesions in this area, reopening internal access to the bleb (Fig. 5-32).

Situations to Avoid During Endoscopic Cyclophotocoagulation

A number of situations to avoid during ECP have already been discussed but they bear reiteration and so are listed in Table 5-3.

Tissue Explosion

Tissue explosion deserves special mention. The transscleral cyclophotocoagulation literature is replete with references to "tissue popping" as a desirable effect or at least one that indicates that some threshold for adequate laser power application is being achieved. This notion is absurd. A tissue "pop" occurs when the power density is so intense that it causes gas bubble formation and tissue explosion (Fig. 5-33). There is also an implication that this phenomenon specifically indicates treatment of the ciliary process. Another incorrect assumption. A tissue explosion is a tissue explosion. One of the exercises in Chapter 7 has the surgeon dramatically increase the laser power during practice of ECP and retinal photocoagulation on a pig's eye. What becomes immediately evident, not only by direct visualization but also by audible and tactile experience, is the effect of overly intensive application of laser power. If this situation were to be repeated numerous times during the course of treatment, especially if the ciliary body were not incor-

TABLE 5-3. SITUATIONS TO AVOID DURING ENDOSCOPIC CYCLOPHOTOCOAGULATION

- Circumvent any intraocular tissues that cannot be gently viscodissected, including lens remnants and dense iridocapsular adhesions.
- Avoid photocoagulating through any prosthetic material in the eye, such as tubes from drainage implants or intraocular lens haptics.
- Avoid putting mechanical stress on sutured intraocular lenses or crystalline lenses that are subluxated or that demonstrate significant phacodenesis.
- Avoid neovascularized tissue.
- Stay away from the conjunctiva adjacent to functioning filtration blebs.
- Avoid eyes with active uveitis.
- Avoid tissue explosion.

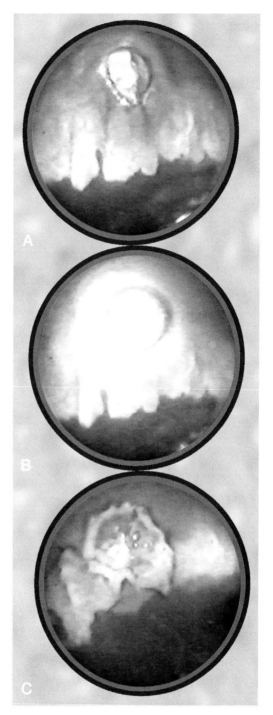

FIGURE 5-33. Endoscopic views of tissue explosions due to over-application of laser. **A:** Early gas bubble formation. **B:** Enlargement of bubble as vaporizing tissue area expands to overtreatment. **C:** "Exploded" laser application site.

porated into the treatment area, complications that are the hallmark of transscleral cyclophotocoagulation, such as hemorrhage, inflammation, pain, cystoid macular edema, and visual loss, might occur. If tissue explosion is avoided, these problems are minimized.

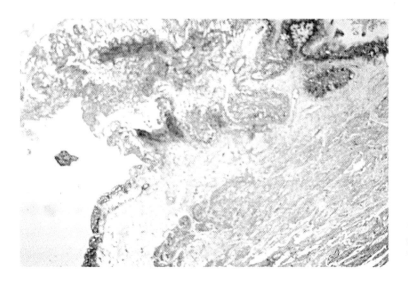

FIGURE 5-34. Histopathologic response to endoscopic cyclophotocoagulation. Specific localization to ciliary body epithelium with sparing of the surrounding tissue can be seen.

HUMAN HISTOPATHOLOGY AND CLINICAL CORRELATIONS

The human histopathology of inflow procedures has been well studied. Cyclocryotherapy damages the sclera, ciliary muscle, and ciliary epithelium. In addition, because of the "blind" nature of its application, surrounding tissues, such as iris and retina, may also be incorporated into the area of destruction. Adjacent nerves and blood vessels are also compromised. An inflammatory response is created. Cell death occurs by two mechanisms, the first being ice crystal formation and thawing, and the second obliteration of the microcirculation with ischemic necrosis of any tissues involved in the treatment site.

Laser transscleral cyclophotocoagulation administered by contact or noncontact methods creates less of a disturbance at the cellular level but still has been demonstrated to effect coagulative necrosis of the ciliary epithelium and, to a lesser extent, the ciliary muscle. There may also be some scleral involvement. Adjacent nonciliary process tissue also experiences these same effects if incorporated into the treatment zone. There is some speculation that involvement of the pars plana may also contribute to reduced aqueous production. Vascular disruption of the ciliary body and the initiation of a chronic inflammatory response likely account

for diminished aqueous production. It has been proposed that increased uveoscleral outflow may also play a role in posttreatment IOP decline.

The human histopathologic response to ECP has been studied as well. This technique has been found to be specifically ablative to the epithelium of the ciliary body only (Fig. 5-34). This epithelium may partially regenerate some time after treatment. The ciliary muscle, sclera, blood vessels, and nerves are typically spared. Interestingly, no inflammatory response, characterized by cellular infiltration, is created by this method, although there may be a disruption of the blood–aqueous barrier. Because the laser is applied under direct visualization, inadvertent inclusion of tissue not involved in aqueous production is minimized at the cellular level.

The distinction between ECP and other inflow procedures is, succinctly, that ECP is *not* a cyclodestructive procedure. It is highly targeted toward the aqueous-producing cells and is *epithelial ablative only* (Table 5-4).

We are now armed with an understanding of the theoretical value of ECP as well as the technology and methods to effect this treatment in any given anatomic situation. One important concept requires emphasis: ECP can precisely control the tissue effect in a given eye under a wide variety of anatomic conditions and glaucoma mechanisms.

TABLE 5-4. COMPARISON OF TISSUE EFFECT OF THE THREE MAIN INFLOW-REDUCING PROCEDURES

Procedure	Cell Damage				
	Sclera	Muscle	Epithelium	Adjacent Tissue	Over- or Undertreatment
Cyclocryotherapy	+	+	+	+	+
TSCPC (diode or Nd:YAG)	−	+	+	+	+
ECP	−	−	+	−	−

TSCPC, transscleral cyclophotocoagulation; ECP, endoscopic cyclophotocoagulation.

This feature is the essence of its value. However, there is no surgical technique that can titrate the clinical outcome. This disconnect accounts for the disparity between a skillfully performed glaucoma surgery (of any type) and what might ultimately prove to be a poor clinical result.

REFERENCES

1. Gayton JL. Traumatic aniridia during endoscopic laser cycloablation. *J Cataract Refract Surg* 1998;24:134–135.

2. Uram M. Ophthalmic laser microendoscopy ciliary process ablation in the management of neovascular glaucoma. *Ophthalmology* 1992;99:1823–1828.

3. Uram M. Endoscopic fluorescein angiography of the ciliary body in glaucoma management. *Ophthalmic Surg Lasers* 1996;27: 174–178.

4. Mochizuki M. Transpupillary cyclophotocoagulation in hemorrhagic glaucoma: a case report. *Jpn J Ophthalmol* 1975;19: 191–198.

5. Merritt JC. Transpupillary photocoagulation of the ciliary processes. *Ann Ophthalmol* 1976;8:325–328.

6. Lee PF. Argon laser photocoagulation of the ciliary processes in cases of aphakic glaucoma. *Arch Ophthalmol* 1979;97:2135–2138.

ENDOSCOPIC CYCLOPHOTOCOAGULATION FOR GLAUCOMA: RESULTS AND COMPLICATIONS

Now that we have a clear understanding of the technology underlying endoscopic cyclophotocoagulation (ECP) as well as the various techniques required to address a given eye with this methodology, perhaps a more specific account of its results and complications in various glaucoma mechanisms is in order. The generalizations about expected outcomes with ECP that follow will serve as a framework for understanding the typical posttreatment course of most eyes treated in this manner.

TITRATABILITY

By enabling direct visualization of the ciliary body, direct monitoring of the tissue effect of each laser application, and delivery of the laser as slowly and precisely as the surgeon desires, ECP is the only inflow procedure in which the outcome of treatment, as far as the tissue effect is concerned, is highly controllable by the surgeon. This advantage should not be confused with the ability to titrate the clinical outcome of this technique. It would be fair to say that there is no glaucoma surgical procedure in which the surgeon can titrate and control the end clinical result. All we can know

is how groups of patients with similar features may respond to our efforts. At this point, then, the best that we can do is control what we do to the tissue and hope that the individual's response fulfills our expectations.

POSTOPERATIVE MANAGEMENT

Endoscopic Cyclophotocoagulation Versus Trabeculectomy

One of the most difficult issues for ophthalmic surgeons is managing the postoperative trabeculectomy patient. It should be evident that in using this approach, the surgical event—trabeculectomy—is just the beginning of a process to defeat the natural course of wound healing, meant ultimately to create a permanent aqueous drainage site. That is why intensive postoperative follow-up is required. Without skillful intervention after surgery, many more filters would fail.

ECP follows a different course. After treatment is completed, little in the way of postoperative treatment is required to optimize the outcome. If a sufficient amount of ciliary epithelium was photocoagulated, the intraocular pressure (IOP) will diminish, and if the treatment was insufficient, the desired outcome will not be achieved.

The intensity of surgical and postoperative management skills are perhaps what deters most ophthalmologists from filtration surgery. The absence of these considerations with ECP may alter this landscape.

Aside from the usual postoperative concerns (e.g., hemorrhage, inflammation, pain, spiking IOP, infection), there are a few perioperative technical points that are peculiar to glaucoma surgery. Table 6-1 compares those of ECP and trabeculectomy.

General Considerations

As with most intraocular surgical procedures, the eye is usually patched postoperatively until the patient is seen the following day. Assuming that there are no alarming problems that demand immediate attention, cycloplegics and topical antibiotic-steroid medications are prescribed. If the patient's status seems to be acceptable at this point, the second visit is usually scheduled for 1 to 2 weeks later. The IOP changes that may evolve over the next month or two will be discussed shortly, but if all is progressing well, the third visit is usually scheduled for 4 to 6 weeks after surgery. Observing the patient closely much beyond this period is not necessary as long as recovery and IOP response seem to be within an adequate range. Certainly, if there are any minor or serious complications, unacceptable changes in IOP, or adjustment in medications required, more frequent visits would be indicated. Typically, no limitations are placed on the patient's

TABLE 6-1. PERIOPERATIVE TECHNICAL ISSUES: TRABECULECTOMY VERSUS ENDOSCOPIC CYCLOPHOTOCOAGULATION

Trabeculectomy	ECP
Intraoperative antimetabolites	None
Postoperative antimetabolites	
Scleral flap suture release	
Internal flap revisions	
Externalized releasable sutures	
Small scleral flap too small	
Thin scleral flap	
Conjunctival flap too small	
Sclerectomy site too posterior	
Sclerectomy adjacent to lateral scleral flap edge	
Bleb failure	
Vitreous through sclerectomy	
Ciliary process in sclerectomy	
Conjunctival buttonhole	
Conjunctival wound leak	
Flat anterior chamber	
Lens–cornea touch	
Choroidal effusion	
Hypotonous maculopathy	
Pupillary block	

ECP, endoscopic cyclophotocoagulation.

activity after surgery, as long as the operated eye is protected from physical trauma and infection.

Intraocular Pressure

If a group of patients is managed by ECP and followed up for months posttreatment, a retrospective analysis will reveal that most of the group will have reached what proved to be their final IOP between the second and eighth postoperative weeks. Following the successes out for years, one will also discover that there typically is not a decremental response. The outcome of surgery will be known to patient and ophthalmologist early in the course and, if successful, will tend to remain so in the long run.

Failures, too, will be known early in the postoperative course, and decisions for the manner in which further treatment will be applied must be considered. The IOP during the first week or two after ECP is mostly irrelevant from a predictive point of view. Hypotony during this period should not be worrisome and is typically due to ciliary body shutdown. This situation usually resolves spontaneously over the course of days.

On the other hand, a marked elevation in IOP demands support. This usually takes the form of administering topical and/or systemic ocular hypotensive agents. Another option that can be used separately or in conjunction with medical therapy is aqueous drainage, usually through a preexisting incision. This is especially useful if clear corneal sutureless incisions were used during ECP. Simply pressing gently on the eye with a cotton-tipped applicator or elevating one lip of the incision will release aqueous and immediately lower the IOP. This maneuver can usually be repeated if necessary (Fig. 6-1). Early IOP spiking does not necessarily indicate failure. Most often, an elevated IOP in

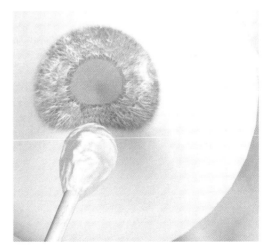

FIGURE 6-1. Postoperative release of aqueous from the anterior chamber through a clear corneal sutureless incision created at the time of surgery. Minimal pressure on the eye with a cotton tipped applicator will usually be sufficient to elicit a prompt decrease in intraocular pressure.

the immediate postoperative period is due to retained viscoelastic in the anterior chamber or sulcus, and resolves promptly with medical treatment or aqueous drainage.

Overall, in most studies, about 90% of ECP patients achieve controlled IOP over an array of glaucoma mechanisms. These perhaps surprisingly good outcomes are associated with another unexpected feature. The great concern most surgeons have with inflow procedures is that they will induce permanent hypotony or phthisis, and so they are fearful of treating "too much" of the ciliary body. What has been learned, essentially by trial and error, is that an entry level treatment is 180 degrees and that in most patients cyclophotocoagulation of 270 to 360 degrees is needed to elicit a significant and permanent effect. As it turns out, it is difficult to "overtreat" with ECP, and the potential for hypotony or phthisis is negligible except in a few situations to be discussed. Perhaps we have been laboring under a misconception that these problems were due to destruction of the target tissue in an overly intensive manner resulting in low aqueous production. Rather, consider what was probably the more likely event. Endoscopic imaging has indicated that a significant amount of non-aqueous-producing tissue has been incorporated into transscleral cyclophotocoagulation (TSCPC) treatment zones and that subsequent inflammation, choroidal hemorrhage, anterior segment vascular compromise, and cyclitic membrane formation with ciliary body detachment may have been the underlying etiologic factors in the development of hypotony and phthisis. Furthermore, one of the most common glaucoma mechanisms managed by cyclodestruction has been neovascular glaucoma, which, as we will discuss, is the form most prone to development of posttreatment hypotony and phthisis.

The eye should be left with either *low or moderate* (within "normal" range) IOP at the completion of surgery. An elevated pressure at this time is unacceptable. This goal is usually simple to achieve by draining aqueous until a satisfactory level has been reached. If the pressure cannot be lowered by this maneuver, even though all of the viscoelastic has been removed from the eye, then it is highly suspicious that a choroidal effusion or hemorrhage is evolving. Management of this problem will be discussed shortly.

If the eye is soft at the conclusion of surgery, cessation of glaucoma medications until the first postoperative visit is reasonable. At that time the surgeon can assess whether restarting some or all preoperative medications would be appropriate. Usually, if the IOP is less than 10 mm Hg and the patient is going to have close follow-up (e.g., weekly), there would be no need to restart medical therapy. This situation would be reassessed at each postoperative visit. As long as the IOP remained at an acceptable level, medical therapy need not be reinstituted. Certainly, if the pressure begins to rise during this period, the medications can be restarted as needed.

If the IOP is in the teens at the conclusion of surgery, very often it seems best to restart all of the preoperative medications and reevaluate the situation at each postopera-

tive visit. This is also helpful if the patient is unable to be followed closely during this period. The medications can then be discontinued according to the IOP response.

Patients must frequently be reminded that during this portion of their recovery, which is approximately 8 weeks in length, the eye is developing its new steady state and the period is often characterized by fluctuations in IOP. Our concern, then, is maintaining control until the final outcome of surgery becomes evident.

There are several different IOP "behavior" patterns that may be discerned following ECP, and it is helpful to recognize them to more effectively anticipate the evolution of each eye's individual response. Certainly, the most desirable response would be to experience an immediate decline in IOP that remains within the low-normal range throughout the postoperative period (Fig. 6-2). One might presume that this effect was due to an appropriately performed ECP that permanently diminished aqueous production in combination with stable outflow obstruction. In this instance, adjustment of medical therapy is straightforward and the patient can be reassured that a successful outcome seems imminent. The trend would also be unlikely to reverse in the future.

A second common scenario would be a slow and more or less steady decline in IOP over the first 8 weeks (Fig. 6-3). Assuming that there has been no change in outflow, this behavior indicates that aqueous production was truly diminished by ECP. As long as the IOP continues to fall, surveillance and medical support are all that would be required. Ultimately, a decision can be made regarding the adequacy of response. Once the IOP has stabilized, it would be expected to remain at that level for an extended period and so if the IOP were still too high for the eye in question, then consideration should be given to further treatment.

Another pattern that may be discerned is characterized by an erratic IOP response with pressure elevations and depressions fluctuating throughout the early postoperative period

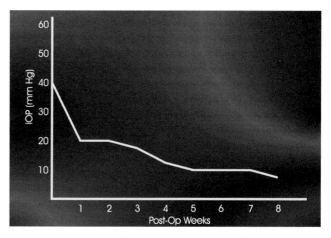

FIGURE 6-2. Intraocular pressure behavior following endoscopic cyclophotocoagulation. In this instance, the intraocular pressure declines promptly after treatment and remains at a low and acceptable level throughout the perioperative period.

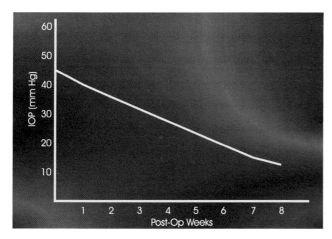

FIGURE 6-3. Intraocular pressure behavior following endoscopic cyclophotocoagulation. A slow but steady decline in intraocular pressure is observed over the perioperative period, ultimately reaching and stabilizing at an acceptable level.

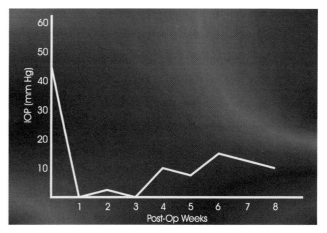

FIGURE 6-5. Intraocular pressure "bottoms out" in the early postoperative period and may remain at that level for several weeks. This is most often due to ciliary body shutdown, with cessation of aqueous production. This response is not indicative of permanent hypotony or phthisis, and often the situation corrects itself over the course of days or weeks.

(Fig. 6-4). As long as the overall trend remains in the acceptable range, then further intervention is not required and the patient can be observed until the situation stabilizes.

This is especially true of neovascular glaucoma, where the early response may be quite erratic and even seems to stabilize at a somewhat unacceptable level. In these eyes, it is important not to gild the lily with another intervention but to follow closely for the overall trend. In some eyes, stabilization may take place over 3 or 4 months rather than the more typical 2 months, and so patience may be rewarded with an excellent outcome that was simply slow to develop.

One of the more disturbing patterns, especially for the novice, is when the IOP immediately "bottoms out" and

the eye remains hypotonous for several weeks (Fig. 6-5). In outflow procedures, a few serious problems will account for this and require intervention to stabilize the eye. With ECP, this finding is typical of ciliary body shutdown, which usually resolves spontaneously. Serous choroidal effusions may develop under these circumstances but mostly do not require treatment. As aqueous production resumes, the IOP rises and the ultimate adequacy of the surgery becomes evident. Even in eyes susceptible to phthisis, such as in neovascular glaucoma, a truly hypotonous state will not become evident for weeks to months; it is certainly not an immediate postoperative event.

Elevated IOP as an initial response is also not a sign of failure. Typically, if the IOP spikes upward during this period, it is due to retained viscoelastic (Fig. 6-6). This

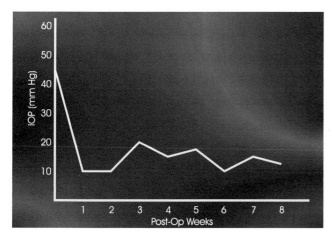

FIGURE 6-4. Erratic intraocular pressure behavior during the perioperative period. As long as the intraocular pressure remains within an acceptable range, patient surveillance is all that is required. This type of behavior pattern can be seen in some of the more difficult to manage glaucoma cases, and such patients may have to be observed for a number of months postoperatively to clearly establish whether the therapeutic goal has been reached or further treatment is needed.

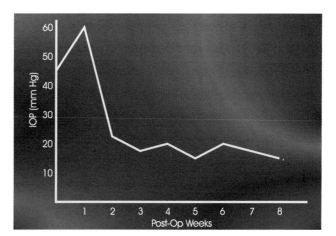

FIGURE 6-6. An immediate spike upward in intraocular pressure after surgery is usually a sign of retained viscoelastic. While this problem may resolve spontaneously, intervention is often required for pain control or for damage protection. This response is not a sign of surgical failure.

problem usually resolves over the course of several days, but if the IOP is quite high or the eye has substantial preexisting field loss and is highly threatened, then immediate intervention is required. Many patients will experience pain from this sudden change and drainage from the corneal incision and medical management will often be required.

The other most common cause of this response is the development of hemorrhagic or serous choroidal effusion. The IOP can spike to a high level in the immediate postoperative period and remain high for an extended time, often until further surgical intervention is applied (Fig. 6-7). This situation can represent a difficult management problem that may ultimately result in treatment failure or visual loss even after their spontaneous or surgical resolution.

Three typical failure patterns may become evident. The first of these is that the IOP seems unaffected by the surgery and hovers more or less at pretreatment levels, or even rises (Fig. 6-8). In this instance, ECP has had an insufficient effect on the ciliary epithelium. This scenario usually becomes apparent between the first and second postoperative months, and further surgery is required.

A second pattern is when the IOP is falling during the first few weeks, although not to a desirable level, and just never achieves the ultimate goal, leveling off at an inadequate response (Fig. 6-9). An insufficient number of ciliary processes were adequately treated resulting in this outcome and further ECP would be expected to attain the desired result.

The third response is perhaps the most disappointing, This is when the IOP initially seems to be responding well but then, suddenly or gradually, reverses direction and rises to an unacceptable level, clearly indicating failure (Fig. 6-

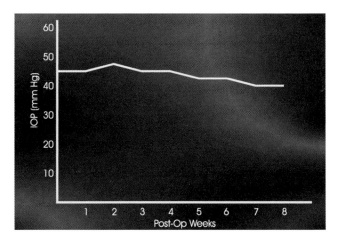

FIGURE 6-8. First failure pattern. intraocular pressure hovers around pretreatment levels. This is indicative of the failure of endoscopic cyclophotocoagulation to substantially diminish inflow. When this pattern becomes apparent, reoperation should be considered.

10). One might conjecture that the initially positive response was actually due to ciliary body shutdown and that as aqueous production returned to a more normal level the IOP responded in kind. Another possible explanation would be that the ECP actually did permanently diminish aqueous production but that progressive drainage obstruction was responsible for reversing the early trend. This would not be surprising, for example, early in the course of acute neovascular glaucoma when the IOP is very high yet only a portion of the angle structures have been affected. If ECP is applied early in the course, it is still likely that further vascularized synechial angle closure will evolve and

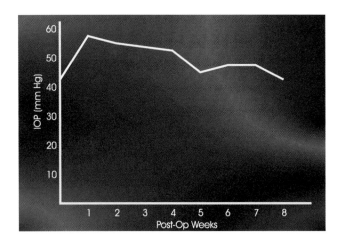

FIGURE 6-7. Early spike in intraocular pressure that remains elevated for an extended period is typical of significant serous, serosanguinous, or hemorrhagic choroidal effusion. Typically medical or surgical intervention is required to reverse this trend. Despite an aggressive response, the potential for a poor outcome is significant.

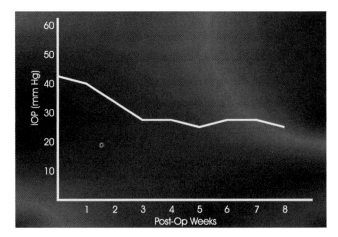

FIGURE 6-9. Second failure pattern. The intraocular pressure drops somewhat during the first weeks following endoscopic cyclophotocoagulation although it does not approach a satisfactory level. It will tend to remain at this unacceptable point for an extended period, as this is the new steady state initiated by treatment. The only option is for reoperation.

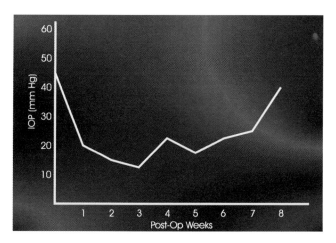

FIGURE 6-10. Third failure pattern. Intraocular pressure response is initially good for days or weeks only to deteriorate and rise again. The only response to this can be additional surgery.

potentially reverse the outcome of an initially successful procedure. Whether this occurs after a few weeks or a few months, additional surgery would be needed.

A group of 347 patients who underwent ECP have been reported and the course of their IOP, grouped by glaucoma mechanism, has been graphed against their follow-up over an extended period (Fig. 6-11). A number of features became evident. First, the IOP response, overall, seemed to be mechanism independent—a critical feature with other glaucoma surgical modalities.

Most forms of glaucoma responded to ECP in a similar fashion and in the manner already described: early decline in IOP that seemed to stabilize over the long term without

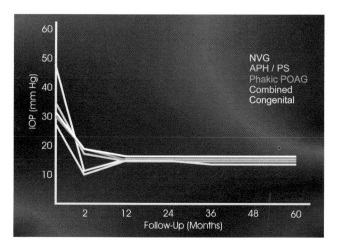

FIGURE 6-11. Various mechanisms of glaucoma intraocular pressure response to endoscopic cyclophotocoagulation. Despite the initial elevation of intraocular pressure or the mechanism of glaucoma, responses were similar with early and significant intraocular pressure decline followed by long-term stabilization and absence of late decremental response.

a late decremental response. This was a unique and surprising observation. It clearly demonstrates that this inflow-reducing procedure is not hampered by anterior segment architectural conditions that promote filtration or tube failure. The surgeon may consider that, with ECP, the difficulty is not so much the mechanism of glaucoma but rather is based on a particular eye's anatomic impediments to accessing the ciliary processes.

Medications

As discussed previously, adjustments to the patient's medical regimen are made during the weeks following ECP, as dictated by the IOP response. Most reports of ECP outcomes indicate that there is a significant decline in use of topical and systemic glaucoma medications, and this should be the expectation. There appears to be some relationship to glaucoma mechanism in this instance, with neovascular glaucoma requiring the least amount of topical and systemic therapy long term and congenital glaucomas responding least well. In one study, about 75% of patients were using systemic carbonic anhydrase inhibitors preoperatively, but ultimately only about 10% required them as continued maintenance (Table 6-2).

Visual Field Loss

The only feature of glaucoma that might be directly controlled by the surgeon is IOP. While the distinction between lowering IOP and preventing visual field loss must be acknowledged, it should be clear to the patient and surgeon that manipulating IOP is the only therapeutic option. What follows from "successful" IOP control is usually, but not always, preservation of visual field.

There are two opportunities for progressive visual field damage in the glaucoma surgical patient. One is in the perioperative period when surgery-associated events, such as IOP spiking or choroidal hemorrhage, result in progressive damage. Failure to control IOP quickly enough can sometimes be associated with progressive field loss in the highly threatened patient. The second opportunity for field loss evolves over time, even in the presence of "good" IOP control, and is a consequence of some of the more subtle and elusive features of glaucoma.

In any event, progressive visual field loss is an uncommon event in the perioperative period and is not to be expected. On the other hand, overall about 10% of patients with "successful" IOP control following ECP exhibit progressive field loss over the long run. The exceptions to this are neovascular glaucoma patients. In this group, about 20% of the patients with adequate IOP response to therapy nevertheless continue with visual loss to blindness. This feature is indicative of some of the other factors affecting vision aside from IOP, such as retinal or optic nerve ischemia.

TABLE 6-2. ENDOSCOPIC CYCLOPHOTOCOAGULATION: PREOPERATIVE AND POSTOPERATIVE MEDICATION REQUIREMENTS

Disease	Topical		CAIs	
	Preoperative	Postoperative	Preoperative	Postoperative
NVG	3.6	0.8	74.1	9.1
Aphatic/Pseudophakic	3.1	1.4	78.7	10.2
Combined	1.9	0.7	65.0	10.0
Phakic POAG	2.4	1.1	73.2	16.1
Congenital	1.7	1.5	88.0	27.7

CAIs, carbonic anhydrase inhibitors; NVG, neovascular glaucoma; APH/PS, ; POAG, primary open-angle glaucoma.

Visual Acuity Loss

It is common in the perioperative period for patients to experience acuity loss for a host of reasons, many of them self-limited. It is important that the surgeon counsel the patient in this regard, especially when operating on the better eye. Transient corneal edema, development of Descemet folds, hyphema, iritis, and vitreous hemorrhage are a few of these not very serious problems that resolve over the short- to mid-term. Permanent visual loss is, therefore, not an expected consequence of ECP.

Cystoid Macular Edema

Any form of intraocular surgery carries with it the potential to incite subtle intraocular inflammation, juxtafoveal capillary leakage, and the development of cystoid macular edema (CME). The long-term incidence of this problem in cataract surgery is approximately 2%. The visual loss from this problem can be troubling to patient and surgeon, whether it is transient or chronic in nature. TSCPC is notorious for inciting this problem, resulting in visual loss in 40% to 50% of treated eyes. Indeed, the proclivity of TSCPC to induce visual loss is one of the primary reasons that it is not a widely useful procedure in glaucoma treatment, being relegated to the management of certain more difficult mechanisms of glaucoma when central vision has already been lost.

This is one of the aspects of ECP that at first was astonishing. It is only natural to conclude that if visual loss and CME are so prevalent following TSCPC, the same must hold true for ECP. As it turns out, this is not the case. In some large studies, the incidence of CME following ECP was about 2%, and in the smaller studies it was not observed at all. The human histopathology of ECP most likely accounts for this. Recall that this technique does not incite an inflammatory cellular reaction, which is a mediator of prostaglandin synthesis and is at the root of CME development. Although this will be discussed later, the expectation is that CME and its associated visual decline will not develop as a consequence of ECP more frequently than it might from any other intraocular surgery, opening the possibility of using this technique for glaucoma management in eyes with good central acuity.

From a treatment viewpoint, CME can be stubborn. Most of the time, surgeons rely on spontaneous resolution as the treatment of choice. When following as a consequence of cataract surgery, the incidence of CME in the immediate postoperative period may be as high as 77% but by the second posttreatment month, the incidence typically declines to about 2%. That is why nontreatment seems to be so successful. The situation is more disturbing when managing chronic CME. Topical and periocular steroids seem to help little, as do topical and systemic non-steroidal anti-inflammatory agents. Some claim success with systemic carbonic anhydrase inhibitors. As most ophthalmologists know, such efforts are not often rewarded.

An approach that demonstrates some efficacy is treating this condition with systemic corticosteroids in a particular manner. Therapy is initiated with prednisone, 40 to 60 mg daily taken with food, either as a single pulse or in divided doses, and is continued for 2 weeks. If subjective acuity, Snellen acuity, or clinical appearance does not improve, then further treatment would be pointless and it is discontinued. On the other hand, if the patient experiences improvement of one of these parameters, then the dosage is diminished and continued for another two weeks. As long as improvement is noted over each 2-week step, treatment is continued. Usually, the course of therapy is 6 to 8 weeks. Once improvement seems to have reached a plateau, a small amount of prednisone (e.g., 5 mg) should be given for 2 more weeks, before discontinuation. This is because some eyes experience a recurrence of the problem over the first or second week following cessation of therapy. If the patient is initially improving on therapy and then seems to be retrogressing, then one might try raising the dosage to see if a proper response can once again be elicited. The key to this regimen is to give enough corticosteroid for long enough to eliminate the biochemical stimulus for the development of CME.

If these efforts fail, the only other option is pars plana vitrectomy. This approach can be helpful if there is an associated derangement of anterior segment architecture, such as vitreous incarceration in a wound or iridovitreal or capsular-vitreal adhesion. Correcting these abnormalities is relatively simple and has a moderate chance of improving the situation. If the eye is quiet and there are no discernible areas of anatomic disruption, it is unlikely that vitrectomy will be of value. The typical eye in this situation does poorly.

Hemorrhage

As in any intraocular surgery, hemorrhage in the eye is a common occurrence following ECP. This may be noted in the anterior or posterior segment. In most studies, the frequency of this event is in the 3% to 10% range. Usually, it is not very important and spontaneous resolution is the rule. Further surgical intervention is rarely required. The most likely source of this problem is bleeding from incision sites, abrasion of intraocular tissue by endoscope manipulation, and overtreatment of one or more ciliary processes resulting in tissue explosion. Neovascularized eyes are also prone to intraocular hemorrhage whether or not ECP is performed. It is common to see a hyphema after treatment of such an eye, this event probably being due to the mechanical features of manipulating the endoscope in the presence of vessels with abnormally weak walls.

Perhaps the most disturbing aspect of this problem is the associated visual loss that may be experienced. Diffuse hyphema and vitreous hemorrhage can markedly, albeit transiently, diminish vision, to the patient's consternation. It is important to inform them of this potential problem before surgery, especially if ECP is to be effected in the better eye.

If the hemorrhage does not spontaneously clear after an appropriate waiting period, then, unfortunately, surgical intervention is required. Still, as complications go, this does not present a difficult treatment problem because most eyes achieve their potential even if surgical evacuation is required.

Inflammation

One of the biggest objections to inflow procedures is their proclivity for inducing significant anterior and posterior segment inflammation. Consequently, a host of problems may arise that may lead to treatment failure, decompensation from the patient's initial status, and general unhappiness. TSCPC deserves to be considered in this manner because it is a fairly uncontrolled and brutish means of diminishing aqueous production. ECP has far less potential for inciting this response; nevertheless, any ablative procedure, even a highly targeted and controlled one as in this instance, creates this possibility. Recall that histopathologi-

cally ECP does not incite an inflammatory response although it may contribute to breakdown of the blood–aqueous barrier. The clinical correlate of this is a noticeable flare without cells by slit-lamp examination.

There are a few circumstances where more than the expected inflammation may arise as a postoperative consequence of ECP. Perhaps the most common cause of this problem is an overly intensive treatment. Usually this takes the form of mild iritis that can be easily managed with topical cycloplegics and steroids. A moderate to intense inflammatory response is quite uncommon and may require the incorporation of systemic steroids in the therapeutic regimen.

Another situation that may incite an inflammatory response is related to mechanical trauma to intraocular tissue by endoscope manipulation. This is especially true if the eye is presenting some technical challenges. Typically, a mild inflammatory reaction evolves that responds well to topical therapy.

Certain eyes are prone to developing an inflammatory response no matter how careful and skillful the surgeon. Clearly, patients with uveitic glaucoma, history of significant uveitis without its secondary glaucoma, and eyes in the pediatric age group are at risk. It would certainly be best to avoid any surgery when active inflammation is present. Best efforts should be made to quiet these eyes preoperatively. Nonetheless, pretreatment or posttreatment with topical or systemic steroids may be a consideration.

Another important factor is related to the method of endoscope sterilization. At this point, there are no autoclavable microendoscopes and the only alternatives are some form of chemical soaking/irrigation or gas sterilization. These approaches are satisfactory as there have been no reported cases of infectious endophthalmitis after ECP. Still, the surgeon must assume responsibility and ensure that there are no residual toxic substances on the intraocular portion of the endoscope. This precaution is quite simply performed. The surgeon merely wipes the distal portion of the endoscope with wet gauze. If these toxic substances are not adequately rinsed from the instrument, they may incite an intense inflammatory reaction that is difficult to control and may lead to a devastating outcome. Table 6-3 lists the causes of post-ECP inflammation.

To be specific about management of inflammation, when the problem is mostly confined to the anterior seg-

TABLE 6-3. MOST COMMON CAUSES OF INFLAMMATION AFTER ENDOSCOPIC CYCLOPHOTOCOAGULATION

- Overly intensive endoscopic cyclophotocoagulation
- Mechanical trauma to intraocular tissue from endoscope manipulation
- Predisposition to inflammatory response
- Toxic residue from endoscope sterilization

ment, then frequent topical steroids and cycloplegics are started and adjustments to initial therapy are made according to the eye's response. It would be quite uncommon for serious anterior segment inflammation to evolve, even after a challenging ECP, and it would be even more uncommon for this not to respond to topical therapy alone. If posterior segment inflammation develops, topical medications alone seem to work poorly. While many ophthalmologists favor periocular steroids for management of vitiritis, it seems that systemic corticosteroids are more effective and their dosage may be adjusted commensurate with the clinical response. Typically, prednisone, 60 mg daily, is initiated to be taken with food either as a single pulse or in divided doses. This regimen is reassessed after 1 week. Diabetic patients must be reminded to follow their blood glucose levels closely and to inform the physician responsible for their management that they now must take steroids. As the eye responds, the dosage may be slowly diminished, usually over the course of a few weeks (not days). Most eyes, even those with intense reaction, seem to respond well to this.

For any scenario in which the surgeon thinks that postoperative inflammation will be out of the ordinary, intraocular steroids can be quite beneficial. Typically, 0.1 to 0.5 mL of dexamethasone (Decadron) can be injected into the eye through one of the preexisting incisions at the conclusion of the procedure. This can be quite effective. It is particularly helpful in the management of pediatric forms of glaucoma, where there is a tendency for inflammation to evolve following any type of intraocular surgery.

If the inflammation is uncontrollable despite these efforts, the surgeon must seriously consider that the patient's problem has arisen from an infectious etiology and intraocular antibiotics, vitrectomy, and systemic therapy must be considered. This degree of difficulty has been virtually unheard of, as far as post-ECP complications are concerned, and furthermore, there has not been a single reported incident of infectious endophthalmitis following ECP.

Pain

Pain is an uncommon response to ECP. Undue pain is such an infrequent experience that the surgeon must first consider that there is some other etiology, such as spiking IOP, choroidal hemorrhage, or unusually intensive inflammation. Typically, the same events that incite an inflammatory response or contribute to marked elevation of postoperative IOP go hand in hand with the experience of pain. Their management is identical. Topical cycloplegics and steroids are usually sufficient to control discomfort from inflammation, and all of the measures previously discussed for management of postsurgical elevated IOP would be appropriate. In the event that these measures prove to be inadequate in a given situation and there are no other reasons why the patient should be experiencing this problem, then narcotic

or nonnarcotic analgesics may be prescribed. It must be emphasized, however, that undue pain is such an infrequent experience following ECP that the surgeon must first consider some other cause.

Serous Choroidal Effusion

Perhaps one of the most annoying problems to arise as a consequence of any type of glaucoma surgery is serous choroidal effusion. This event may evolve at any time, potentially compromising the execution of the procedure. Alternatively, it may present at any point during the immediate postoperative course, sometimes to the extreme detriment of the patient. The causative factors are rarely apparent and so consciously attempting to prevent its occurrence is not possible. As the choroid bulges into the ocular interior it may increase the IOP, causing pain and visual loss. This situation may alternatively be associated with hypotony, again being associated with visual loss. In outflow procedures this may even initiate failure. Fortunately, as far as ECP is concerned, the evolution of this problem has little to do with the final IOP response. Still its presence may demand intensive follow-up and medical therapy or even further surgical intervention. Intraoperatively, it may be recognized as shallowing of the anterior chamber or by observing the ciliary processes rotating upward and bulging forward. Hypotony during the course of surgery, venous congestion, and inflammation are considered to be possible etiologic factors. This can be especially troublesome because a cycle may be established wherein a low IOP initiates a reduction in aqueous production and an increase in uveoscleral outflow, exacerbating the inciting event, that is, hypotony.

Usually, this problem resolves spontaneously over the course of a few days to a few weeks. If the etiology is considered to be inflammatory, intervention may consist of moderate doses of systemic corticosteroids. However, some eyes do not respond to conservative measures. In these situations it is necessary to surgically drain the effusions. Some indications for surgical drainage are outlined in Table 6-4.

Intervention would rarely be required intraoperatively but would be appropriate if the sudden development of this problem were deemed severe.

The surgical goal is straightforward, being directed to reforming the anterior chamber combined with drainage of the effusion. A paracentesis is created (or previous site reopened) and balanced salt solution (BSS) or viscoelastic

TABLE 6-4. INDICATIONS FOR SURGICAL DRAINAGE OF CHOROIDAL EFFUSION

- Persistence of a significant effusion
- Lens–cornea touch
- Failure of medical therapy
- Presence of a hemorrhagic component to the effusion

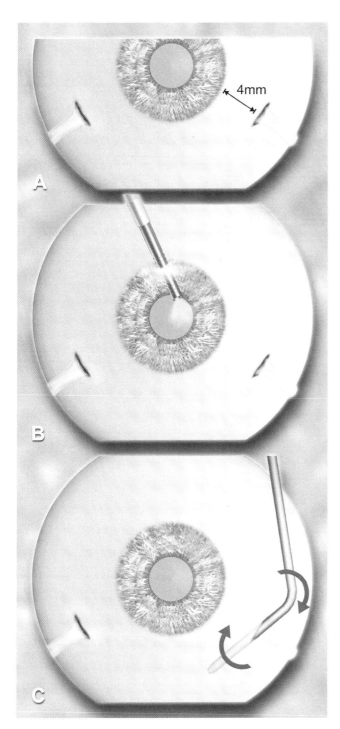

FIGURE 6-12. Technique for draining choroidal effusion. **A:** Sclerotomy sites are fashioned approximately 4.0 mm from the limbus in one or both inferior quadrants. Not infrequently, suprachoroidal fluid drains spontaneously. **B:** The anterior chamber is then perfused with balanced saline solution through an anterior chamber maintainer or 22-gauge needle. **C:** If the effusion has still not drained adequately, a cyclodialysis spatula may be inserted parallel to the limbus and gently manipulated by lifting with its tip or depressing with its heel to express suprachoroidal fluid.

injected, or an anterior chamber maintainer with BSS infusion is established, with care taken not to traumatize the iris or lens. Then a scleral incision is made, usually in one but sometimes in both inferior quadrants, that is several millimeters in length starting from a point about 4.0 mm from the limbus. Laceration of the underlying uvea should be avoided although typically, once the sclerotomy has been fashioned, the suprachoroidal fluid drains immediately. The cycle of anterior chamber reformation and fluid drainage may be repeated as necessary.

There are a few key points to bear in mind. It is best to maintain a more or less constant IOP during the procedure and to limit, as much as possible, hypotonous periods during the surgery; otherwise, a hemorrhagic component may evolve, exacerbating the situation. Establishing a constant infusion with an anterior chamber maintainer or a 22-gauge needle is a simple and effective way to limit this complication. Some surgeons insert a cyclodialysis spatula through the sclerotomy into the suprachoroidal space paralleling the limbus. The tip of the spatula may then be gently elevated in the hope that more fluid will drain through the sclerotomy. Alternatively, the "heel" of the instrument, which remains on the external surface of the sclerotomy, may be depressed at the edge of the wound to effect additional drainage. At the conclusion of the procedure, the sclerotomies are usually left open although the overlying conjunctiva is closed (Fig. 6-12).

Choroidal Hemorrhage

Glaucoma surgery is fraught with hazard and one of the more difficult problems to engage is choroidal hemorrhage. It is in some ways the worst complication that may be experienced by the patient and surgeon. Although it may occur in about 2% of eyes undergoing filtration surgery, it is an exceedingly uncommon event associated with ECP. The major risk factors for the development of this problem are outlined in Table 6-5.

Patients with eyes that are aphakic or that have undergone vitrectomy, patients with uncontrolled hypertension at the time of surgery, patients whose eyes experience intraoperative hypotony, or those using anticoagulants are at an increased risk for the development of choroidal hemorrhage.. It may develop at any point along the course of surgery or perioper-

TABLE 6-5. RISK FACTORS FOR THE DEVELOPMENT OF PERIOPERATIVE HEMORRHAGIC CHOROIDAL EFFUSION

- Aphakia
- Previous vitrectomy
- Uncontrolled hypertension at surgery
- Anticoagulated at surgery
- Intraoperative hypotony

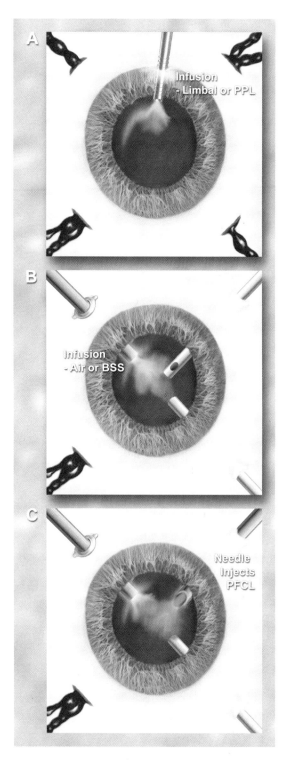

FIGURE 6-13. Treatment of choroidal hemorrhage. **A:** Initiate anterior chamber infusion. Fashion sclerotomies in all affected quadrants (usually all four). Place drainage sites as if they were going to be used for a pars plana vitrectomy. **B:** If drainage is insufficient, consider pars plana vitrectomy using a high infusion pressure of either balanced saline solution or air to assist in expression of the hemorrhage through the sclerotomy sites. **C:** If this maneuver proves to be insufficient, injection of perfluorocarbon liquid will force the choroidal blood out of the eye through the incision sites.

atively. Signs are similar to choroidal effusion, with shallowing of the anterior chamber along with forward rotation and bulging of the ciliary body and posterior segment. If this problem can be detected intraoperatively, it seems best to expeditiously discontinue surgery. Postoperatively the patient may experience severe pain, nausea and vomiting, and markedly diminished vision. Typically, but not necessarily always, the IOP is dramatically elevated. Sometimes this event does not become a threatening problem, and no treatment or medical management is required.

On the other hand, if the eye's status is in jeopardy, then surgical drainage, as previously described, would be in order. Usually, blood clots undergo lysis in the 1 to 2 weeks after their appearance, and so, theoretically, this might be the best time to intervene. If the usual approach to choroidal drainage is not successful, a somewhat complicated vitrectomy technique can be applied. In this instance, the basic concept remains the same, which is maintaining IOP at a constant level while simultaneously draining the choroid. The anterior chamber is deepened with infusion. Drainage sclerotomies are fashioned in each involved quadrant (usually four). Then a pars plana vitrectomy is performed. Realize that the sclerotomy sites for vitrectomy may serve as choroidal drainage sites as well. If a pars plana infusion line is desired, the surgeon must take great care to know with certainty that it is placed within the vitreous cavity and not underneath the pars plana. Endoscopy can be quite helpful in this regard because often in this situation anterior segment conditions preclude a posterior view. Typically, there is little vitreous to remove because the bulging choroid compresses it centrally and anteriorly. Raising the IOP by BSS or gas infusion may force the choroidal hemorrhage through the sclerotomy sites and open the funnel created by the internally bulging choroid. If this approach fails, it may be helpful to inject a perfluorocarbon liquid into the vitreous cavity and slowly "push" the choroidal hemorrhage through the drainage incisions. Once completed, any retinal breaks or areas of detachment can be photocoagulated (Fig. 6-13). Even after a successful surgery most of these patients do poorly with profound visual loss and subsequent development of hypotony or phthisis.

This complication has not yet been observed in any eye with open-angle, pseudophakic, or pseudoexfoliative glaucoma managed by ECP or in association with combined cataract surgery and ECP. Careful preoperative medical preparation, deliberate attention to blood pressure control and surveillance of coagulation parameters, as well as avoidance of intraoperative hypotony in patients with known risk factors such as aphakia and/or previous vitrectomy, may limit the potential for this difficult problem to evolve.

Devastating Complications

Devastating complications are the most emotionally stressful for patients and surgeons. It is difficult to help the patient with a devastating complication, not just from a medical or surgical management viewpoint but also on an emotional level as well. Choroidal hemorrhage has been discussed previously, and it should be clear that when this problem develops to a significant extent the overall prognosis is quite poor, despite the most skillful treatment. Many of these eyes ultimately become hypotonous or phthisical. It is frustrating to treat an eye that has uncontrolled high pressure only to develop a surgical complication that in short order evolves into a low-pressure blind eye. This roller-coaster effect can be daunting and the unfortunate truth is that the surgeon cannot do much to reverse it.

Infectious endophthalmitis has never been reported as a consequence of ECP although certainly it will become an eventuality. Still the overall incidence will be a small fraction of a percentage point, so that undue concern on the part of the surgeon or patient is not necessary. One of the specific advantages that ECP has over any outflow procedure is its lack of propensity for the development of this problem. Compare this with the 1% cumulative risk per year for the development of endophthalmitis in any eye with a filter. The management of endophthalmitis will be discussed in greater detail later.

Retinal detachment is considered by many to be a devastating complication of intraocular surgery. With the exception of two pediatric eyes, this problem has not been reported as a complication in any series of ECP patients. Perhaps this is because of the fact that the bulk of the ECPs that have been performed worldwide have been executed at the time of phacoemulsification. Recalling the techniques available to the surgeon for the performance of ECP in this situation, one should realize that there is no vitreous in the area that can be manipulated to create vitreoretinal traction and subsequent retinal break formation and detachment. Compare this with the 2% to 5% incidence of this problem after trabeculectomy and the 1% to 3% occurrence rate following phacoemulsification alone. The treatment would be the same as under more typical circumstances, usually scleral buckling. This would result in approximately 80% of the patients experiencing retinal reattachment with a single surgery. With subsequent interventions 90% reattachment rates may be achieved. Ultimately, about 10% of those treated in this manner would fail and therefore experience blindness in the eye. Most of these patients would have proliferative vitreoretinopathy as a consequence of their rhegmatogenous detachment and would require extensive vitreous and retinal surgery to achieve reattachment. Visual potential in these patients as a group is quite poor.

Crystalline lens or intraocular lens dislocation is another theoretical complication of ECP, especially when one considers the considerable physical stresses placed on the zonules and capsule by their posterior displacement with viscoelastic, instrumentation in their vicinity, and laser application at the attachment of the zonules to the ciliary body. Amazingly, not a single case of this potential problem

has been reported. Probably it is just a matter of time before this serious condition evolves after an ECP; however, from a statistical point of view, its incidence would seem to be less than a fraction of 1%. Treatment of dislocated crystalline lens will be discussed in detail later, but briefly, the patient must undergo pars plana vitrectomy and phacofragmentation to rectify the situation. The prognosis for these patients, even after extensive surgery, is quite good. Management of dislocated intraocular lens is more controversial. If the implant is not causing much of a visual disturbance and is not creating a retinal problem such as hemorrhage, tear formation, or CME, then it may be left in the posterior segment and another lens implanted. At other times, it is best to perform a pars plana vitrectomy and reposition the lens implant with or without sutures, or to remove the IOL altogether from an anterior or posterior segment approach and replace it with another implant. Again, most of these patients do well despite numerous surgical interventions. None of this would have much of an effect on the IOP outcome of ECP.

Hypotony and Phthisis

Hypotony and phthisis are among the most devastating outcomes that the patient and surgeon can experience. In the instance of outflow surgery, issues related to "overfiltration," wound leak, conjunctival hole and leak, choroidal effusion, and others may result in a hypotonous state that can be addressed in some way. The hypotony or phthisis following TSCPC or cyclocryotherapy is more ominous. Assuming that the low pressure is not being transiently created by the treatment's induction of inflammation, temporary ciliary body "shutdown," or choroidal effusion, not much can be done to reverse the situation.

These problems are rarely associated with ECP but may present under a few conditions. Eyes affected by neovascular glaucoma, pediatric forms of glaucoma, or that are aphakic and vitrectomized are at risk and should be managed accordingly. If hypotony develops, there are only a few, not very effective, choices remaining. First, it is important to ensure that one of the more reversible causes of this problem is not active. Intraocular inflammation should be aggressively managed with topical and systemic steroids, as previously discussed. Choroidal effusions or hemorrhage should be drained. If it is remotely possible to inadvertently create a cyclodialysis cleft during previous surgery, then this entity should be sought. Treatment consists of photocoagulation to the cleft (either endoscopically or by slit-lamp delivery), cryotherapy, or suturing. Cleft closure does not ensure success. Cyclitic membranes may develop post treatment or as a consequence of an underlying condition that results in ciliary body detachment, such as severe diabetic retinopathy or silicone oil in the eye. This may be impossible to detect clinically but may be easily ascertained endoscopically. Surgical excision of the contracting membrane

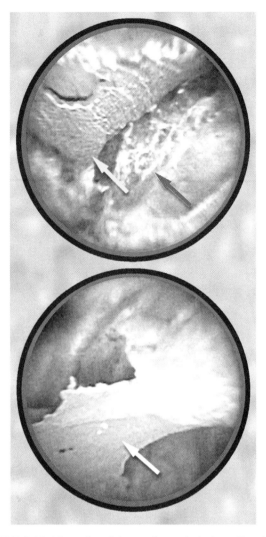

FIGURE 6-14. View of cyclitic membrane inducing ciliary body detachment requiring excision for reattachment. Overall prognosis is poor. The (orange arrow) indicates the membrane on the peripheral retina and pars plana. The (yellow arrow) shows the connection to the ciliary body with associated detachment. The membrane indicated by the white arrow is detaching the ciliary body.

may result in reattachment of the ciliary body allowing the production of aqueous to ensue (Fig. 6-14). If it is ultimately determined that the ciliary body is nonfunctional and there are no underlying problems that might be addressed to reverse the situation, the prognosis for the eye is exceedingly poor. Even though it may seem that the entities listed in Table 6-6 might offer some hope for potential resolution, usually it is clear that none of these factors are important and that, basically, low IOP indicates that the ciliary body is "dead."

As an act of desperation, the occasional patient with nonfunctional ciliary body may undergo vitrectomy and silicone oil injection, with complete filling of the vitreous. Usually the presence of silicone oil is associated with low IOP. It might seem, therefore, that this approach would not

TABLE 6-6. CAUSES OF HYPOTONY AND PHTHISIS

Potentially Repairable
- Wound leak
- Serous choroidal effusion
- Hemorrhagic choroidal effusion
- Anterior or posterior uveitis
- Cyclodialysis cleft
- Cyclitic membrane with ciliary body detachment

Irreparable
- Dead ciliary body

be helpful, and often it is not. However, some patients may maintain a low IOP but not develop phthisis or at least the cosmetic appearance of this problem by using this approach. Even when this approach is "successful," the vision is poor to nonexistent in these eyes and the major reason to proceed is mostly to maintain adequate cosmesis.

PATIENT SELECTION

It should be clear that the technical difficulty of performing ECP is based not on the severity or mechanisms of glaucoma but rather on the anatomic status of the eye. There are three primary concerns. The most important of these is lens status. Second is whether the surgeon will use an anterior or a posterior segment approach. The final consideration is presence or absence of vitreous in the "work area." Based on these features, a hierarchy can be established for patient selection, which is important for the novice endoscopist.

Certainly, the most straightforward situation is that in which cataract surgery is combined with ECP. The eye is already open with a relatively large incision and the surgeon has several choices of when, along the way, ECP may be performed. The degree of safety is high because most of these eyes are fairly healthy, there is usually no vitreous in the treatment zone, and the space between iris and capsule can be widely expanded. This is fortunate because most ECP procedures have been performed in combination with phacoemulsification.

Next on the list would be eyes with posterior chamber lens implants using an anterior approach. In this situation, the working area can be easily expanded and usually there are no vitreous considerations or other anatomic impediments. The risks are slightly greater in this situation because the surgeon must avoid trauma to the IOL and its capsular support, be cautious if there is any preexisting instability of the lens, and avoid overinflation of the posterior iris region with viscoelastic in the presence of a capsulotomy to prevent vitreous extrusion.

Following this situation, eyes with previous vitrectomy that are pseudophakic are quite simple to treat from a pars plana incision. No viscoelastic is required and there are often no physical impediment to accessing the ciliary processes. The degree of difficulty is slightly increased because a posterior segment entry site is used and because at times ECP must be combined with scleral depression. These two features are quite easily mastered by most surgeons. Finally, infusion may be required to maintain IOP intraoperatively.

Aphakic eyes that have previously undergone vitrectomy are actually quite simple to manage, although sometimes scleral depression may be required. It is easier to access the ciliary processes from a pars plana incision than from the anterior segment. Nevertheless, the anterior approach is still relatively simple and easily learned. Curved endoscopes are expeditious in this situation. It is important to recall that there is an increased risk for developing choroidal hemorrhage, and so control of hypertension and correction of any coagulopathy should be effected preoperatively to minimize the potential for this problem to evolve. It is also desirable to prevent intraoperative hypotony from developing and so infusion may be required.

Of slightly greater technical difficulty is the anterior chamber pseudophakic eye with previous vitrectomy approached from the anterior segment. Residual lens material opacified capsule, and other physical impediments may demand multiple incisions and the use of scleral depression. Infusion may be required to maintain a satisfactory intraoperative IOP. If vitreous in the anterior chamber is present, then it must be removed either by an anterior or pars plana approach, adding somewhat to the difficulty of the procedure. Also, by removing the vitreous, infusion may be required during ECP, again increasing the degree of difficulty associated with this situation.

Finally, the most difficult eyes in which to perform ECP are those that are phakic, for reasons that were discussed previously. The degree of difficulty is increased if vitrectomy is required in order to adequately displace the lens to permit access to the ciliary processes.

It is important for the novice endoscopist to be aware of these issues to ensure proper patient selection and enhance the potential for a successful experience. Table 6-7 lists these permutations according to their degree of difficulty. Although this list may appear to be daunting, most patients who have undergone ECP fall into the first or second group. Moreover, once the surgeon has become skillful with endoscope manipulation and laser delivery, none of these situations is particularly difficult to manage.

Finally, review of these permutations makes it clear that if surgery is to proceed expeditiously, an infusion line and vitrector should be available. Still, it would be highly unlikely to require these in combined phacoemulsification and ECP and with an anterior approach in the pseudophakic eye, which is by far the most common scenario under which ECP is performed.

REOPERATION

One of the most common experiences for the novice following execution of an ECP is eliciting an inadequate IOP-lowering effect. One phenomenon that will become clear to the surgeon in short order is that, excepting ischemic eyes, extensive ECP must be performed to achieve any lasting and significant IOP decline. Entry level treatment is 180 degrees, and many eyes require 360-degree applications. When initially using ECP, many surgeons treat "lightly," which is a satisfactory approach until some experience and confidence has been gained. On the other hand, the surgeon must plainly understand that light treatment will not induce a dramatic result.

Even when first treating eyes for 270 to 360 degrees, many do not experience the outcome that was hoped for. One might wonder how 360-degree treatment can result in little effect. The answer is that a good deal of viable functioning ciliary epithelium may remain after treatment. It seems that the surgeon's first group of patients treated by, for example, 270 degrees of ECP do not exhibit the same IOP response that the same 270-degree ECP elicits from the next group. As with any other surgical procedure, patience during the initial learning and practice phase will be rewarded.

TABLE 6-7. ENDOSCOPIC CYCLOPHOTOCOAGULATION: DEGREE OF DIFFICULTY OF SURGICAL EXECUTION

Rank	Lens Status	Approach	Vitreous	Difficulty
1	Combined procedure	Anterior	With/without previous vitrectomy	Minimal
2	PC IOL	Anterior	With/without previous vitrectomy	Minimal
3	PC IOL	Pars plana	Previous vitrectomy	Minimal
4	AC IOL	Pars plana	Previous vitrectomy	Minimal–moderate
5	Aphakic	Pars plana	Previous vitrectomy	Minimal (caution)
6	AC IOL	Anterior	Previous vitrectomy	Minimal–moderate
7	Aphakic	Anterior	Previous vitrectomy	Minimal–moderate (caution)
8	Aphakic	Pars plana	Needs vitrectomy	Moderate
9	AC IOL	Anterior	Needs vitrectomy	Moderate
10	Phakic	Anterior	No vitrectomy	Moderate–difficult
11	Phakic	Anterior	Needs vitrectomy	Difficult

PC, posterior chamber; AC, anterior chamber; IOL, intraocular lens.

TABLE 6-8. FREQUENCY OF ENDOSCOPIC CYCLOPHOTOCOAGULATION REOPERATIONS BY MECHANISM OF GLAUCOMA IN ONE LARGE SERIES[a]

Type	No. of Eyes	No. of Reoperations
Neovascular	143	12 (8%)
Aphakic and pseudophakic	108	19 (17.6%)
Phakic POAGI	56	7 (12.4%)
Combined phaco/IOL/ECP	20	3 (15%)
Congenital	18	7 (34.4%)
ROP	2	0 (0)
Total	347	48 (13.8%)

[a]With the exception of congenital glaucomas, the need for further surgery is about the same across these glaucoma mechanisms. POAGI, primary open-angle glaucoma; Phaco, phacoemulsification; IOL, intraocular lens; ECP, endoscopic cyclophotocoagulation; ROP, retinopathy of prematurity.
From Uram M. Endoscopic cyclophotocoagulation in glaucoma management: indications, results, and complications. *Ophthal Pract* 1995;13:173–185.

Ophthalmic endoscopy combined with fluorescein angiography has provided some insight into this phenomenon. Although the details will be discussed later, it has been clearly demonstrated in eyes that have failed ECP and TSCPC, for that matter, that there are missed portions of what was initially thought to be adequately treated processes. These areas continue to produce aqueous, contributing to treatment failure.

If one of the typical failure curves seems to be evolving, repetition of ECP should be considered. The surgeon must photocoagulate what ultimately proves to be enough ciliary epithelium to achieve a successful outcome (Table 6-8).

One of the advantages of ECP is that most failures are evident during the first 8 weeks post treatment and, if the patient has been informed and prepared for this possibility, then it is usually not very difficult for him or her to understand why another operation might be needed "so soon." From a technical viewpoint, there are two approaches that may be considered. One is to access the same ciliary processes that were already treated. Photocoagulated processes appear to be shrunken and white. Untreated processes are clearly evident. Untreated portions of an individual process appear to be brown, whereas the treated portions appear to be white and shrunken (Fig. 6-15). Fluorescein angiography clearly demonstrates treated versus untreated portions of individual processes. Once the untreated portions are identified, they can be lasered. The tissue will whiten and shrink. If a considerable amount of viable ciliary process tissue is photocoagulated in the previous treatment area, perhaps a small amount of a new area can be lasered as well, or the surgeon may elect not to proceed any further.

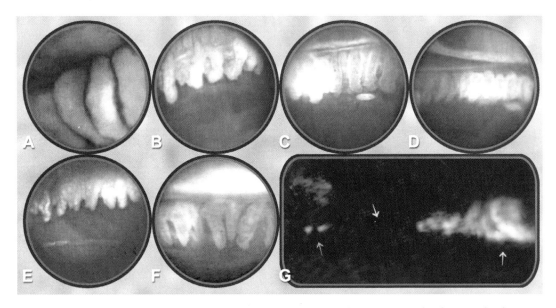

FIGURE 6-15. Failure to control intraocular pressure may be related to incompletely treated individual ciliary processes or simply because the extent of endoscopic cyclophotocoagulation (ECP) along the ciliary ring was inadequate. **A,B:** Partially treated ciliary processes. **C–F:** Border of white treated processes and brown untreated ones. **G:** Endoscopic fluorescein angiogram of ciliary body. The yellow arrow indicates completely treated processes; the orange arrow, partially treated processes; and the blue arrow, untreated processes. The green hyperfluorescent zones represent the portions that have not been affected by ECP.

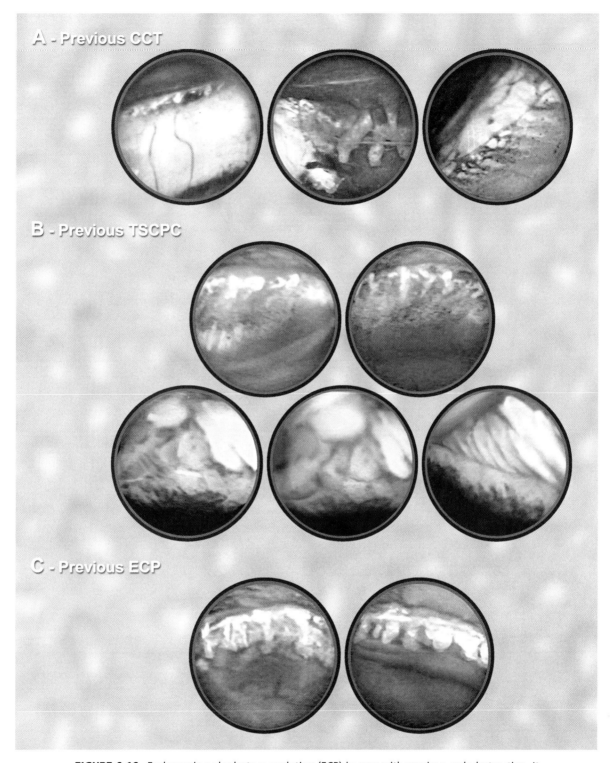

FIGURE 6-16. Endoscopic cyclophotocoagulation (ECP) in eyes with previous cyclodestruction. It is straightforward to identify treated and untreated zones in order to determine the extent of previous application. **A:** Previous cyclocryotherapy. There is massive destruction of the ciliary processes and pars plana. **B:** Previous transscleral cyclophotocoagulation (TSCPC). The processes have been overtreated, and the adjacent non-aqueous-producing tissue has also been incorporated into the treatment zone. **C:** Previous ECP. The ciliary processes are white and shrunken in appearance. The adjacent pars plana and iris are clearly not incorporated into the treatment zone.

TABLE 6-9. SUMMARY OF HISTORICAL TREATMENT "SUCCESS" RATES BY PROCEDURE AND GLAUCOMA MECHANISM

Procedure	Glaucoma Mechanism (%)							
	OAG	OAG with Failed Surgery	CAGC	CAGC with Failed Surgery	NVG	Pediatric Glaucoma	Phaco and Uncontrolled Glaucoma Surgery	Phaco and Controlled Glaucoma Surgery
Trabeculectomy	90	50	50	30	NA	<50	70	NA
Tube	NA	50–70	50–70	50–70	50–70	<50	NA	NA
TSCPC	NA	NA	30–50	30–50	30–50	<50	NA	NA
ECP	90	90	90	90	90	>50	90	>90

OAG, open-angle glaucoma; CAGC, chronic angle-closure glaucoma; NVG, neovascular glaucoma; Phaco, phacoemulsification; TSCPC, transscleral cyclophotocoagulation; ECP, endoscopic cyclophotocoagulation.

On the other hand, if little ciliary process tissue was missed initially, then a more extreme zone of ECP must be created at the surgeon's discretion, up to 360 degrees. How much to treat depends on the patient's response to initial therapy. As an example, 180 degrees of ECP performed in a pseudophakic, glaucoma eye would be unlikely to achieve an adequate IOP effect. Let us say that the IOP barely changed from baseline. Subsequent endoscopic inspection reveals that only about 120 degrees, or 4 clock hours, of ciliary process tissue was actually affected. This eye would require completion of the untreated areas from the first surgery and at least an additional 90 degrees, or 3 clock hours, more for a total of 270 degrees in order to approach a satisfactory outcome.

Another scenario might be that a similar eye had 300 degrees of initial ECP with modest IOP response postoperatively. Endoscopic evaluation at reoperation indicates numerous missed portions of ciliary process tissue. In this instance, it may be effective to complete the initial 300-degree treatment and not expand the ECP zone.

A more puzzling situation is that in which an experienced ECP surgeon treats 360 degrees completely on two occasions and still the IOP does not respond in a satisfactory manner. In this scenario, a scatter photocoagulation treatment to the pars plana region for 180 to 360 degrees often is helpful.

These same basic concepts hold true for eyes that have had previous laser TSCPC or cyclocryotherapy. The previously affected areas are fairly straightforward to identify, and missed or untreated portions of the ciliary process may be addressed (Fig. 6-16, Table 6-9 and Table 6-10).

The following chapters will address some specific mechanisms of glaucoma and the role that ECP might have in their management.

TABLE 6-10. COMPARISON OF INFLOW PROCEDURE OUTCOMES

Inflow Procedure	Complications (%)				
	Visual Loss	Pain	Inflammation	Phthisis	Success Rate
CCT	50	+	+	30	50
TSCPC (diode or Nd:YAG)	40	+	+	10	50–70
ECP	–	–	–	–	90

CCT, cyclocryotherapy ; TSCPC, transscleral cyclophotocoagulation; ECP, endoscopic cyclophotocoagulation.

7

PRACTICING ENDOSCOPIC CYCLOPHOTOCOAGULATION

One of the interesting features of endoscopic cyclophotoco-agulation (ECP) is that the surgeon can acquire a good deal of facility by practicing in an animal eye. Pig eyes seem to be readily available and inexpensive. Unlike other practice situations, a bare minimum of equipment is required. Aside from the laser and endoscopy components, the only essential materials are some nonsterile gloves, 4 × 4 inch gauze pads for endoscope wiping, any blade, and some sodium hyahironale viscoelastic (which can be expired). Pig eyes require a lot of viscoelastic, so at least several syringes will be necessary. It is best to obtain several eyes per surgeon, just in case the eyes are not in good condition.

GETTING STARTED

First, set up the laser and endoscopy componentry. If using an integrated system, the light intensity may be controlled by the same foot switch as the laser. It is best to be seated and to adjust the placement of the video monitor for most comfortable viewing. Hold the endoscope in your hand and establish proper image rotation. Then practice raising and lowering the light with the foot switch. This will become important in practicing ECP. The laser parameters are set typically at 200 to 500 mW of power on continuous wave. When you are comfortable and in control of the image and illumination, and laser parameters have been established, you can begin practicing.

ANTERIOR APPROACH

Hold the pig eye wrapped in a 4 × 4 gauze in one hand, and make a very generous incision in the peripheral cornea with

the other hand. Pig eye Descemet membrane is very tough, so make sure that the blade enters the anterior chamber. This incision should be at least 2 mm in length, not just externally but internally as well. Otherwise the wound will be "too tight" and the laser endoscope might be damaged on insertion. Once the incision is fashioned, pass the needle of the viscoelastic syringe across the anterior chamber and place it beneath the iris. Inject the viscoelastic. You should see the iris move forward, the pupil dilate, and the lens displace posteriorly. Use a lot of viscoelastic; a wide-open working area will make it easier to learn. Also recall that this situation will simulate ECP in the phakic eye, the most difficult of paradigms. Usually, 1 to 2 mL is needed. When adequate inflation of the working space has been achieved, remove the viscoelastic needle and insert the endoscope.

The first view is of the anterior chamber, a ballooned iris, ciliary processes, and lens (Fig. 7-1). Direct the aiming beam toward the ciliary processes. When about 5 mm from the target, you can begin laser application. Three or four ciliary processes are usually in the field of view at this time. If the process turns white and shrinks in a fraction of a second, decrease the laser power setting or move further away from the target. It is best to have the reaction develop over a few seconds. In that way, you will gain some experience in controlling the tissue response to laser delivery. One of the tissue treatment goals is to laser the entire length of each ciliary process. This may not be possible in the pig eye because the processes are much longer than in the human eye and extend well posteriorly. Apply the laser to what can be seen from this approach. Move around the ciliary ring, completing one process at a time.

The next maneuver is to practice manipulating the laser power density components (power, duration, and probe

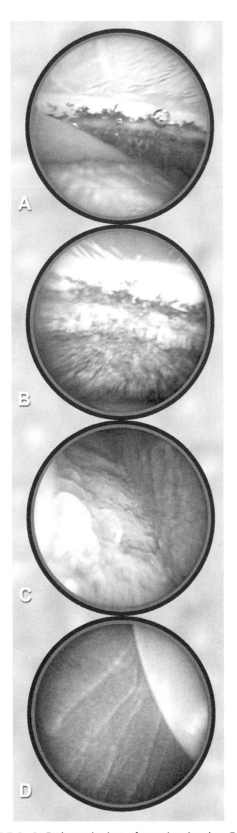

FIGURE 7-1. **A:** Endoscopic view of anterior chamber, **B:** iris, **C:** inflated sulcus, and **D:** "heads" of the ciliary processes.

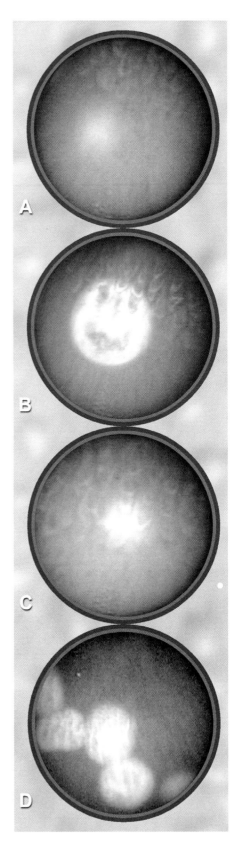

FIGURE 7-2. Endoscopic view of laser lesions created by varying laser power, duration, and distance from the target tissue.

distance) to create variable-intensity lesions: hot spots, barely visible spots, and rapidly and slowly evolving spots (Fig. 7-2). Again, the purpose of this experience is to learn how to control the tissue effect by manipulating these variables.

Once you have achieved some facility, practice the painting technique by moving the laser endoscope laterally, from ciliary process to ciliary process, while continuing to fire the laser. At first you might observe that the tissue effect varies as the endoscope is maneuvered. This is because the ciliary processes are in a circle, and the distance of the target from the tip of the instrument changes around the circumference. To create a smoother pattern, try subtle adjustments to the working distance.

In a brief time, most surgeons can become quite comfortable with these maneuvers and will be prepared to execute treatment in human eyes.

POSTERIOR APPROACH

Strictly speaking, it is not necessary for most anterior segment surgeons to practice the posterior approach, but it can be interesting and may help to hone some newly acquired skills.

To begin, find an area about one third the distance from the limbus to the optic nerve. The pig pars plana is very wide compared with that in humans. Find an area without overlying conjunctiva, or remove it by scraping with the blade. Again, make a generous incision internally and externally. If the eye is soft, it can be squeezed a bit during the incision to offer more resistance. It is not a problem if vitreous extrudes; finding the incision sites becomes easier.

When first inserting the probe, do not advance it very far. Rather, tip it anteriorly. The view will be slightly hazy because vitreous is present and diffuses the illumination of the endoscope. If the incision was made in a sufficiently posterior position, anteriorly directed viewing will reveal the spherical nature of the lens, ciliary ring, posterior aspect of the iris, and ambient light entering through the pupil.

Next, tip the endoscope in a posterior direction to view the retina, its vessels, and the optic nerve (Fig. 7-3). Advance the endoscope toward the optic nerve, and then follow one of the vessels from posterior to anterior until the retinal insertion is reached. The pig eye has a vessel that runs circumferentially around this border (Fig. 7-4). Continue to tip the probe anteriorly and view the pars plana and ciliary processes. It may be observed that the pig eye processes are quite long and extend well behind the lens. If the illumination is proper, one can see fine with the attachment between the edge of the lens and the ciliary body. These are the zonules (Fig. 7-5).

You can practice cyclophotocoagulation from this vantage point in a fashion similar to the anterior segment approach.

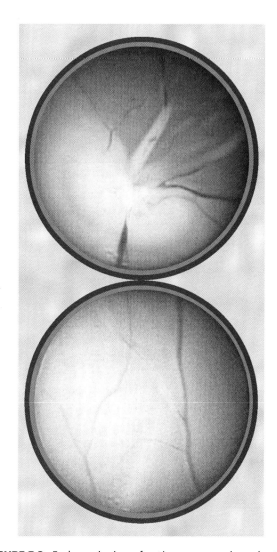

FIGURE 7-3. Endoscopic view of optic nerve, vessels, and retina.

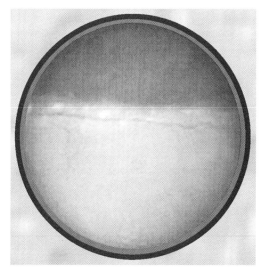

FIGURE 7-4. Endoscopic view of retinal insertion at pars plana.

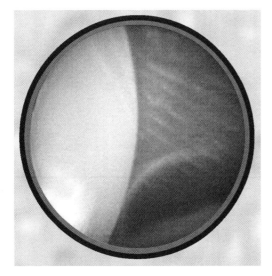

FIGURE 7-5. Endoscopic view of lens and zonules.

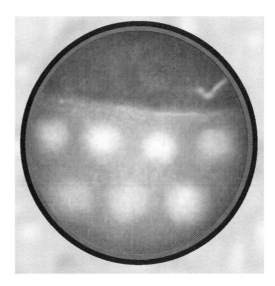

FIGURE 7-6. Endoscopic view of laser applications to the peripheral retina.

This would also be a good opportunity to try peripheral retinal photocoagulation. The laser parameter settings need to be changed. Start with 810-nm diode laser power at 500 to 700 mW and decrease the duration from continuous wave to 0.2 or 0.3 second. Adjust aiming beam intensity accordingly. Next, apply rows of laser burns in a circumferential or radial fashion (Fig. 7-6). Anterior segment surgeons may at first feel that this still would not be helpful in their practice, and perhaps that assertion is correct. How-

ever, if they will be treating eyes with schemia-driven glaucoma, a situation in which completing peripheral retinal ablation may present itself at the time of ECP, it would then be beneficial to the eye to execute this maneuver.

One final exercise illustrates the concept of "overtreatment" and is instructive regarding the upper limits of the laser power density equation. Raise the laser power from 700 to 1,000 mW and reset the duration to continuous wave. Advance the tip of the endoscope to a distance a few

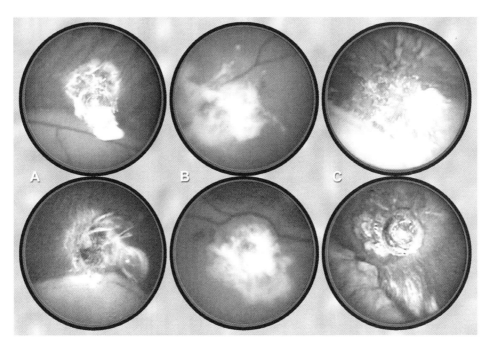

FIGURE 7-7. A: Endoscopic view of exploded ciliary process. **B:** Retina. **C:** Iris.

millimeters from the ciliary processes (not too close; this will damage the instrument). Fire the laser and observe a rapidly evolving burn. Continue to apply the laser energy, and suddenly a "pop" will be heard and felt. This is a tissue explosion. Observe the results, as it will become clear why transscleral cyclophotocoagulation (TSCPC) can be so damaging and associated with an array of severe complications whereas ECP is not. Next, direct the endoscope posteriorly and try to create the same effects with the retina as the target tissue (you may have to raise the laser power) (Fig. 7-7). This will serve to illustrate that tissue explosions do not necessarily indicate that the ciliary process was ablated, albeit in an overly intensive manner, but rather that any intraocular tissue treated in such a way can produce the same effect. Again, TSCPC tissue explosions incite compli-

cations by incorporating nonciliary process tissue in the treatment zone.

During the course of the practice session, or when in the operating room, it is important to frequently wipe the tip of the endoscope with dry gauze or other material to maintain image clarity and prevent instrument damage. If the view is hazy from blood or debris, it should be removed from the tip and cleaned prior to laser application. Otherwise this film may attenuate laser delivery and also may serve as a heat sink, "baking" the material onto the endoscope tip and ruining the instrument.

With a little bit of practice in these eyes, the surgeon can become fairly adept at intraocular endoscope manipulation and photocoagulation. Armed with this ability, the management of glaucoma in humans can be addressed.

8

ENDOSCOPIC CYCLOPHOTOCOAGULATION FOR OPEN-ANGLE GLAUCOMA

Now that an understanding of the technology behind endoscopic cyclophotocoagulation (ECP) and its technical application in various anatomic scenarios has been gained, attention should be directed to its use in specific clinical situations. One way to approach this is to evaluate ECP results and complications when applied to specific glaucoma mechanisms. These discussions are not offered as an in-depth analysis of glaucoma pathogenetic features and treatment outcomes analysis but rather to convey the experience attained to date using this approach to glaucoma therapy.

One of the most commonly encountered statistical treatments of outcome data in this context is the Kaplan-Meier survival curve. Essentially, it measures the amount of time it takes for a specific event to occur. In terms of glaucoma surgery, "survival" refers to the length of time the surgical procedure (e.g., ECP or trabeculectomy) will continue to function (survive). This analysis can overcome some of the difficulties encountered in the "real world" by including subjects in a study who may not completely cooperate with its design, such as being lost to follow-up before completion. The analysis is graphically displayed in a manner that looks somewhat like a staircase. The vertical axis of the graph represents the percentage "surviving," the maximum being 1.0 (100%) and the minimum being 0.0 (0%). The horizontal axis represents time from treatment.

It is also possible to compare the Kaplan-Meier survival curves of one or more treatment modalities with others. The distinction between methods represented in this manner is readily apparent (Fig. 8-1).

Clearly, open-angle glaucoma is the most common glaucoma mechanism encountered by ophthalmologists. For the purposes of this discussion, all of the ECP patients were phakic. Those eyes that were pseudophakic or aphakic or that had previously failed filtration surgery are discussed elsewhere because these features are associated with a worse prognosis under any treatment scenario. To mix them with cases of phakic open-angle glaucoma in previously unoperated eyes would distort the data and the inferences that may be derived from them.

When phakic open-angle glaucoma is uncontrolled, it is typically managed with filtration surgery (with or without antimetabolites), which, as an initial procedure, has a high degree of success. Although there is some debate as to the optimal timing for surgical intervention and despite a host of perioperative and long-term problems that have been discussed, the underlying concept and its variations have been a standard of ophthalmic surgery for many years. Long-term outcome data of trabeculectomy in open-angle glaucoma reveals variable success. However, most studies indicate that 40% to 70% of these patients will maintain good IOP control over the 5- to 10-year range. Progressive visual loss is, however, another matter. Despite controlled intraocular pressure (IOP), progressive visual loss over a 5- to 10-year period is between 30% and 60%. Cataract development subsequent to trabeculectomy occurs in 20% to 40% of eyes treated. Despite the apparent widespread acceptance of filtration surgery, inquiry among most ophthalmologists would indicate a strong disinclination to perform this procedure under any circumstances. This attitude reflects not so much on this straightforward surgical technique itself or on its ultimate efficacy, but rather on the experience that

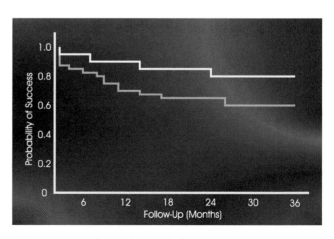

FIGURE 8-1. Kaplan-Meier survival curve comparing two treatment modalities.

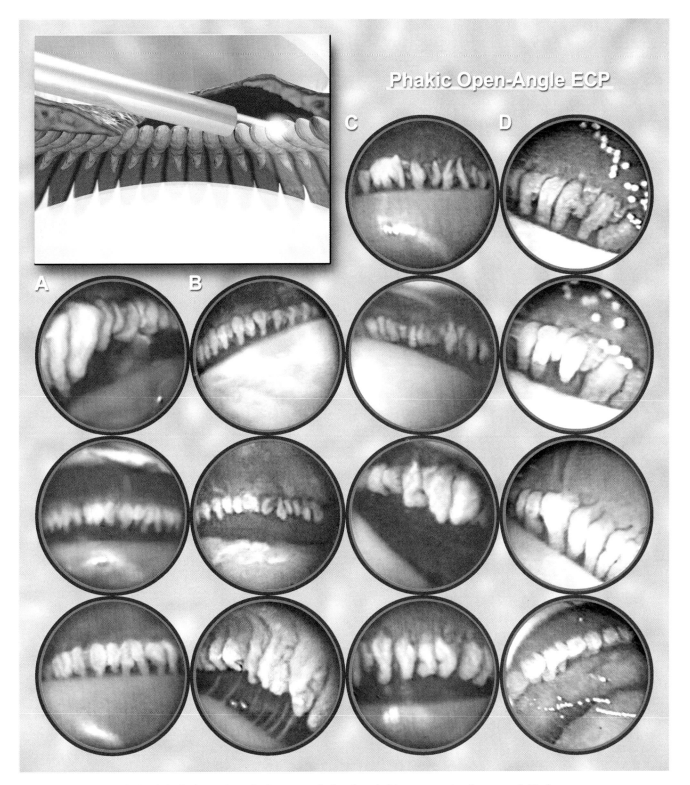

FIGURE 8-2. Endoscopic cyclophotocoagulation for phakic open-angle glaucoma. **A–D:** Course of treatment is four phakic eyes

the "work" actually begins after the operation, when intensive management addressing both minor and major complications seems to be the rule. Variable outcomes despite best efforts even in the best-scenario open-angle glaucoma further discourage many ophthalmologists from using this procedure.

As previously discussed, issues such as mechanism of glaucoma, angle status, number of previous surgeries and failures, status of the conjunctiva, and a host of other parameters may certainly increase the difficulty of performing filtration surgery and thereby limit its potential for a successful outcome. On the other hand, the most significant technical challenge for ECP relates to the status of the lens and the approach selected by the surgeon. The most difficult situation to manage is the phakic eye because there is only one treatment method paradigm (Fig. 8-2). This situation demands that the surgeon have the skill to displace the lens well posteriorly and the iris anteriorly, creating a generous zone within which the endoscope must be manipulated. The situation further requires that the surgeon be facile in maneuvering the endoscope while avoiding lens contact. These issues are far less important in the other lens/vitreous approach scenarios for accessing the ciliary body, as previously discussed. In addition, otherwise "healthy" open-angle glaucoma eyes most often require 270 to 360 degrees of ECP (usually requiring at least two incisions) to achieve any therapeutic effect. Somewhat paradoxically, then, eyes that have undergone many interventions and demonstrate marked anatomic abnormalities and have a poor prognosis with filtration surgery are actually relatively simple to treat with ECP while the anatomically "correct" open-angle glaucoma clear lens eye, with the best prognosis from filtration surgery, is the most demanding situation when using ECP.

In the initial report of ECP in phakic open-angle glaucoma management (1), 56 eyes with mean preoperative IOP of 29.8 mm Hg were treated for 270 to 360 degrees. Postoperatively mean IOP decreased to 16 mm Hg, representing a 46.3% absolute decrease. The mean number of preoperative topical medication was 2.4 and the postoperative was 1.1. Systemic carbonic anhydrase inhibitor usage diminished from 73.2% to 16.1% by the final postoperative visit. None of the patients demonstrated perioperative visual field loss, although this became evident in 8.9% when evaluated 1 year post treatment

A total of 12.4% of patients underwent a second ECP. Overall, 88% achieved successful IOP control, defined as less than or equal to 22 mm Hg. Lens dislocation, cystoid macular edema, phthisis, or endophthalmitis did not evolve. None of the patients demonstrated cataract formation immediately following surgery, although 14.3% developed this complication by the last follow-up visit. In this study, follow-up ranged from 6 to 33 months with a mean of 21 months. It was noted that a minimum of postoperative care was required. The study was retrospective in nature with a relatively large study group and medium-term follow-up.

In another study (2), 16 eyes with open-angle glaucoma that failed maximum medical therapy and surgery were treated with ECP. The mean IOP was 21.3 mm Hg preoperatively and 15.6 mm Hg postoperatively ($p = 0.0001$), with 90% achieving "successful" control with a mean follow-up of 13 months. No devastating complications evolved. These outcomes mirror the experience reported by others.

One of the arguments that can be made about much of the glaucoma literature is that most reports are uncontrolled, retrospective, and noncomparative in nature, incorporating small study groups with short-term follow-up. It is actually quite difficult to do otherwise. A comparative randomized trial of ECP versus trabeculectomy in the management of phakic open-angle glaucoma is currently under way (3). Until its completion, it is only possible to contrast ECP with the historical results of trabeculectomy (Table 8-1).

Nevertheless, ECP compared favorably with filtration surgery in the management of phakic open-angle glaucoma. This set of circumstances represents the best prognosis group

TABLE 8-1. COMPARISON OF HISTORICAL TRABECULECTOMY AND ENDOSCOPIC CYCLOPHOTOCOAGULATION OUTCOMES (%)

Procedure	Decrease in IOP	IOP Successfully Controlled		Intensity of Postop Care	Visual Field Loss			Cataract	Devastating Complication	Peculiarities
		2 yr	5 yr		Periop	1 yr	5 yr			
Trabeculectomy	50	80	30–60	Extreme	Small	10	30–60	20–40	5–10	1% risk per year of endophthalmitis
ECP	40	90	80	Minimal	0	10	30	20–30	0	Difficult to obtain a low IOP in 5–10 mm Hg range

IOP, intraocular pressure; ECP, endoscopic cyclophotocoagulation.

for filtration surgery but is perhaps the most difficult for ECP. Cataract formation was the most significant postoperative complication of ECP that one might argue would represent a limitation to its use, particularly in younger patients, with a clear lens preoperatively. On the other hand, it should be recalled that there is a greater than 20% risk of cataract development in phakic trabeculectomy, that postoperative management is more intensive with trabeculectomy, and that there are inherent long-term risks with filtration surgery (e.g., a 1% per year incidence of endophthalmitis) that do not apply to ECP.

Finally, consider that there has never been a reported case of phthisis, hypotony, or other devastating outcome in this mechanism of glaucoma. The theoretical objection to managing this problem with an inflow-reducing technique is moot.

REFERENCES

1. Uram M. Endoscopic cyclophotocoagulation in glaucoma management. *Current Opinion in Ophthalmology* 1995;11:19–29.
2. Chen J, Cohn RA, Lin SC, et al. Endoscopic photocoagulation of the ciliary body for treatment of refractory glaucomas. *Ophthalmol* 1997;124:787–796.
3. ECP Study Group. In progress. Unpublished data.

9

ENDOSCOPIC CYCLOPHOTOCOAGULATION FOR APHAKIC AND PSEUDOPHAKIC GLAUCOMA

Aphakia and pseudophakia are factors that present adversity to potential treatment options when uncontrolled glaucoma is present. The angle may be open or there may be nonvascularized synechial angle closure, or a combination of both. The first-line surgical treatment option that one might consider is trabeculectomy. Unfortunately, this fairly common situation of uncontrolled glaucoma in the aphakic or pseudophakic eye does not respond as well to filtration surgery as the phakic open-angle glaucoma eye. This is particularly true in aphakic patients undergoing trabeculectomy, with about 30% exhibiting failure within the first 3 years, necessitating further surgery. The situation is compounded by previous filtration failure. In this scenario, less than 50% of treated eyes would be expected to achieve even short-term success, yet the potential for complications increases substantially.

One might theorize that adding antimetabolites to the treatment plan would enhance the potential for success; however, it appears that this is not the case. It has been clearly demonstrated that fluorouracil and mitomycin-C fail to increase the efficacy of this approach to glaucoma management while increasing some of the more serious risks of the procedure.

It is also important to recall that the highest risk group for the development of immediate and delayed onset hemorrhagic choroidal effusion is the aphakic vitrectomized eye.

As an alternative, one might consider tube implantation. This method can be somewhat more successful in controlling glaucoma, typically achieving controlled intraocular pressure (IOP) in 50% to 70% of treated eyes. However, the involved technique, postoperative management, and potential for significant complications make this a less attractive option.

Transscleral cyclophotocoagulation (TSCPC) can effect adequate IOP control in the 50% to 70% range, albeit after multiple procedures, but its utility is limited because of the brutality of the technique and its potential for inducing visual loss and other severe complications. This approach is certainly not indicated in a quiet eye with useful central acuity, which many of these eyes demonstrate.

Assessing the reality of the situation, there are many patients who fall into this category of uncontrolled glaucoma in the presence of aphakia or pseudophakia. Yet it would be fair to say that, despite the plethora of literature on the subject, most ophthalmologists do not regularly perform filtration surgery, trabeculectomy reoperations, tube implantations, or any type of cyclodestruction, and do not use antimetabolites.

On the other hand, it is technically simple to perform endoscopic cyclophotocoagulation (ECP) in the aphakic or pseudophakic eye, even in the presence of functioning or failed filters, tube implants, previous transscleral cyclodestruction, or other structural impediments by a limbal and/or pars plana approach (Figs. 9-1 to 9-6). Indeed, when the surgeon is first acquiring the skills to perform ECP these are the types of cases that are preferred due to their relative anatomic simplicity. Once facility with this technique has been acquired, the entire procedure may be performed within minutes, enhancing the potential for a quiet eye postoperatively. Most ophthalmologists who manage this form of glaucoma by ECP incorporate 270 to 360 degrees of ciliary process tissue in the treatment zone.

A number of reports have appeared addressing ECP in this situation. In one study (1), 108 aphakic and pseudophakic eyes were treated by 270 to 360 degrees of ECP from a limbal approach. Mean IOP was 34.6 mm Hg preoperatively and 15.2 mm Hg postoperatively, representing an absolute decrease of 56.1%. "Successful" IOP control was recorded in 89% of these eyes. Visual acuity and perioperative visual field loss did not evolve, but 8.3% demonstrated progressive visual field loss at least 1 year after treatment. Prior to ECP, 3.1 topical medications were used by these patients, and at the last

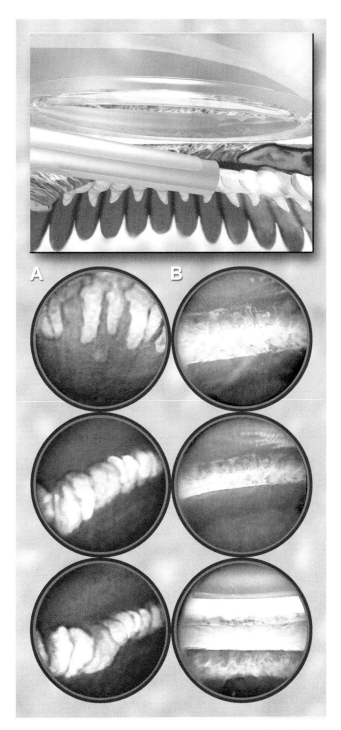

FIGURE 9-1. ECP: limbal approach in an anterior chamber pseudophakic eye. **A:** After a limbal incision is fashioned, the laser endoscope is directed beneath the anterior chamber intraocular lens (IOL) and iris, enabling imaging and cyclophotocoagulation. Some viscoelastic can be placed over the anterior surface of the IOL to protect the corneal endothelium. **B:** Images of six eyes treated in this fashion. There is considerable variability in the appearance of the ciliary processes. The bottom right photo is captured at the level of the pupil. From the top down, the structures visible in this photo are the anterior chamber IOL optic, anterior chamber and angle, pupillary edge, whitened ciliary processes, and pars plana.

postoperative visit a mean of 1.4 medications were used. Systemic carbonic anhydrase inhibitor (CAI) usage diminished from 78.7% to 10.2%. Cystoid macular edema (CME), either clinical or angiographic, was not observed. Reoperations were performed in 17.6% of these patients. Follow-up ranged from 6 to 50 months, with a mean of 35 months.

These findings were corroborated by another report of ECP for aphakic and pseudophakic glaucoma in which ten refractory patients who had not obtained success with maximal medical therapy and previous surgery underwent ECP (2). The mean IOP was 24.7 mm Hg preoperatively and 16.2 mm Hg ($p = 0.004$) postoperatively, with 90% achieving an IOP equal to or less than 21 mm Hg, yet there were no devastating complications.

Table 9-1 outlines some of the historical results obtained from various treatment methodologies when applied in the context of aphakic and pseudophakic glaucoma. It should be noted that data from pediatric populations have been excluded because they present a much more challenging situation despite being labeled with a similar pathogenetic mechanism.

A multicenter, community ophthalmologist–based, randomized, comparative study of ECP versus trabeculectomy in the management of CACG in aphakic and pseudophakic eyes with and without previously failed filter is currently under way (Table 9-2). In the subset that did not have previous glaucoma surgery, 25 patients treated by trabeculectomy were compared with 25 patients treated by ECP (270 to 360 degrees). Among the data collected so far, with a mean follow-up of 25 months (range, 8 to 41 months), 88% of ECP patients achieved IOP control (defined as 22 mm Hg or less) compared with 44% of the trabeculectomy treated group ($p = 0.05$). Visual acuity loss was recorded in 0% of the ECP group and in 12% of the trabeculectomy group ($p = 0.05$). Progressive visual field loss at last evaluation was 20% in the ECP group and 64% in the trabeculectomy patients ($p = 0.01$). Considering other parameters such as the development of CME or minor or devastating complications, there was no significant difference between the groups.

In a second subset of patients with aphakic or pseudophakic CACG with at least one previously failed filter, 25 patients were treated by repeating the trabeculectomy while 25 patients underwent ECP (270 to 360 degrees). Mean follow-up at this juncture has been 23 months (range, 6 to 47 months). Under these circumstances, 84% of ECP patients achieved IOP control compared to 24% of the trabeculectomy group ($p = 0.05$). Visual acuity loss was not observed in the ECP group but presented in 72% of the trabeculectomy group ($p = 0.01$). Progressive visual field loss evolved in 28% of the ECP patients and in 80% of the trabeculectomy patients ($p =$

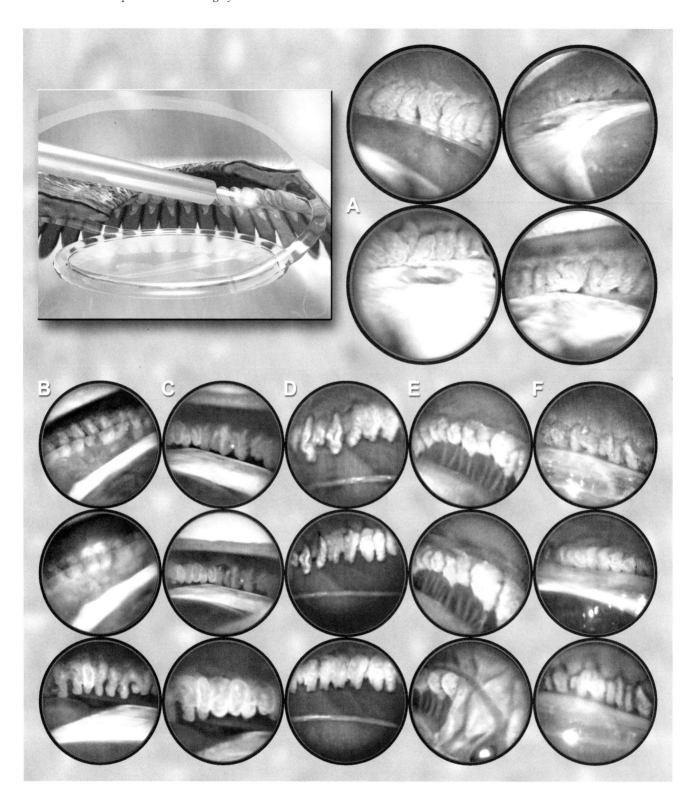

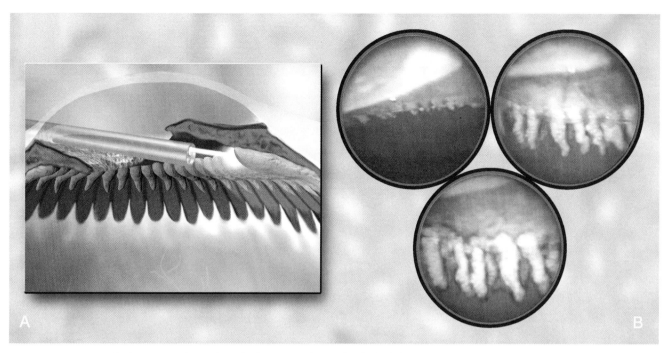

FIGURE 9-3. Endoscopic cyclophotocoagulation (ECP): limbal approach in the aphakic eye. **A:** After a limbal incision is created, the laser endoscope is inserted through the pupillary space to access the ciliary processes and laser application can begin. Recall that there may be residual lens material, opacified capsular remnants, membranes, and other impediments to accessing the ciliary processes, increasing the technical difficulty of ECP in this setting. It is also important to prevent hypotony from developing in these eyes. This situation increases the potential for choroidal hemorrhage to evolve. **B:** Views of the ciliary processes in the aphakic eye. Portions of the ciliary ring can be retracted anteriorly presenting obstacles for adequate ECP. Either scleral depression with the surgeon's second hand or the use of a curved endoscope will surmount this problem.

FIGURE 9-2. Endoscopic cyclophotocoagulation (ECP): limbal approach with a posterior chamber intraocular lens (IOL). A limbal incision is fashioned, and the sulcus is inflated with viscoelastic. This severs most iridocapsular adhesions and displaces the posterior chamber IOL and capsule posteriorly. The laser endoscope is then inserted for viewing and photocoagulation of the ciliary processes. **A:** Images of the ciliary processes in an eye with a plate-haptic silicone IOL. Note the capsular fibrosis around the positioning hole. **B:** From top to bottom represents the progress of ECP in this eye. The sulcus is not well inflated here, so that photocoagulation takes place through the capsular bag. The white line is the edge of the capsulorrhexis. At the bottom of the figure, the same eye now has a well-inflated sulcus, simplifying imaging and photocoagulation of the ciliary processes. The translucent white area in the lower left corner is residual cortex within the capsular bag. **C:** A well-inflated sulcus provides a simple opportunity for ECP demonstrating before, after, and close-up images. **D:** In this eye, the sulcus is inflated well and an IOL haptic can be seen within the capsular bag. The haptic is relatively distant from the ciliary processes and so will not be incorporated into the treatment zone, eliminating it as a source of inflammation postoperatively. **E:** A well-displaced posterior chamber IOL and capsule reveals stretched but intact zonules. The IOL haptic is "out of the bag" and resting in the sulcus. Care must be taken to avoid direct photocoagulation of the haptic, but adjacent ciliary epithelium can be treated. **F:** One portion of the sulcus can be inflated to only a moderate degree **(upper two photos)** while a different area in the same eye may permit wider exposure **(bottom photo)** for ECP.

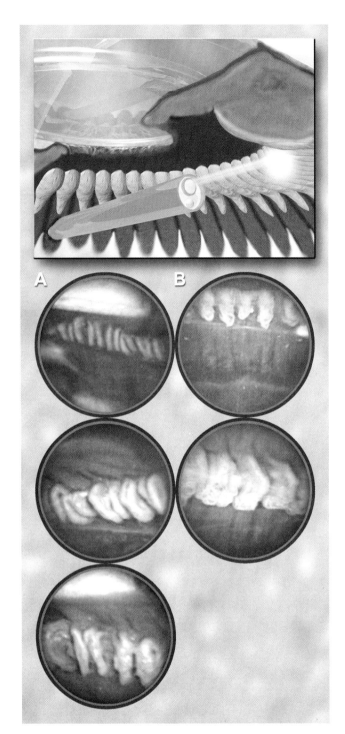

FIGURE 9-4. Pars plana approach to the ciliary processes in apha-kic or pseudophakic glaucoma. **A:** This approach is quite simple with insertion of the laser endoscope 4.0 mm from the limbus. This instrument is passed across the vitreous cavity and tilted slightly anteriorly. If the processes are retracted anteriorly, scleral depres-sion with the surgeon's second hand or the use of a curved endo-scope will resolve the difficulty so that endoscopic cyclophotoco-agulation (ECP) can be performed. It is best to remove at least the anterior vitreous before ECP to prevent vitreoretinal traction and its potential complications. **B:** Typical appearance of the ciliary processes in the aphakic or anterior chamber pseudophakic eye when approached from the pars plana.

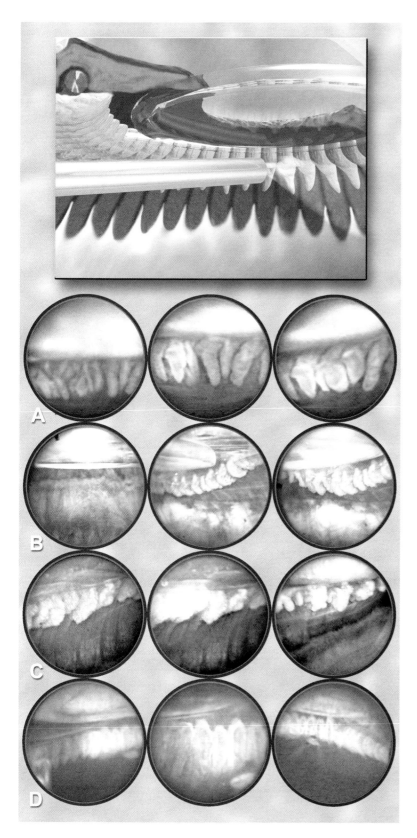

FIGURE 9-5. Pars plana approach in posterior chamber pseudophakic glaucoma. The laser endoscope is inserted about 4.0 mm from the limbus and directed anteriorly and across the vitreous cavity to image and laser the ciliary processes. The anterior vitreous should be removed prior to ECP. **A:** Typical view of the ciliary processes in this scenario with subsequent laser application. **B:** Ciliary processes are more anterior than expected. Scleral depression permits complete ECP. **C:** Adequate access to ciliary processes for straightforward ECP. **D:** Haptic on the superior pole of the ciliary processes. ECP was well executed, yet the haptic was not incorporated into the treatment zone, limiting the potential for postoperative inflammation.

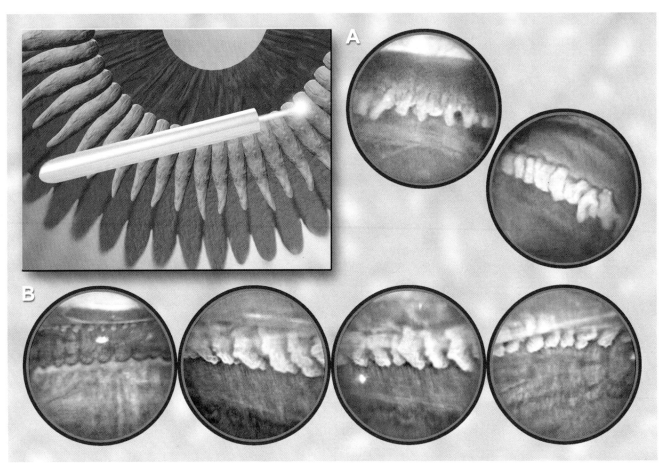

FIGURE 9-6. Pars plana approach in aphakic glaucoma. The laser endoscope is inserted through the pars plana sclerotomy and directed anteriorly for ECP. The vitreous in this region must be removed prior to endoscope manipulation. **A:** In these two eyes, there is no residual lens material or other physical obstruction to the ciliary processes, so that ECP is quite simple. It is important to prevent hypotony by placing some sort of infusion line prior to treatment. **B:** Four eyes with aphakic glaucoma undergoing ECP from a pars plana approach.

TABLE 9.1. COMPARISON OF HISTORICAL OUTCOMES OF GLAUCOMA TECHNIQUES USED IN THE MANAGEMENT OF APHAKIC AND PSEUDOPHAKIC GLAUCOMA[a]

Technique	Success Rate (%)	Severe Complication Rate (%)	Surgical Time	Postoperative Care
Trabeculectomy	50–70	10–20	Extensive	Extensive
Tube implant	50–70	30	Extensive	Extensive
TSCPC	50–70	40–50	Minimal	Minimal
ECP	80–90	<1	Minimal	Minimal

[a]Data from pediatric populations have been excluded because they present a much more challenging situation despite being labeled with a similar pathogenetic mechanism.
TSCPC, transscleral cyclophotocoagulation; ECP, endoscopic cyclophotocoagulation.

TABLE 9.2. DATA FROM COMPARATIVE STUDY OF ENDOSCOPIC CYCLOPHOTOCOAGULATION VERSUS TRABECULECTOMY IN APHAKIC AND PSEUDOPHAKIC GLAUCOMA

	IOP Control	Visual Acuity Loss	Visual Field Loss	CME	Minor Complications	Devastating Complications
No previous glaucoma surgery						
ECP ($n = 25$)	88% ($p = 0.05$)	0 ($p = 0.5$)	24% ($p = 0.01$)	0	4%	0
Trabeculectomy ($n = 25$)	44%	12%	64%	0	4%	0
Previous failed filter						
ECP ($n = 25$)	84% ($p = 0.05$)	0 ($p = 0.01$)	28% ($p = 0.05$)	0	8%	0
Trabeculectomy ($n = 25$)	24%	72%	80%	0	8%	12% ($p = 0.05$)

CME, cystoid macular edema; ECP, endoscopic cyclophotocoagulation; IOP, intraocular pressure.

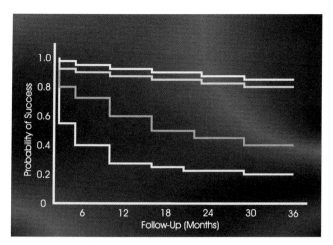

FIGURE 9-7. Comparative study of ECP vs. trabeculectomy in the management of aphakic or pseudophakic (CACG). This Kaplan-Meier survival analysis predicts successful IOP control by 36 months following treatment. The top, yellow line represents CACG patients without previous filtration surgery who were managed with ECP. The second, pink line represents the CACG patients who had failed at least one previous filtration surgery and who were then managed by ECP. The third, orange line represents the CACG patients without previous surgery treated by filtration, and the fourth, blue line the CACG patients with previously failed filtration surgery who underwent an additional filtration procedure. These data indicate that, compared with filtration surgery as a first or subsequent procedure, ECP effected the better long-term outcome for CACG treatment, regardless of whether the patient experienced a previously failed filter.

0.05). Devastating complications were not seen in the ECP group but presented in 12% of the trabeculectomy eyes ($p = 0.05$).

Kaplan-Meier survival analysis (Fig. 9-7) graphically demonstrates two points:

1. There does not appear to be a difference in the response of aphakic or pseudophakic closed-angle glaucoma eyes managed by ECP, regardless of previously failed filtration surgery.
2. ECP appears to achieve superior outcomes to trabeculectomy under this set of conditions.

Ongoing analysis of these data will be important as follow-up continues from the mid- to long term. Still, it seems significant that the comparative study data mirror the experience reported in noncomparative studies.

REFERENCES

1. Uram M. Endoscopic cyclophotocoagulation in glaucoma treatment. *Curr Opin Ophthalmol* 1995;11:19–29.
2. Chen J, Cohn RA, Lin SC, et al. Endoscopic photocoagulation of the ciliary body for treatment of refractory glaucomas. *Ophthalmology* 1997;124:787–796.

10

ENDOSCOPIC CYCLOPHOTOCOAGULATION FOR PSEUDOEXFOLIATION GLAUCOMA

When pseudoexfoliation glaucoma fails to respond to medical and laser therapies, surgical intervention is required. Although these cases have not been studied extensively in this regard, filtration seems to have about the same effect or better as it does for open-angle glaucoma. Although the role of lens removal in pseudoexfoliation is unclear, it probably does not affect the resolution of this problem.

A few physical peculiarities might be observed endoscopically in pseudoexfoliation. First, white, flaky material may be seen on the posterior aspect of the iris; it might then extend into the sulcus, onto the anterior lens surface or capsule, and onto zonules. Second, the zonules in many of these eyes appear to be markedly thicker than normal. They do not appear to be "weak," nor do their attachments to the ciliary body or lens capsule. They do not break when stretched with viscoelastic during endoscopic cyclophotocoagulation (ECP). The zonules may be coated with a dense accumulation of white material, although a minimal amount is more usual. This same range of accumulation applies to the posterior iris surface (Fig. 10-1). Finally, this white material can be found not infrequently during ECP in pseudophakic eyes without a history of pseudoexfoliation. This physical finding suggests that there was an undiagnosed element of pseudoexfoliation (Fig. 10-2).

On a practical level, another oddity may be observed in some of these eyes. During the course of ECP, it might seem that there is no tissue response to laser application. Naturally, the surgeon raises the laser power, but there may still seem to be no tissue response. As the power is further increased, a "pop" (tissue explosion) suddenly occurs. This can be puzzling, since at one setting there seems to be no response, but a small increase in power results in "overtreatment" (Fig. 10-3). As it turns out, the ciliary processes of pseudoexfoliative eyes often do not whiten and shrink during ECP, making it difficult to titrate treatment. The best approach seems to be raising the laser power sufficiently to create one or two pops, indicating the threshold for overtreatment, then lowering the power slightly. Treatment should then proceed in the usual manner. Although the surgeon does not benefit from visualizing the tissue response during surgery, ECP often results in the desired outcome.

A corollary of this situation is when no pseudoexfoliative material is visible yet the tissue does not respond physically to ECP in the expected manner, although the surgeon confirms that the laser is functioning properly. Under this scenario, one might suspect the reason for this is pseudoexfoliation, even though the physical evidence may have been removed, such as by cataract surgery.

Several studies have addressed the management of this form of glaucoma by ECP. In one small study (1), five patients uncontrolled by maximum medical therapy and surgery underwent 180- to 360-degree ECP. The intraocular pressure (IOP) was 29.2 mm Hg preoperatively and 15.2 mm Hg postoperatively (p = 0.058), with 90% of the patients experiencing IOP of 21 mm Hg or less at last follow-up (mean, 13 months). No devastating complications were encountered.

In another study (2), 26 eyes with pseudoexfoliative glaucoma and cataract underwent combined phacoemulsification and ECP for 180 to 300 degrees. The preoperative mean maximal IOP was 20.4 ± 4.45 mm Hg. The postoperative IOP was 19.9 ± 9.3 mm Hg at 1 day, 17.4 ± 2.6 mm Hg at 1 month, and 19.11 ± 3.2 HG at 2 months. The best corrected visual acuity was 20/60 ± 5.7 preoperatively and 20/40 ± 7.2 postoperatively. The mean number of antiglaucoma medications was 1.68 ± 0.95 preoperatively and 0.63 ± 0.7 postoperatively. There were no complications of significance.

In this situation, all patients experienced an improvement in Snellen acuity. ECP effectively reduced the number of antiglaucoma medications needed to control IOP, perhaps improving patient compliance and quality of life. Indeed, the authors advocated the use ECP in a more aggressive fashion, with ablation of 300 to 360 degrees of the ciliary processes, to better control IOP and reduce the need for antiglaucoma medications and the monetary burden associated with them.

Although these studies cannot be used to make grandiose inferences, the outcomes seem to fall into line with the results obtained in other larger groups of patients with various mechanisms of glaucoma that were followed up more extensively.

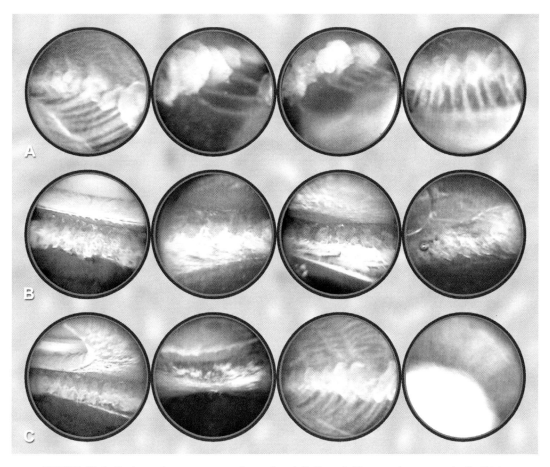

FIGURE 10-1. Endoscopic appearance of pseudoexfoliation. **A:** The zonules are markedly thickened compared with normal eyes and may also appear to be lax. **B:** White debris is often scattered over the surface of the ciliary process. This accumulation can be quite dense. **C:** White material can also be seen, to varying degrees, on the posterior aspect of the iris.

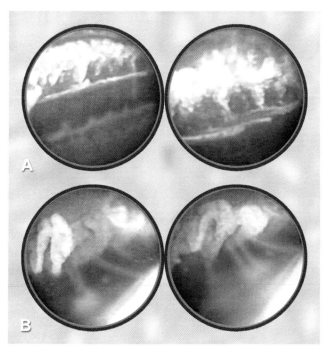

FIGURE 10-2. A: White material may be so dense that whitening of the ciliary process surface during endoscopic cyclophotocoagulation (ECP) cannot be perceived endoscopically. **B:** At times, the ciliary processes seem to be resistant to laser application in that they do not whiten or shrink. Nevertheless, ECP still seems to be effective in these eyes, despite their apparent lack of visible response to laser application.

Finally, pseudoexfoliative eyes do not seem to experience any greater risk of complications or less efficacy from ECP than do eyes with other glaucoma mechanisms despite their unique response to laser application.

REFERENCES

1. Chen J, Cohn RA, Lin SC, et al. Endoscopic photocoagulation of the ciliary body for treatment of refractory glaucomas. *Ophthalmology* 1997;124:787–796.
2. Berke SJ, Cohen AJ, Sturm RT, Nelson, DB. Endoscopic cyclophotocoagualtion and phacoemulsification in the treatment of medically controlled primary open-angle glaucoma. *J Glaucoma* 2000;9:129.

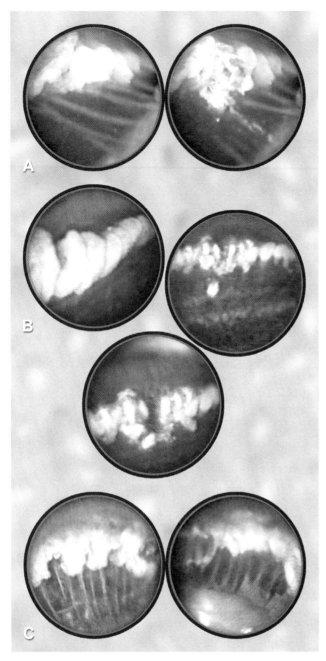

FIGURE 10-3. Endoscopic cyclophotocoagulation overtreatment as a result of pseudoexfoliation. **A:** Typical appearance of eye with pseudoexfoliation intensely thickened zonules and "unresponsive" ciliary processes. As the laser power is raised to achieve an "adequate" treatment level, the tissue is exploded. In this situation, the laser power is diminished and the remainder of the processes are treated, whether or not they appear to whiten or shrink. **B:** Relatively high laser power level used to whiten process. Still, tissue explosion occurs. A few minutes later, this site starts to bleed. **C:** Pseudoexfoliation eye with thickened zonules. A ciliary process is exploded with pigment dispersion along the course of the zonules, stopping at its attachment to the lens capsule. Note the resilience of the zonules; even in this situation, they do not rupture.

ENDOSCOPIC CYCLOPHOTOCOAGULATION FOR NEOVASCULAR GLAUCOMA

Management of neovascular glaucoma (NVG) challenges the surgeon to define the therapeutic goal. Is treatment directed to pain control alone, preservation of useful vision, or even recovery of good visual function—all with lowered and stabilized intraocular pressure (IOP)? A number of factors determine the potential for each eye, particularly the cause of NVG.

Consider that the most common disorder precipitating NVG is diabetic retinopathy. Some of these eyes have the potential not only to be pain free and demonstrate good cosmesis but also to recover excellent visual function. Aggressive and prompt retinal ablation (diminishing ischemic drive and therefore effecting stabilization or regression of iris neovascularization) combined with rapid IOP control (limiting optic nerve damage and perhaps increasing vascular perfusion) can be quite effective.

The second most common etiologic event is central retinal vein occlusion (Fig. 11-1). In these patients, recovery of central acuity is a remote possibility under any circumstance. Retinal ablation to prevent the onset of NVG is routine, and even if the patient initially presents with NVG, such treatment is indicated. In a way, IOP control in this group is more important because the primary therapeutic goal is to maintain the integrity of the eye and perhaps retain some measure of useful peripheral vision. Regardless of the cause, in the presence of long-standing NVG, recovery of useful vision is rarely an option, and the primary goal of treatment would be to lower the IOP to achieve pain control and improved cosmesis.

NVG responds poorly to standard glaucoma procedures. Trabeculectomy is associated with a 30% success rate. Most of these procedures fail early in the postoperative course. Adjunctive antimetabolites are of little value, with high risk for failed filtration, poorly controlled IOP, loss of light perception, and development of phthisis bulbi. Success with drainage implants varies widely, but overall they have proved moderately efficacious in controlling IOP. Substantial complications, including phthisis and loss of light perception, are not uncommon.

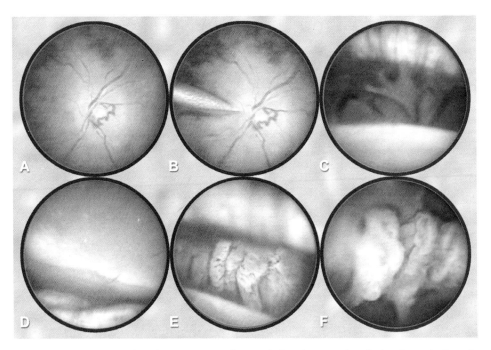

FIGURE 11-1. Neovascular glaucoma secondary to ischemic central retinal vein occlusion. **A:** Note optociliary collateral vessels. **B:** Radial optic neurotomy with MVR blade. **C:** Hemorrhage "dripping" from extensive iris neovascularization posteriorly into sulcus region. Note anterior capsule of crystalline lens. **D:** Angle with blood and vessels. **E:** Endoscopic cyclophotocoagulation (ECP) with anterior segment hemorrhage migrating posteriorly. **F:** ECP.

An alternative approach to NVG management is to lower IOP by diminishing aqueous inflow. Cyclocryotherapy has been reported to give moderate success in controlling IOP in this situation, but it is brutal and associated with a high incidence of devastating complications. Transscleral laser cyclodestruction achieves a moderate rate of success in the management of NVG but still suffers from the complications associated with cyclocryotherapy, albeit to a lesser degree. Prominent among these are an 11% to 29% risk of phthisis and 40% to 56% incidence of visual loss. This approach has been generally reserved for eyes with poor visual potential. Inability to view as well as to apply laser energy to the ciliary process epithelium and titrate it accurately characterizes the failure of the transscleral approach to cyclophotocoagulation (TSCPC), regardless of the type of laser used. Treatment that incorporates tissue not involved in aqueous production also contributes to these significant complications. Using fluorescein angiography intraoperatively to study the ciliary processes of eyes that failed to respond to one or more TSCPC treatments, it was observed that most patients demonstrated far less cycloablation than expected by the treating surgeon (1). This considerable disadvantage is addressed by ECP.

It would be fair to say that the standard methods for managing NVG are poorly to moderately effective, can be technically difficult, and are associated with an array of severe complications. Most ophthalmologists do not end up managing this problem, the typical patient being treated by a subspecialist.

ECP was first described in a small group of NVG patients as demonstrating a high degree of efficacy and safety (2). A larger group of these patients studied retrospectively has been reported (3). A long-term prospective study is under way comparing ECP, TSCPC, and tube implantation.

INTRAOCULAR PRESSURE

Substantially lowered IOP can be expected during the first 8 postoperative weeks in about 90% of NVG patients treated with ECP. This outcome is consistent with all the ECP trials to date, as well as the IOP response observed in other glaucoma mechanisms, and with photocoagulation of the ciliary processes after vitrectomy and lensectomy and using scleral depression while viewing through the operating microscope. An absolute decrease in IOP of 60% to 70% can be anticipated with this approach.

Early IOP elevations, primarily occurring during the first postoperative day, may be observed in up to 25% of eyes when an anterior segment approach is elected, undoubtedly as a result of residual viscoelastic. IOP spikes are infrequent when a pars plana approach has been used.

Late IOP elevations are distinctly uncommon. Most patients maintain lowered IOP level throughout the lengthy follow-up. Long-term assessment of patients treated for NVG with tube implants, with or without antimetabolites, indicates a substantial level of decompensation (4,5). Similar observations have been attributed to the transscleral route of cyclodestruction.

Hypotony and phthisis were not observed in any study group or in reports of transvitreal ciliary body photocoagulation. Personal communications have indicated a small number of patients who have unfortunately developed this problem, but the overall incidence seems to be far less than 1%. This remarkable finding illustrates one of the major distinctions between the transscleral route of cyclodestruction and ECP. When the ciliary process epithelium can be directly viewed and titratably photocoagulated without involvement of nonciliary process tissue or prosthetic material, the risk of overtreatment becomes greatly reduced. Clinically, this advantage translates into a wide margin of safety, mostly eliminating hypotony or phthisis as a complication of the procedure.

GLAUCOMA MEDICATIONS

A substantial decline in the use of both topical and systemic glaucoma medication can be observed after ECP for NVG. Typically, patients believed to have the potential for useful vision should be maintained on their preoperative regimen until they have achieved an IOP in the middle teens. Then these drugs can be eliminated as long as the IOP remains at an acceptable level. If the IOP does not achieve this target, the preoperative medications should be maintained. If the ultimate result was a limited success or frank failure, usually observed by the eighth postoperative week, reoperation might be considered. In those treated for pain control, the bar is set at a lower level, an IOP in the 20s or perhaps 30s being acceptable. It is desirable to use as few medications as possible to maintain this IOP.

VISUAL ACUITY

Neovascular glaucoma eyes can be stratified into three groups: those with Snellen acuity of 20/100 or better, those between 20/200 and 5/400, and those with visual function lower than 5/400. The therapeutic goal in the first two groups is to achieve an IOP conducive to maintaining the presenting acuity. In the third group, pain control and acceptable cosmesis is the desired end point. Even when the first two groups have been "successful," progressive visual loss may be expected in up to 25% of patients, and they should be forewarned. Compromised retinal or optic nerve perfusion due to the underlying etiologic process of NVG is the most likely explanation and should be differentiated from visual loss associated with ongoing glaucomatous damage or resulting from a surgical complication. Visual outcome after ECP appears to be better than has been reported following tube implantation or transscleral cyclodestructive surgery; these approaches are typically associated with a 24% to 56% incidence of visual loss (Table 11-1).

PANRETINAL PHOTOCOAGULATION

Panretinal photocoagulation (PRP) is used to diminish ischemic drive and to prevent or arrest the development of iris neovascularization (NVI). Ideally, a complete PRP would effect regression of NVI (Fig. 11-2). Unfortunately, the extent and duration of NVI at the time of presentation can vary widely. It may not be possible to effect adequate retinal ablation in eyes with corneal opacification, hyphema, miotic pupils, dense cataract, or vitreous hemorrhage. Indeed, it may not be possible to perform PRP in up to half of NVG patients because of these obstacles to visualization. Furthermore, the extreme effort that is required to accomplish panretinal ablation under these circumstances may be impractical, considering the advanced disease state encountered at presentation. This would be especially true if the goal of therapy was directed to pain control and preservation of acceptable cosmesis.

Fortunately, extensive retinal ablation is not a prerequisite for achieving adequate IOP control from ECP. Recall that there are really two issues here: The first is the iris vessels themselves, and the second is their effect, that is, uncontrolled glaucoma. Retinal ablation may eliminate or stabilize the growth of vessels but will not reverse glaucoma once it has been established. On the other hand, ECP can lower the IOP but will not stabilize or reverse NVI. These

TABLE 11.1. HISTORICAL OUTCOMES IN THE MANAGEMENT OF NEOVASCULAR GLAUCOMA (%)

Outcome	Trabeculectomy	Trabeculectomy + Antimetabolites	Tube Implant	Cyclocryotherapy	TSCPC	ECP
Success (%)	30	30–50	50–70	50	50–70	90
Visual loss (%)	5–20	5–20	20	50	40	0–5
Phthisis (%)	5	5	10	30	10	0–2

TSCPC, transscleral cyclophotocoagulatin; ECP, endoscopic cyclophotocoagulation.

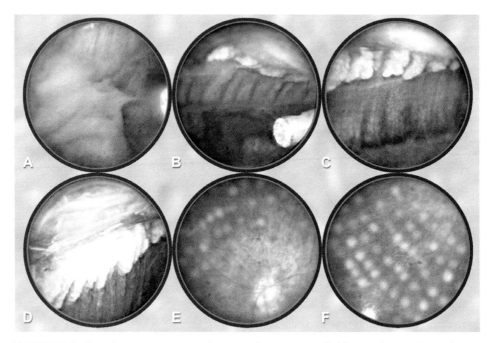

FIGURE 11-2. Complete management of neovascular glaucoma. **A:** Vitreous hemorrhage obscuring peripheral retina, pars plana, and ciliary body. **B:** Vitrectomy removes obstruction, allowing visualization of treatment area. **C:** Ciliary processes are now clearly visible. **D:** Endoscopic cyclophotocoagulation. **E:** Panretinal photocoagulation posterior retina. **F:** Complete ablation of peripheral retina.

must be considered as independent events. As an example, two curious situations may present themselves. A painful blind NVG eye with lush NVI and opaque media may undergo ECP and achieve good IOP control and resolution of pain yet suffer from the long-term consequences of neovascularization, such as recurrent hyphema or vitreous hemorrhage. These problems do not require treatment because the eye is already blind; removing the blood and ablating the ischemic retina will not improve visual function. Only ECP is necessary. Alternatively, consider a diabetic eye with 20/20 vision that develops acute NVG. It would be extremely important in this situation to effect dense retinal

ablation as well as control IOP by ECP. The specter of permanent visual loss, recurrent intraocular hemorrhage, and worsening glaucoma intensifies the level of intervention required.

IRIS NEOVASCULARIZATION

Clearly, ECP does not affect the course of NVI. Resolution of ocular schemia resulting from retinal ablation (in diabetic retinopathy or central retinal vein occlusion) or from an increase in ocular perfusion (by carotid endarterectomy

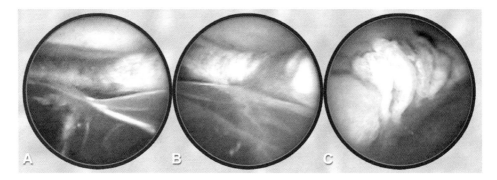

FIGURE 11-3. Neovascular glaucoma and hyphema. **A:** Pseudophakic eye with bleeding iris neovascularization extending over papillary edge. **B:** Magnified image. **C:** Endoscopic cyclophotocoagulation in progress.

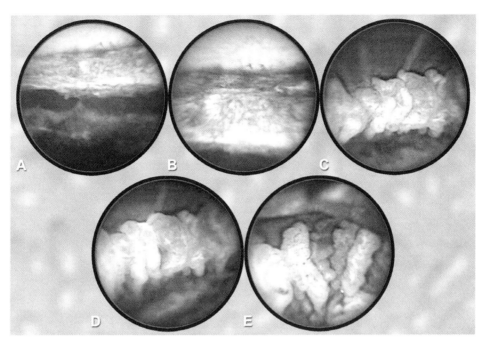

FIGURE 11-4. Neovascular glaucoma. **A:** View at the level of the pupil. Note blood vessels in the angle and extensive iris fibrovascular proliferation extending over the papillary edge and continuing in a posterior direction. The ora serrata and some vitreous hemorrhage can be seen. **B:** Magnified view of iris vessels with abnormal angle in background. **C:** Ciliary processes. **D:** Treated and untreated ciliary processes. **E:** Hemorrhage on the ciliary process surface that migrated anteriorly from the vitreous cavity.

in ocular ischemic syndrome) theoretically diminishes ischemic drive, causing the regression of ocular proliferation. It should not be surprising that perhaps half of the patients presenting with NVG are beyond the point where it would be straightforward to ablate the retina or rehabilitate their vision. Specifically addressing the NVI would not be indicated. Nevertheless, it is important to appreciate that if retinal ablation can be accomplished without resorting to extraordinary means (vitrectomy, lensectomy, or "blind" panretinal cryoablation), it may be beneficial to control

NVI. As Ritch has suggested (6), patients with treated retinal disease fare better with filtration surgery as treatment for NVG than do those who have not. Similarly, many ECP patients requiring reoperation demonstrate persistent NVI and inadequate retinal treatment. Late-onset hyphema is a common occurrence in eyes with untreated NVI but is not seen often in those with totally regressed NVI (Figs. 11-3 to 11-5). Insufficient retinal ablation in the presence of successful ECP may result in the rather peculiar combination of clinically florid NVI, a clear cornea, and normal IOP.

PAIN CONTROL

Many NVG patients, perhaps up to half, require treatment primarily for pain control. The ideal of achieving a long-term IOP in the low teens is not as important in this group. Often, a qualified success with IOP in the high 20s, 30s, or 40s is sufficient to completely control pain and maintain adequate cosmesis. Even in the presence of late hyphema secondary to persistent NVI, recurrence of pain is not often observed. ECP is highly effective in achieving this goal because a modest decrease in IOP often proves sufficient. For such a patient, it seems foolish to recommend enucleation or some other aggressive procedure when 180-degree ECP will most likely achieve the desired goal with little morbidity.

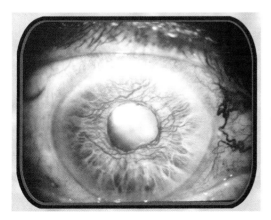

FIGURE 11-5. Extensive iris neovascularization in the presence of normal intraocular pressure.

LENS DISLOCATION

The theoretical potential for lens dislocation would seem inherent to the procedure, especially when one considers that all the surgical manipulation occurs within a small space bounded by the iris superiorly, the lens or lens implant inferiorly, and the ciliary body laterally. This is of particular concern in this situation because many eyes with NVG are phakic. It is also well known that it is better to preserve this lens barrier between the anterior and posterior segment, which conceptually "blocks" the diffusion of "angiogenesis factor" from the ischemic retina to the iris. Nevertheless, this problem has not been encountered. The zonules are quite resilient, being able to withstand stretching by the introduction of viscoelastic as well as by retraction of the ciliary process at the time of photocoagulation (Figs. 11-6 to 11-8).

CATARACT FORMATION

Cataract formation seems to be an inherent component of anterior segment schemia and NVG. Add to this the additional potential for lens opacification associated with intraocular surgery and it should come as no surprise that significant cataracts ultimately develop in many ECP-treated NVG patients. The risk of cataract development after ECP is about 30% by the second postoperative year across all mechanisms of glaucoma. This compares favorably with the statistics associated with phakic trabeculectomy (with or without antimetabolites) and phakic vitrectomy. Schuman (7) has reported a greater frequency of cataract formation in NVG eyes compared with non-NVG eyes treated by neodymium:yttrium-argon-garnet (Nd:YAG) laser transscleral cyclodestruction, perhaps testimony to the proclivity for NVG eyes to develop lens opacification. Many of the patients in whom cataract evolves following ECP experience this within the first few postoperative weeks. This is most likely due to the anterior lens capsule becoming gouged during manipulation of the laser endoscope under the iris. This technical problem can generally be avoided by using enough viscoelastic to displace the lens into a suitable posterior position, thus protecting the capsule from trauma.

INFLAMMATION

A hallmark of transscleral cyclodestruction, and to a lesser degree filtration surgery, is the evolution of significant inflammation. A chronic inflammatory response is not unusual. ECP has been associated with scant inflammatory reaction in NVG. Recall that human histopathologic study has indicated that ECP is specifically ablative to the ciliary epithelium only and that it does not incite an inflammatory response at the cellular level. Avoiding overtreatment, incorporation of non-aqueous-producing tissue, or prosthetics such as IOL haptics in the treatment zone further limits the potential for producing this reaction, unlike transscleral cyclodestructive techniques..

NONDEVASTATING COMPLICATIONS

Glaucoma surgery of any type is frequently associated with postoperative complications, although many may be transient. Eyes undergoing filtration surgery may experience intraocular hemorrhage, serous choroidal effusion, flat chamber, overfiltration or underfiltration, and hypotonous maculopathy. Intensive postoperative care is the rule. Tube implants may be associated with strabismus, pain, blockage, and corneal decompensation. Transscleral cyclodestructive procedures are painful and are associated with the development of choroidal effusion, hemorrhage, and cystoid macular edema. ECP, on the other hand, is infrequently associated with the complications experienced after other forms of glaucoma surgery. Transient vitreous or anterior segment hemorrhage is the most common of these (3% to 8%) followed

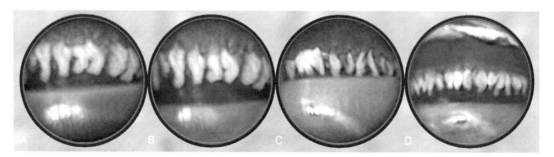

FIGURE 11-6. Endoscopic cyclophotocoagulation (ECP) in neovascular glaucoma. **A:** In this phakic eye, the sulcus is well inflated with viscoelastic. **B:** The aiming beam of the laser is placed on the ciliary process surface. **C:** ECP is initiated. White processes have been treated while brown ones have not. **D:** More panoramic view of completed ECP.

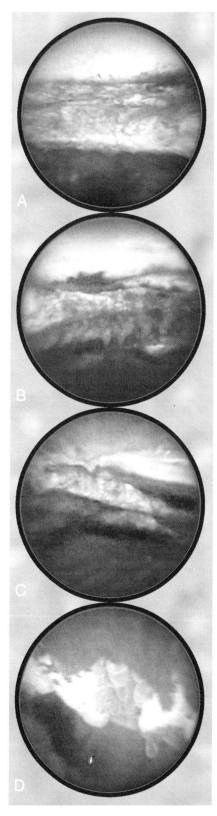

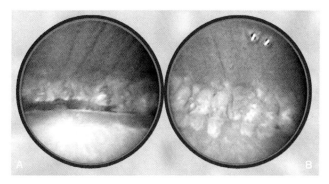

FIGURE 11-8. Endoscopic cyclophotocoagulation (ECP) in neovascular glaucoma. **A:** Posterior chamber pseudophakic eye with well-inflated sulcus. Blood obscures view of processes but does not prohibit ECP. **B:** Pseudophakic eye in which posterior aspect of ciliary processes is now seen through the lens capsule. ECP can be applied through the peripheral lens or capsule without damaging it.

by pain of one to several days duration (5%) (2). Choroidal effusion, flat chamber, cystoid macular edema, and hypotonous maculopathy have notably been absent. The number of follow-up visits required to manage these conditions is small compared with the other treatment modalities (about four during the first 2 postoperative months). This intensity of postsurgical care seems to be considerably less than required by other glaucoma procedures, although this issue has not been specifically studied. In effect, either ECP is effective during the first 8 postoperative weeks or it isn't, but minor complications rarely contribute to ultimate treatment failure, and their presence is of less concern and significance than with other surgical approaches to the treatment of NVG.

DEVASTATING COMPLICATIONS

Perhaps the greatest pitfall of filtration, tube implantation, and transscleral cyclodestructive procedures rests with their potential for devastating complications, specifically massive choroidal hemorrhage, retinal detachment, sympathetic uveitis, endophthalmitis, hypotony, and phthisis. NVG represents a special situation for some of these problems because these eyes are compromised in ways other than simply having elevated IOP as a consequence of obstructed outflow.

Infectious endophthalmitis has never been reported following ECP for any glaucoma mechanism, although it would not be an unexpected event given enough surgical interventions. Compare this with the cumulative risk associated with filtration surgery, which is 1% per year. It would appear, then, that late bleb-associated endophthalmitis or seton infections are risks not inherent to ECP, making it a safer procedure insofar as this issue is concerned.

FIGURE 11-7. Neovascular glaucoma and endoscopic cyclophotocoagulation (ECP). **A:** Image of anterior segment with extensive iris neovascularization and hemorrhage in the angle. **B:** Same area viewed at the level of the pupil. The eye is aphasic. **C:** Same area while imaging from posterior to iris. Although extensive neovascularization is present on the anterior iris surface, it is notably absent posteriorly. **D:** Anomalous appearance of the ciliary processes at ECP may be a consequence of previous cataract surgery.

Because vitreous is not encountered in the phakic and posterior chamber pseudophakic eye during ECP, retinal detachment as a consequence of vitreous manipulation would not be expected and has not been observed. In those with aphakia or anterior chamber pseudophakia, the anterior vitreous is usually removed at the time of previous surgery or before ECP, theoretically and practically limiting the potential for retinal detachment. There have only been two reported cases of retinal detachment following ECP, and both have been associated with pediatric glaucoma. It was not clear whether their etiology was rhegmatogenous in nature. It would be fair to say that retinal detachment is at most a rare consequence of ECP for NVG, its incidence being far less than 1%.

The mechanism of massive choroidal hemorrhage following transscleral cyclodestructive procedures has not been elucidated. However, consideration must be given to the possibility of overtreatment rupturing a choroidal vessel. Similarly, transection of a choroidal vessel at the time of filtration surgery or mechanical erosion from an implant tube may be responsible for the evolution of this complication. Because ECP is performed under direct visualization and laser delivery is substantially more titratable, the potential for overtreatment is reduced. There is no mechanical cutting of ciliary tissue nor are any prosthetics implanted that might ultimately erode it. There has never been a reported case of this problem in the management of NVG.

HYPOTONY AND PHTHISIS

Hypotony and phthisis represent a potentially devastating adverse response to transscleral cyclodestructive surgery. Overtreatment of aqueous-producing ciliary processes is the presumed mechanism. Cyclocryotherapy is associated with a higher incidence of this complication (30%) than is transscleral laser cycloablation (11% to 29%) (8,9).

Endoscopic and fluorescein angiographic examination suggests another possibility. Many eyes previously treated transsclerally that did not experience an adequate IOP response were observed to have extensive areas of non-ciliary process tissue incorporated into the treatment zone. Although phthisical eyes have not been studied in this fashion, one may conjecture that substantial cryotherapy or laser application to the peripheral retina, pars plana, and iris may initiate anterior segment schemia, excessive inflammation, or cyclitic membrane formation with ciliary body detachment resulting in phthisis. Therefore, it does not appear to be the straightforward case of simply ablating "too many" ciliary processes. There is an additional consideration specific to NVG. In virtually all mechanisms of chronic glaucoma, one can assume that the inflow side of the equation is fully operational and that 100% of the "problem" is obstructed outflow. (This does not mean that

the inflow side of the equation cannot be manipulated.) With NVG, however, it has been demonstrated that in certain eyes there is also an element of diminished inflow. As a simplistic example, such an eye might have only 40% function of the ciliary epithelium (inflow) and 20% unobstructed drainage system (outflow). The overall IOP is quite high as a result of this imbalance. If 50% of the ciliary epithelium is then ablated (cyclocryotherapy, TSCPC, ECP, disease-induced progression of schemia, and ciliary body death), the already compromised production of aqueous is pushed over the cliff and the IOP plummets. Compare this with an open-angle glaucoma eye with 100% functioning ciliary epithelium and 20% functioning drainage. Lowering aqueous production by 50% will certainly not result in hypotony or phthisis, and it may not lower the IOP at all! Being able to measure aqueous production with a simple noninvasive test would make decision making simple, but this technology does not exist. We can only go by our clinical experience and hope that there are not too many unhappy surprises.

Furthermore, as alluded to previously, there may be a roller coaster effect with IOP in NVG. The pressure may be extremely high and then spontaneously become quite low, heralding the eye's demise. Surgical intervention further confounds the issue. In the end, there does not appear to be a clear answer as to how extensive treatment should be based on IOP and other characteristics in a given eye. For most patients, 180 degrees of ECP seems to be the safest initial approach. If aqueous production is within the normal range, this minimalist treatment will not be effective and it will be clear that further surgery is required. If, on the other hand, aqueous production is low to begin with, 180 degrees of treatment will have a profound effect on the IOP. Most patients with post-ECP hypotony or phthisis have had NVG with more extensive treatment (270 to 360 degrees). Starting with a 180-degree ECP has dramatically lowered the incidence of this uncommon yet severe problem at the cost of necessitating reoperations in those who, in the end, prove to have more healthy inflow.

REOPERATION

If an inadequate response has been attained, a second ECP should be performed. The decision for further intervention is typically made early in the postoperative course and is based on the following: (a) the IOP response to initial ECP is poor; (b) after an initially good response, the trend reverses; or (c) by the 8-week posttreatment mark, the therapeutic goal was not achieved. Late failures do occur, but they are uncommon. Overall, 20% of these eyes require a second treatment. When the IOP responds poorly to initial therapy, one may proceed with confidence at reoperation because it should then be clear that the eye in question has adequate aqueous production. The risk of hypotony or phthisis becomes remote.

INTRAOCULAR VERSUS TRANSSCLERAL TECHNIQUE

Why should an intraocular procedure (ECP) be performed when a "noninvasive" one (TSCPC or cyclocryotherapy) exists? This question speaks to the issue of risk. It should be clear from the previous discussion that the noninvasive approach has far more serious complications than the invasive one. It is mystifying that some might consider, even for a moment, that the blind external approach could be comparable to ECP. In view of the facts that laser treatment can be selectively delivered to the ciliary epithelium, that the surgeon can choose the number of ciliary processes to be treated, and that nonciliary epithelial tissue can be excluded from the treatment zone, the most frequent and devastating complications of transscleral cyclodestruction can be avoided with ECP. It is this selectivity that renders ECP a benign operative procedure, whereas the noninvasive transscleral approach is not.

REFERENCES

1. Uram M. Endoscopic cyclophotocoagulation in glaucoma management. *Curr Opin Ophthalmol* 1995;11:19–29.
2. Uram M. Endoscopic cyclophotocoagulation in glaucoma management: indications, results and complications. *Ophthalmic Pract* 1995;13:5.
3. Uram M. Ophthalmic laser microendoscope endophotocoagulation. *Ophthalmology* 1992;99:1829–1832.
4. Tsai JC, Feuer WJ, Parrish RK II, Grajewski AL. 5-Fluorouracil filtering glaucoma surgery and neovascular glaucoma: long-term follow-up of the original pilot study. *Ophthalmology* 1995;102: 887–893.
5. Mermoud A, Salmon JF, Alexander P, et al. Molteno tube implantation for neovascular glaucoma: long-term results and factors influencing the outcome. *Ophthalmology* 1993;100:897–902.
6. Ritch R. 5-Fluorouracil filtering surgery and neovascular glaucoma. [Discussion] *Ophthalmology* 1995;106:892–893.
7. Schuman JS, Puliafito CA, Allingham RR, et al. Contact transscleral continuous wave Nd:YAG laser cyclophotocoagulation. *Ophthalmology* 1990;97:571-580.
8. Bellows AR. Cyclocryotherapy for glaucoma. *Int Ophthalmol Clin* 1981;21:99–111.
9. Krupin T, Mitchell K, Becker B. Cyclocryotherapy in neovascular glaucoma. *Am J Ophthalmol* 1978;86:24–26.

COMBINED CATARACT SURGERY AND ENDOSCOPIC CYCLOPHOTOCOAGULATION

Cataract and glaucoma are common ophthalmic disorders that are not uncommonly seen together; up to one third of patients undergoing cataract surgery have some element of these problems. Combining procedures to address both of these issues can be, at least theoretically, a reasonable course of action, although there is significant controversy as to the specific indications and operative technique. When maximal medical therapy has effected only borderline control, or in the presence of unacceptable medication side effects despite good control, or when the intraocular pressure (IOP) is frankly uncontrolled in the presence of significant cataract, most would agree that the combined approach should be given serious consideration. The decision to intervene depends on a number of factors, including the surgeon's comfort in managing these diseases and their impact on the patient's life.

Opinion certainly varies as to the precise indications for the combined approach. Some assert that failure of medical control is the threshold, whereas others think that if two or more glaucoma medications are required to maintain adequate IOP, the combined procedure should be considered. Another suggested indication is such significant optic nerve damage that the eye might not sustain a postoperative cataract surgery IOP spike without progression.

It is well known that cataract surgery in and of itself does not effect long-term IOP control but that, on the other hand, early postoperative IOP spikes can be quite significant and that eyes with glaucoma tend to have higher postcataract surgery IOP elevations than nonglaucomatous eyes. When an eye with previous trabeculectomy undergoes subsequent phacoemulsification, IOP and medication requirements typically do not diminish. Indeed, the IOP may rise.

Finally, in the presence of severe glaucomatous visual field loss before surgery, up to 10% of patients experience progression following cataract and glaucoma surgery. Bearing this in mind, there are a few combined procedure issues to examine.

GENERAL CONSIDERATIONS IN COMBINED CATARACT–FILTRATION SURGERY

There are three important areas in which combined cataract and filtration surgery differs from cataract surgery and filtration surgery performed separately: wound closure, visual loss, and clinical "success."

Wound Closure

Combining filtration surgery with cataract extraction and intraocular lens (IOL) implantation is the standard for treating patients with uncontrolled glaucoma and visual loss due to lens opacification. Enhancing aqueous outflow results in lowering of the IOP. Doing so is inconsistent with the wound closure requirements of cataract surgery. Recall that a nonleaking wound is the expected end point of cataract surgery, whereas a "controlled" wound leak is the anticipated outcome of filtration. Immediate postoperative complications, such as flat anterior chamber, choroidal effusion/hemorrhage, hypotony, and visual loss, are the consequences of this paradox.

To further complicate matters, the amount of filtration is unpredictable in a given eye. Variables such as mechanism of glaucoma, race, previous ophthalmic surgery, and use of antimetabolites may profoundly affect the outcome. Postoperative overfiltration or underfiltration is common.

While overfiltration can create a host of complications, underfiltration (too "tight" a closure) results mainly in failure of the glaucoma portion of the procedure as well as IOP spikes and resultant progressive field loss.

Despite this seeming wound closure contradiction, a balance must be struck by these competing interests for the procedure to be successful, and that is the crux of the problem. These issues are typically beyond the control of the surgeon and may present despite best efforts and great skill.

Visual Recovery

Another significant deterrent to combining cataract and filtration surgery is the longer interval to visual recovery postoperatively compared with cataract surgery alone. This phenomenon may arise from a number of causes. Hypotony from overfiltration may result in loss of acuity. Secondarily, choroidal effusion/hemorrhage, corneal edema (especially Descemet folds), flat anterior chamber, and maculopathy may evolve as a consequence, resulting in diminished vision.

There is certainly an increased risk for transient intraocular hemorrhage when procedures are combined. If confined to the vitreous, it may not be terribly symptomatic. Patients may complain of diffuse blurring of vision or of floater-type symptoms. Hyphema, on the other hand, especially when diffuse, can result in markedly diminished vision. These problems most often resolve spontaneously and are of transient concern and annoyance, but occasionally surgical intervention may be necessary.

Operative Success

It is well known that eyes treated with combined cataract/filtration surgery have longer postoperative recovery and higher risk of failure, immediate and long-term complications, and endophthalmitis than those treated with cataract surgery alone. Even if these two procedures were to be performed separately, many of these difficulties would be experienced less frequently than when the procedures are performed concomitantly. Filtration surgery alone typically results in a better outcome than the combined approach. The operative technique used for cataract surgery seems to have little effect on the outcome when combined with filtration.

Reported outcomes of combined filtration/cataract surgery demonstrate a variable reduction in IOP, ranging from 5 to 10 mm Hg at 2-year follow-up.

Numerous studies have addressed the issue of antimetabolites used in conjunction with filtration and cataract surgery. Although results and conclusions vary in regard to their value, it seems that adjunctive 5-fluorouracil and mitomycin-C are not particularly helpful in improving the long-term success of combined procedures and, rather, enhance the long-term potential for complications such as bleb leak and endophthalmitis.

Considering all of these obstacles, it should come as no surprise that most ophthalmologists shun combined surgery and that it is infrequently employed at best.

COMBINING CATARACT SURGERY WITH INFLOW REDUCTION

It would be inconceivable to combine delicate intraocular microsurgery with brutal transscleral cyclodestruction, and this, no doubt, accounts for the absence of historical precedent. To be conceptually accurate, prior to endoscopic cyclophotocoagulation (ECP), there were no reports of cataract surgery combined with an inflow-reducing glaucoma procedure. Theoretically, there would be no reason that this approach would not work (aside from the obvious known drawbacks of transscleral cyclophotocoagulation (TSCPC), cyclocryotherapy, and diathermy); indeed, this method would circumvent some of the major flaws associated with current cataract and filtration techniques. The efficacy and safety of ECP demonstrated in intractable forms of glaucoma confirm the theoretical assertion that inflow can be surgically manipulated in a minimally invasive fashion that may be appropriately combined with cataract microsurgery.

There are two broad areas in which phacoemulsification or extracapsular surgery has been combined with ECP. The first is in the presence of "uncontrolled" glaucoma, and the second is in eyes with medically controlled glaucoma that are undergoing cataract surgery for visual rehabilitation.

Techniques

Three approaches can be taken to access the ciliary processes when combining ECP with cataract surgery, and use of one does not necessarily exclude use of the others. Perhaps the safest is the "over-the-bag" technique. In this situation, the cortical and nuclear material is removed from the capsular bag and viscoelastic is injected between the anterior capsule and posterior iris. This inflates the region of the sulcus, collapsing and posteriorly displacing the bag. The laser endoscope is inserted through the cataract incision or a side port, and the processes are photocoagulated (Fig. 12-1). Advantages to this method are that the capsular bag can be inspected for residual lens material, areas of capsular tear, or zonular dehiscence. Detection permits an appropriate response. Finally, the theoretical potential for IOL dislocation is obviated by placement of the lens implant following ECP.

The second technique is the "through-the-bag" approach wherein the empty capsular bag is inflated with viscoelastic. The laser endoscope is inserted into the bag, and laser application is made to the ciliary processes

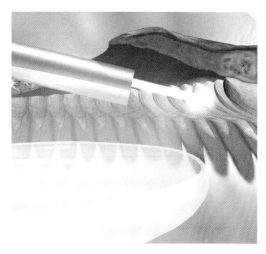

FIGURE 12-1. Over-the-bag approach.

through the capsule (Fig. 12-2). The advantages of this approach are that the capsule can be inspected for tears or dehiscence as well as residual cortical or nuclear material before IOL insertion. This approach requires fewer exchanges of viscoelastic. As a further advantage, scleral depression can be added to this technique, splaying open the "valleys" between the ciliary processes to allow more complete photocoagulation of the ciliary epithelium as described by Francisco Lima, M.D. (personal communication). The theoretical safety feature of placing the lens implant after ECP may be a factor in the surgeon's choice.

The third technique is to perform ECP after completion of cataract surgery and placement of the posterior chamber (PC) IOL and removal of all viscoelastic. In this "over-the-PC IOL" approach, new viscoelastic is placed between the anterior capsule and posterior iris, inflating the region for laser endoscope insertion (Fig. 12-3). The viscoelastic used for the phaco-IOL component of the surgery is removed for two reasons. The main purpose is

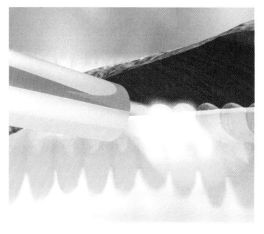

FIGURE 12-2. Through-the-bag approach.

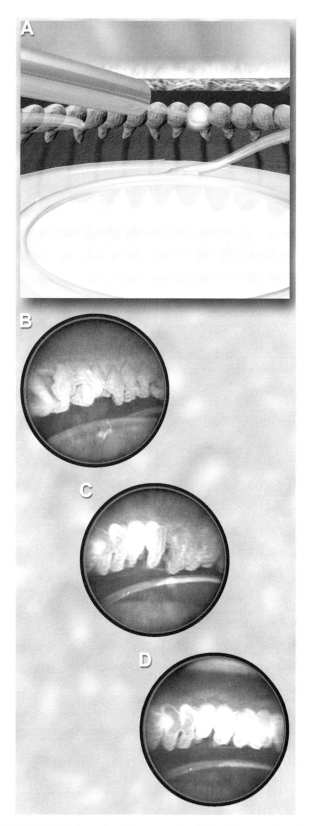

FIGURE 12-3. Over-the-IOL approach. **A:** In this scenario, the entire sequence of phacoemulsification, intraocular lens (IOL) insertion, and removal of viscoelastic is performed. Then the sulcus is inflated with viscoelastic and endoscopic cyclophotocoagulation (ECP) proceeds. **B:** IOL is well placed in capsule and the sulcus is inflated, maximizing access to the ciliary processes. **C:** ECP is initiated. **D:** ECP continues along the ciliary ring.

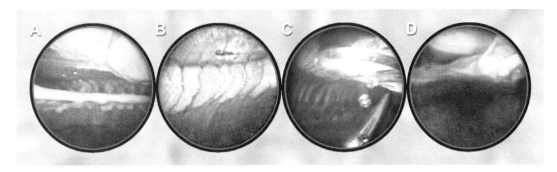

FIGURE 12-4. Capsular rupture. **A:** Capsular rupture with retraction of posterior capsule. Sulcus-placed lens is malpositioned. Note edge of optic and extent of pupillary space without intraocular lens (IOL) posterior to it. **B:** Very small rent in the posterior capsule being pierced by haptic tip. **C:** Old rupture of posterior capsule and retraction observed years after surgery in a patient undergoing vitrectomy. **D:** Old capsular dehiscence with roll-up edge in anterior chamber pseudophakia.

to maximize sulcus inflation for ECP, which may be hindered by residual material within the capsular bag. In addition, more complete viscoelastic removal seems to result when removal takes place in stages. Care must be taken to avoid injecting viscoelastic into the capsular bag. When this does occur it is certainly not a serious problem, but the surgeon will have inadvertently converted the over-the-IOL technique into the through-the-bag approach with the added task of ultimately having to remove viscoelastic from the capsular bag with an IOL in place. While this technique has the theoretical disadvantages of not being able to detect residual lens material or capsule/zonule damage before IOL insertion, it is nevertheless by far the most commonly employed approach. This method is usually the most time efficient, and the potential complications with capsule, zonule, and IOL are, in reality, rarely encountered.

Capsular tears do not necessarily preclude combining ECP with cataract surgery. Indeed, this problem may come to light only during endoscopy. The surgeon should manage this complication before ECP, if possible, so that the judgment to continue with the glaucoma portion of the surgery can be made using all of the information at hand (Fig. 12-4).

COMBINED CATARACT SURGERY AND ENDOSCOPIC CYCLOPHOTOCOAGULATION FOR UNCONTROLLED GLAUCOMA

The first reported study combining these two treatment modalities included ten patients (1). A number of issues were addressed, including final postoperative IOP, change between preoperative and postoperative glaucoma medications, early and late postoperative inflammation, postoperative cystoid macular edema (CME), 1-month and 1-year postoperative visual field loss, IOL dislocation, and visual acuity, as well as assessment of minor and devastating complications (Table 12-1).

TABLE 12-1. COMBINED PHACOEMULSIFICATION, ENDOSCOPIC CYCLOPHOTOCOAGULATION, AND POSTERIOR CHAMBER INTRAOCULAR LENS INSERTION: PREOPERATIVE AND POSTOPERATIVE STATUS

	IOP (mm Hg)		Visual Acuity		Topical Meds		CAIs		Inflammation		CME	VF Loss				Follow-up (mo)
	Preop	Final Postop	Preop	Final Postop	Preop	Final Postop	Preop	Final Postop	1 day Postop	2 mo Postop	2 mo Postop	1 mo Postop	1 yr Postop	IOL Disl	VA Loss	
1	30	12	20/70	20/25	3	1	+	−	Trace	−	−	−	−	−	−	20
2	35	17	20/100	20/50	3	1	+	−	+1	−	−	−	−	−	NEMD	20
3	28	14	20/200	20/25	3	0	−	−	Trace	−	−	−	−	−	−	20
4	30	11	20/80	20/20	2	0	+	−	Trace	−	−	−	−	−	−	20
5	30	8	20/200	20/40	3	0	−	−	+ 1	−	−	−	−	−	NEMD	20
6	27	14	20/80	20/20	2	1	+	−	+ 1	−	−	−	−	−	−	20
7	34	10	CFs	20/25	4	0	+	−	+ 1	−	−	−	−	−	−	18
8	41	26	HMs	20/80	4	4	+	+	Trace	−	−	−	+	−	BRVO	18
9	28	15	20/70	20/40	2	1	−	−	Trace	−	−	−	−	−	NEMD	18
10	31	8	20/100	20/25	3	0	+	−	+ 1	−	−	−	−	−	−	18

IOP, intraocular pressure; Meds, medications; VA, visual acuity; CAIs, carbonic anhydrase inhibitors; VF, visual field; NEMD, nonexudative macular degeneration; BRVO, branch retinal vein occlusion; CME, cystoid macular edema; CFs, counts fingers; HMs, hand movements; IOL, intraocular lens.
Data from Uram M. Combined phacoemulsification, endoscopic cyclophotocoagulation, and intraocular lens insertion in glaucoma management. *Ophthal Surg* 1995;26:346–352.

All of the study patients experienced a decrease in IOP and need for topical and systemic glaucoma medications. All demonstrated improved visual acuity. No cases of chronic inflammation, CME, visual field loss, IOL dislocation, or devastating complication were observed. This early report clearly indicated the safety of this combination of procedures. Furthermore, it has added to the evidence that in a practical sense, there is not an inherent risk to visual acuity if an inflow-reducing procedure is performed.

In this study, analyses of patients with less than desired visual acuity outcomes were due to preexisting disease, specifically nonexudative macular degeneration and branch retinal vein occlusion. It should be apparent that the visual loss associated with other inflow-reducing procedures (cyclocryotherapy, TSCPC, cyclodiathermy) is a consequence of their "blind" application and nontitratability rather than an inherently negative feature of reducing aqueous production.

Another issue related to this first study bears some scrutiny. The incidence of chronic CME after cataract surgery is about 2%, resulting in a disappointing outcome for the patient and surgeon. Certainly, it would be a nonstarter to combine any procedure with cataract surgery if this were likely to enhance the potential for this problem to develop. In this study, clinical and angiographic evidence of CME was sought 2 months after surgery, the dividing line between transient spontaneously resolving CME and chronic nonresolving CME. No such evidence was found. Much larger groups of patients treated in this fashion have also addressed this issue and will be discussed.

Of particular concern was the integrity of the zonules during and after ECP. Could the zonules withstand the manipulation required and then retain sufficient stability to support IOL implantation? From this and subsequent reports, it is apparent that the zonules are highly resilient and zonular rupture from viscoelastic injection, extrusion, and infrared laser application is not an issue.

Most zonular dehiscences that have been observed arise from two distinct situations. The first is a consequence of direct trauma from an intraocular instrument. It is not difficult to envision tearing the zonules if a phacoemulsifier tip or endoscope is literally pushed through the equator of the lens capsule or through a row of zonules when they are stretched during the over-the-bag approach to ECP. Extensive damage can arise from this situation, rendering the capsular bag too unstable for IOL insertion (Fig. 12-5). This situation can be easily avoided by recognizing the potential for this problem and taking care while working near the zonules.

A second potential cause of dehiscence is overly intensive laser application to the ciliary process adjacent to its connection with the zonule, so that a tissue explosion literally tears the zonular attachment form the process (Fig. 12-6). In this situation, usually only a few zonules are involved, and so often this focal damage serves as a warning rather than creating sufficient capsular instability to preclude posterior chamber IOL implantation.

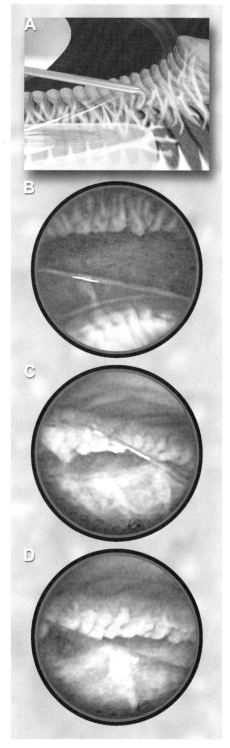

FIGURE 12-5. Zonular dehiscence. **A:** Drawing of ruptured zonules. This usually results as a consequence of mechanically tearing them with an instrument. **B:** Image of capsular dehiscence. Note posterior dislocation of intraocular lens (IOL)–capsular complex and residual white cortex within the bag. The wide separation between edge of capsule and the ciliary processes are indicative of this situation. Peripheral retina can be seen in the background. **C:** IOL haptic pierces capsule. Maneuvers to reposition have apparently ruptured adjacent zonules. **D:** Haptic now in capsular bag. Note that the posterior capsule has a V-shaped appearance because a few zonules have remained intact (creating the apex) while adjacent ones have ruptured.

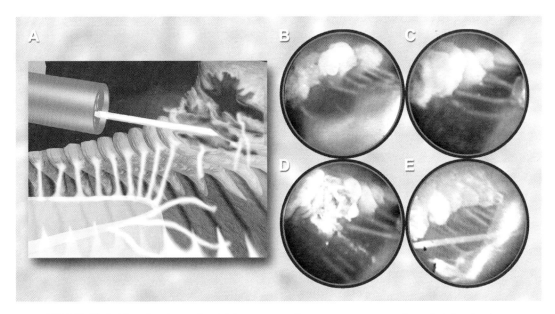

FIGURE 12-6. More focal zonular dehiscence, usually as a consequence of overly intensive laser application to a ciliary process with resultant tissue explosion tearing zonule from process surface. **A:** Drawing of focal zonular rupture. **B:** Focal zonular rupture after overly intensive endoscopic cyclophotocoagulation (ECP). **C:** Second case of same event. **D:** Third case of focal zonular rupture. **E:** Instance of focal zonular rupture from haptic trauma observed during ECP.

In another study (2), 20 patients were treated by this approach and the data were accumulated over a mean period of 29 months (range, 6 to 40 months). Once again, the safety and efficacy of this combination of surgical procedures was demonstrated by improved IOP control and no significant complications, with all experiencing improvement in visual acuity (Table 12-2). About 50% of these patients achieved the "ideal" outcome of maximized visual potential, controlled IOP, and no need for glaucoma medications.

In another report (3), uncontrolled glaucoma and cataract were managed by combined phacoemulsification and ECP (phacoemulsification/ECP). In this study, 12 patients underwent a mean of 271 degrees (± 88 degrees) of ciliary process photocoagulation. Mean IOP decreased from 27.0 (±13.7) mm Hg to 14.0 (± 3.9) mm Hg (p = 0.01). Eighty-eight percent achieved an IOP of 21 mm Hg or less. The mean number of glaucoma medications decreased from 2.8 (± 0.6) to 2.2 (± 0.9) (p = 0.03). Visual acuity improved in all patients, and there were no devastating complications (Table 12-3).

These results appear to be similar to the other reports of phacoemulsification/ECP in the setting of cataract and medically uncontrolled glaucoma.

Of particular interest are the results of the only randomized comparative study of phacoemulsification/ECP versus

TABLE 12-2. SUMMARY OF DATA ON 20 EYES TREATED BY PHACOEMULSIFICATION AND ENDOSCOPIC CYCLOPHOTOCOAGULATION

Intraocular pressure	
Preoperative	29.1 mm Hg
Postoperative	14.3 mm Hg
Absolute decrease	50.1%
Topical medications	
Preoperative	1.9%
Postoperative	0.7%
Carbonic anhydrase inhibitors	
Preoperative	65%
Postoperative	10%
Visual field loss	
1 mo postoperative	0
1 yr postoperative	10%
Improved visual acuity	100%
Devastating complications	0

Data from Uram M. Endoscopic cyclophotocoagulation in glaucoma management. *Curr Opin Ophthalmol* 1995;11:19–29.

TABLE 12-3. ENDOSCOPIC CYCLOPHOTOCOAGULATION IN THE MANAGEMENT OF UNCONTROLLED GLAUCOMA AND CATARACT

N	12
Follow-up	2 yr
ECP extent	271 degrees (±88 degrees)
Intraocular pressure	
Preoperative	27.0 mm Hg (±13.7 mm Hg)
Postoperative	14.0 mm Hg (±3.9 mm Hg)
Successful control (≤21 mm Hg)	88%
Visual acuity improvement	100%
Devastating complications	0

Data from Chen J, Cohn RA, Lin SC, et al. Endoscopic photocoagulation of the ciliary body for treatment of refractory glaucomas. *Ophthalmology* 1997;124:787–796.

TABLE 12-4. RANDOMIZED COMPARATIVE STUDY OF PHACOEMULSIFICATION PLUS TRABECULECTOMY AND PHACOEMULSIFICATION PLUS ENDOSCOPIC CYCLOPHOTOCOAGULATION IN THE MANAGEMENT OF CATARACT AND UNCONTROLLED *GLAUCOMA*[A]

Procedure	IOP Control Without Meds (%)	IOP Control With/Without Meds (%)	Postoperative Inflammation	Postoperative Hyphema	Postoperative Manipulation (%)	Devastating Complications
Phaco/Trab (n = 29)	40	92	More	Day 1—59% Week 1—26%	52	0
Phaco/ECP (n = 29)	30	95	Less	0	0	0

[a]Mean follow-up of 2 years.
IOP, intraocular pressure; ECP, endoscopic cyclophotocoagulation; Phaco, phacoemulsification; Trab, trabeculectomy.
Data from Gayton JL. Combined cataract and glaucoma surgery: trabeculectomy vs. endoscopic laser cyclophotocoagulation. *J ASCRS* 1999;25:1212–1219.

phacoemulsification/trabeculectomy (4). Here, 58 patients with mean follow-up of 2 years were randomly assigned to undergo either phacoemulsification/ECP or phacoemulsification/trabeculectomy. The 29 phacoemulsification/ECP eyes underwent 240 to 270 degrees of cyclophotocoagulation after phacoemulsification and posterior chamber IOL implantation. The 29 phacoemulsification/trabeculectomy procedures were performed in the usual manner, with 14 eyes also receiving adjunctive mitomycin-C. Uncontrolled glaucoma was defined as IOP greater than 30 mm Hg, progressive visual field loss, progressive optic nerve cupping, or any combination of these factors. Success was defined as IOP below 19 mm Hg without associated optic nerve cupping or field loss.

In the phacoemulsification/ECP group, 95% of the patients achieved success and 30% of them required no glaucoma medications to achieve this level of control (Table 12-4). In the phacoemulsification/trabeculectomy group, as expected, there was no significant difference between patients who were treated with antimetabolites and those who were not. Success was achieved in 92% of these patients, with 40% of the eyes requiring no glaucoma medications. There were no devastating complications in either group. Postoperative inflammation was more profound in the phacoemulsification/trabeculectomy group than in those who underwent ECP. In addition, 59% of the phacoemulsification/trabeculectomy eyes demonstrated hyphema on the first postoperative day and 26% continued with this problem at 1 week. No ECP patients developed hyphema. Of the phacoemulsification/trabeculectomy patients, 52% required bleb needling to maintain function. Hypotony did not evolve in any eye.

Overall, the potential for achieving good IOP control by phacoemulsification/ECP or phacoemulsification/trabeculectomy is excellent and of similar frequency. However, phacoemulsification/ECP is associated with a lower incidence of inflammation and hyphema, as well as a lower requirement for further postsurgical intervention, such as bleb manipulation. In addition, the operative technique was noted to be

simpler and the operative time shorter with phacoemulsification/ECP than phacoemulsification/trabeculectomy.

Keratometric changes following ECP also have been studied in the setting of this combined procedure (5). Mean postoperative keratometry remained within 0.25 diopter of the preoperative readings throughout a 3-month follow-up period.

Considering minor complications (transient hemorrhage, inflammation, pain, blurred vision), most reports indicate a 3% to 8% incidence. These problems are typically self-limited and require little or no management.

Phacoemulsification/ECP never been reported to be associated with a devastating complication (choroidal hemorrhage, hypotony, phthisis, endophthalmitis, loss of the eye). Despite the theoretical objections of combining an inflow procedure with cataract surgery, experience has illuminated the safety of this combination.

COMBINED PHACOEMULSIFICATION AND ENDOSCOPIC CYCLOPHOTOCOAGULATION FOR MEDICALLY CONTROLLED GLAUCOMA

What initially might seem like an avante garde use of this technology has actually proved to be the most widely applied inflow-reducing procedure in ophthalmology. Well over 10,000 such procedures have been performed worldwide.

Up to 30% of patients undergoing cataract surgery are simultaneously afflicted with glaucoma. Available medications are effective in treating this condition. Still, issues of expense and patient compliance remain. Certainly, when medical management proves to be inadequate, few would argue against combining these procedures, despite the increased risk. On the other hand, phacoemulsification/trabeculectomy would be considered inappropriate in the setting of cataract and medically controlled glaucoma because of the inherent difficulties and complications associated with this approach.

What if there were a procedure that could be combined with cataract surgery that could diminish the patient's long-term need for glaucoma medications, add little to the operative time, but not contribute to postoperative management requirements and complications? Previous experience with ECP in the management of more intractable forms of glaucoma has indicated a surprisingly safe track record, and so it was theorized that a vast number of patients might benefit from the combination of these two modalities if, indeed, the operating hypothesis proved to be true. As an aside, the longstanding belief among many ophthalmologists that the act of cataract surgery alone results, to some degree, in the long-term reduction of IOP required attention.

Mackool (unpublished data) performed a comparative randomized study of phacoemulsification/ECP versus phacoemulsification alone for the management of cataract and medically controlled glaucoma, the completion of which is nearing. Data analyzed thus far indicate a number of important points. The patients in his study underwent 180 degrees of ECP through their phacoemulsification incision, typically after posterior chamber IOL implantation. This added a few minutes to the operative time. It was observed that 87% of the phacoemulsification/ECP patients experienced at least some long-term decrease in their postoperative glaucoma regimen, whereas only 9% of the phacoemulsification-alone patients had a similar outcome. This was a highly significant difference. Furthermore, 61% of the phacoemulsification/ECP eyes required no glaucoma medications by the end of the follow-up period, compared with 5% of the phacoemulsification-alone group. Again, this was a highly significant difference. There were no instances of serious complications, visual loss, or CME.

One arm of the ECP Study Group (unpublished data) has a large number of patients with cataract and medically controlled glaucoma assigned in a randomized prospective fashion to either a phacoemulsification/ECP or phacoemulsification-alone group. This is a long-term study intended to run for a mean follow-up of 5 years. Analysis to date has demonstrated findings remarkably similar to those of Mackool (Table 12-5). Specifically, 80% of the phacoemulsification/ECP group experienced at least some decrease in their glaucoma medication requirement, as opposed to only 14% of the phacoemulsification-alone group. In addition, 54% of the phacoemulsification/ECP group discontinued all glaucoma medications long term, which was highly significant compared with the phacoemulsification-alone patients at 9%. Again, there were no devastating complications. Furthermore, the incidence of CME and major complications was not statistically different between the two groups.

In a noncomparative study by Berke and colleagues (6), 180- to 360-degree ECP was performed at the time of phacoemulsification in the setting of medically controlled glaucoma. Some of the results are recorded in Table 12-6. Their findings were similar to those of the comparative studies that were previously discussed. Again, there was a significant decrease in glaucoma medications without an associated downside of added intraoperative or postoperative complications.

Furthermore, they supported the use of ECP in a more aggressive fashion of 300 to 360 degrees for better control of IOP and medication reduction. This was an interesting notion considering that the initial studies elected 180 degrees as the treatment zone because this is typically the largest extent of the ciliary process ring that is accessible through a single incision. With the development of the curved laser endoscope that can access up to 300 degrees of the processes through a single incision, the simplicity of the approach (no additional incisions) can be maintained yet more extensive treatment achieved.

TABLE 12-5. PHACOEMULSIFICATION PLUS ENDOSCOPIC CYCLOPHOTOCOAGULATION VERSUS PHACOEMULSIFICATION ALONE IN THE MANAGEMENT OF CATARACT AND MEDICALLY CONTROLLED GLAUCOMA: COMPARISON OF TWO STUDIES

Factor	ECP Study Group[a]			Mackool[b]		
	ECP	Control	p	ECP	Control	p
n	512	501	—	24	22	—
Mean follow-up (mo)	24 (10–62)	22 (12–62)	—	24 (16–36)	44 (13–117)	—
Mean change in IOP (mm Hg)	−2.0	−1.8	0.48	−3.3	−2.4	0.48
Medications (%):						
Decrease	80	14	0.001	87	9	0.01
Same	16	68	0.01	13	73	0.01
Increase	4	18	0.01	0	18	0.001
None	54	9.4	0.01	61	5	0.01
Cystoid macular edema (%)	2.8	2.2	0.56	0	0	—
Major complications (%)	1.6	2.0	0.48	0	0	—

[a]ECP Study Group (unpublished).
[b]R.J. Mackool (unpublished).
IOP, intraocular pressure; ECP, endoscopic cyclophotocoagulation.

TABLE 12-6. PHACOEMULSIFICATION PLUS ENDOSCOPIC CYCLOPHOTOCOAGULATION IN THE MANAGEMENT OF CATARACT AND MEDICALLY CONTROLLED GLAUCOMA

N	26
Follow-up	2 yr
Extent of ECP	180–360 degrees
Mean IOP decrease	15%
Medications	
Mean preoperative	1.68 ± 0.95
Mean postoperative	0.63 ± 0.7 (*p* = 0.0005)
Mean reduction	68%
Postoperative visual loss	0
Major complications	0

IOP, intraocular pressure; ECP, endoscopic cyclophotocoagulation. Data from Berke SJ, Cohen AJ, Sturm RT. Endoscopic cyclophotocoagulation and phacoemulsification in the treatment of medically controlled primary angle glaucoma. *J Glaucoma* 2000;9:129.

DECISION MAKING

The decision to perform filtration combined with cataract surgery is a complex one, not only with respect to the myriad of technical and anatomic considerations but also with regard to weighing the substantial risks against the potential to benefit from this approach. ECP in combination with cataract surgery does not share this burden. Anatomic variables do not affect the procedure to nearly the same degree, and the additive complications seen with filtration are not relevant with ECP. This technique appears to be effective in controlling glaucoma in this setting as well as diminishing the need for glaucoma medications. Finally, it is clear that the act of cataract surgery alone only occasionally results in long-term improved IOP control or limits long-term use of glaucoma medications.

For these reasons, the decision-making process is far less grave. Because ECP does not contribute significantly to the inherent risks of cataract surgery alone, ophthalmologists have the opportunity to simultaneously address glaucoma in a simple, effective, low-risk fashion.

REFERENCES

1. Uram M. Combined phacoemulsification, endoscopic cyclophotocoagulation, and intraocular lens insertion in glaucoma management. *Ophthalmic Surg* 1995;26:346–352.
2. Uram M. Endoscopic cyclophotocoagulation in glaucoma management. *Curr Opin Ophthalmol* 1995;11:19–29.
3. Chen J, Cohn RA, Lin SC, et al. Endoscopic photocoagulation of the ciliary body for treatment of refractory glaucomas. *Ophthalmology* 1997;124:787–796.
4. Gayton JL. Combined cataract and glaucoma surgery: Trabeculectomy vs. endoscopic laser cyclophotocoagulation. *Journal of the American Society on Cataract & Refractive Surgery* 1999;25:1212–1219.
5. Gayton J. Combined surgery with an endoscopic laser. In: *Maximizing results: strategies in refractive, corneal, cataract and glaucoma surgery.* Thorofare, NJ: Slack, 1996:224–234.
6. Berke SJ, Cohen AJ, Sturm RT. Endoscopic cyclophotocoagulation and phacoemulsification in the treatment of medically controlled primary angle glaucoma. *J Glaucoma* 2000;9:129.

ENDOSCOPIC MANAGEMENT OF
PEDIATRIC GLAUCOMA

TREATMENT CHOICES

The treatment of pediatric glaucoma is challenging because of an array of factors, including dysgenesis of ocular structures, acquired disease processes resulting in intraocular structural anomalies, and surgically induced anatomic abnormalities. These eyes defy routine surgical correction, and, typically, no single management approach is effective in all or even most cases. The treatment paradigm shifts from the more orderly methodology used in adult glaucoma to one of sampling from the small array of surgical procedures that are at our disposal to achieve the best outcome. These choices include trabeculectomy, trabeculotomy, tube implantation, transscleral cyclophotocoagulation (TSCPC), standard and endoscopic goniotomy, and endoscopic cyclophotocoagulation (ECP).

Primary congenital glaucomas, characterized by inherent abnormalities in the angle structures, can be effectively addressed with goniotomy and trabeculotomy. Goniotomy is perhaps the treatment of choice in this group. Typically, a goniolens is placed on the eye to view the angle, and then the goniotomy blade is used to incise the abnormal membrane that obstructs the flow of aqueous to the angle structures. Most often, 4 or 5 clock hours are incised. Results can be quite good, with excellent outcomes in about 90% of those treated with one or several procedures during the first year of life.

In trabeculotomy, Schlemm's canal is entered through an external approach and a trabeculotome is passed in such a fashion as to break in to the anterior chamber, creating a permanent communication. The historical success rate of this procedure has been variously reported between 70% and 100% (1,2). One advantage is that it can be used despite the presence of an opaque cornea.

Considering the relative simplicity and excellent treatment outcomes associated with these techniques, it is clear that they represent the treatments of choice for initial management of primary congenital glaucomas.

Secondary glaucomas are a different matter. They can develop in association with aphakia, aniridia, Sturge-Weber syndrome, or anterior segment dysgenesis. Glaucoma has been reported in 5% to 41% of patients following congenital cataract surgery. Anterior segment dysgenesis is a consequence of abnormal neural crest cell migration and presents as an array of ophthalmic disorders, including posterior embryotoxin, Axenfeld and Reiger's anomaly and syndrome, posterior keratoconus, and Peter's anomaly. Glaucoma develops in more 50% of these patients. Aniridia can manifest a spectrum of findings, including iris anomalies, macular and optic nerve hypoplasia, nystagmus, and corneal degeneration. It is a bilateral disorder, with glaucoma occurring in 50% to 75% of patients. Sturge-Weber syndrome is one of the phakomatoses, presenting most often as a facial nevus flammeus (usually with upper eyelid or conjunctival involvement) and, among other abnormalities, hemangiomas of the conjunctiva, episclera, choroid, and retina. Glaucoma is present in about 30% of those affected.

When goniotomy or trabeculotomy has failed, so that the congenital glaucoma can now be considered refractory, or in the presence of aphakic glaucoma or other secondary forms of pediatric glaucoma, trabeculectomy, tube implantation, or ECP can be considered.

Under these circumstances, trabeculectomy performs poorly, demonstrating a significant long-term failure rate. These disappointing outcomes can be attributed to a variety of factors, including the presence of a thick Tenon's capsule, strong wound closure response, and compliance issues. Addition of mitomycin-C has enhanced the efficacy of filtration, with most reports indicating 1- to 2-year successful outcomes in 40% to 50% of those treated (3–5). Unfortunately, the cost of this success is a substantially increased the incidence of serious complications, such as visual loss (10%), bleb-related endophthalmitis (8%), and wound leaks (12%). Undoubtedly, the incidence of these problems will increase as a result of progressive thinning of avascular blebs.

Tube implantation offers some theoretical advantages in these patients. However, most studies indicate a 30% to 40% probability of success during the first year (6—8), declining after that. Major complications, such as strabismus, retinal detachment, hypotony, corneal decompensation, and tube migration or erosion, are not uncommon. Up to 32% of pediatric patients experience a decline in vision, in some cases progressing to the extreme of loss of light perception (7). In one series (6), only 44% of the patients maintained adequate intraocular pressure (IOP) control after the second postoperative year. In this study of 18 eyes, a total of 69 minor and severe complications developed during the follow-up period.

It would seem that outflow surgery in this setting can be summarized as poorly to moderately effective and associated with a significant risk for major and minor complications.

Cyclodestructive procedures, particularly cyclocryotherapy (CCT) and TSCPC, have achieved limited success in the management of primary and secondary pediatric glaucomas. In most studies, successful IOP control was achieved in 20% to 40% of the patients in three to seven treatments. The development of cataract, retinal detachment, hypotony, or phthisis is a frequent consequence of these procedures and has been reported in about one third of the patients. Indeed, phthisis may eventually occur in 10% of these eyes. Visual loss is common, typically in the 40% to 60% range. Historically, inflow procedures seem to share the same outcomes as those manipulating outflow, with poor to moderate success in controlling IOP yet with a substantial risk for the evolution of major complications. To say the least, this is not a good situation.

ENDOSCOPIC CYCLOPHOTOCOAGULATION

The first report of ECP in the management of congenital glaucoma included 18 patients who had already failed multiple surgical interventions, including goniotomy, trabeculotomy, trabeculectomy, tube implantation, and TSCPC (9). In this group, 40% presented with opaque cornea. All patients were initially treated over 180 to 240 degrees. The data are summarized in Table 13-1.

Virtually all of the patients had undergone previous TSCPC, reportedly 270 to 360 degrees. They were in fact found to have had essentially no actual treatment of the ciliary processes! In all cases, this area was missed. Many of these eyes demonstrated anomalous location of the

TABLE 13-1. OUTCOMES OF FIRST REPORT OF ENDOSCOPIC CYCLOPHOTOCOAGULATION FOR REFRACTORY CONGENITAL GLAUCOMA

N	18
Follow-up	17 mo (6–28 mo)
Intraocular pressure	
Preoperative	31.5 mm Hg (±11.2 mm Hg)
Postoperative	15.8 mm Hg[a] (±6.8 mm Hg)
Absolute decrease	49.8%
Successful control (≤2 mm Hg)	55.5%
Topical medications	
Preoperative	1.7
Postoperative	1.5[b]
Carbonic anhydrase inhibitors	
Preoperative	88.8%
Postoperative	27.7%[c]
Severe complications	11.1%[d]
Hypotony/phthisis	0
Reoperation	34.4%

[a]$p = 0.01$.
[b]$p = 0.57$.
[c]$p = 0.05$.
[d]Two patients had hemorrhagic choroidal effusion.
Data from Uram M. Endoscopic cyclophotocoagulation in glaucoma management. *Curr Opin Ophthalmol* 1995;11:19–29.

processes, most of them being very anterior, seemingly on the posterior aspect of the iris. Even during application of TSCPC guided with transillumination, it would be impossible for the surgeon to appropriately place the TSCPC probe to achieve effective treatment. As a disclaimer, it is critical to understand that the eyes in this study were previous treatment failures; there would be no need for further intervention, and therefore assessment, in eyes that were successfully treated with TSCPC.

In another study of refractory adult and pediatric glaucomas (10), 12 children were treated by 300 degrees of ECP. The mean IOP was 30.1 mm Hg preoperatively and 20.3 mm Hg postoperatively ($p = 0.001$). No devastating complications were observed.

Perhaps the most significant work in this area was reported by Neeley and Plager (11) (Tables 13-2 and 13-3).

TABLE 13-2. CHARACTERISTICS OF DIFFICULT PEDIATRIC GLAUCOMA CASES MANAGED BY ENDOSCOPIC CYCLOPHOTOCOAGULATION

N	36
Bilateral treatment	24%
Eyes with any previous surgery	94%
Mean no. previous procedures	2.75 ± 2.39 (0–11)
Eyes with previous glaucoma surgery	50%
Mean no. previous glaucoma surgeries	1.89 ± 2.45 (0–8)
Previous transscleral cyclophotocoagulation	11%

Data from Neeley DE, Plager DA. Endocyclophotocoagulation for the management of difficult pediatric glaucomas. *Journal of American Academy of Pediatric Ophthalmolgy & Strabismus* 2001;5:221–229.

TABLE 13-3. OUTCOMES OF ENDOSCOPIC CYCLOPHOTOCOAGULATION FOR DIFFICULT PEDIATRIC GLAUCOMAS: COMPARISON OF SUCCESSFUL AND UNSUCCESSFUL TREATMENTS

	Successful ECP	Unsuccessful ECP	p
n	15	20	
Follow-up (mo)	30.19 ± 24.44	11.97 ± 9.05	0.0137
Intraocular pressure			
Preoperative (mm Hg)	32.53 ± 7.83	36.42 ± 8.68	0.1804
Final (mm Hg)	16.67 ± 3.44	28.85 ± 11.98	0.0003
Reduction (mm Hg)	15.87 ± 8.17	7.68 ± 15.38	0.0562
Absolute decrease (%)	46.54 ± 15.18	15.57 ± 41.371	0.0060
ECP treatment			
No. procedures	1.20 ± 0.041	1.60 ± 1.10	0.1467
Degrees of treatment	248 ± 62	268 ± 56	0.3204
Medications			
Preoperative	1.53 ± 0.64	1.60 ± 0.82	0.7889
Final	0.60 ± 0.83	1.30 ± 1.03	0.0330

ECP, endoscopic cyclophotocoagulation.
Data from Neely DE, Plager DA. Endocyclophotocoagulation for the management of difficult pediatric glaucomas. *Journal of American Academy of Pediatric Ophthalmolgy & Strabismus* 2001;5:221–229.

In this study, refractory primary congenital glaucomas as well as aphakic and secondary pediatric glaucomas were managed by ECP. The cumulative success rate was 43%, indicating that over a mean of 1.2 treatment sessions, successful intermediate-term IOP control was achieved. Complications were few; inflammation and cystoid macular edema were notably absent. Four patients experienced significant complications. Their descriptions are summarized in Table 13-4.

Neeley and Plager make some observations regarding various outcomes following ECP. Specifically, they experienced only one instance of hypotony in the management of this difficult group of patients. Combining their data with the historical information presented in the world literature, the incidence of hypotony or phthisis following ECP is less than 1%. This is quite a remarkable result considering hypotony or phthisis has been reported as a complication of in up to 34% of CCT patients and in 10% of TSCPC patients.

Although there was some concern about the lens status in the phakic ECP patients, progressive cataract or zonular weakness was not detected.

Another issue was the potential for initiating chronic inflammation as a consequence of ECP, as observed with CCT and TSCPC. This problem did not arise as might be expected, given the histologic features of ECP. As previously explained, this technique is specifically ablative to the epithelium of the ciliary body only, without involvement of adjacent tissue, and there appears to be no tissue cellular inflammatory response. The clinical manifestation of this is a transiently increased flare on slit-lamp examination.

A vexing problem that seems to be peculiar to pediatric intraocular surgery is the postoperative development of

TABLE 13-4. COMPLICATIONS ASSOCIATED WITH ENDOSCOPIC CYCLOPHOTOCOAGULATION IN DIFFICULT PEDIATRIC GLAUCOMAS

Glaucoma Diagnosis	No. Previous Glaucoma Surgeries	Complications	Associated Data
Congenital	8	Retinal detachment Vision decrease 20/400 to LP	Aphakic Previous TSCPC
Anterior segment dysgenesis	0	Hypotony	Aphakic Complicated PKP with lensectomy
Congenital	4	Vision decrease from HMs to NLP	Aphakic Preoperative IOP 40 mm Hg
Aphakic	0	Retinal detachment	Aphakic Marshall syndrome High risk for retinal detachment

LP, light perception; TSCPC, transscleral cyclophotocoagulation; PKP, penetrating keratoplasty; HMs, hand motions; NLP, no light perception; IOP, intraocular pressure.
Data from Neeley DE, Plager DA. Endocyclophotocoagulation for the management of difficult pediatric glaucomas. *Journal of American Academy of Pediatric Ophthalmolgy & Strabismus* 2001;5:221–229.

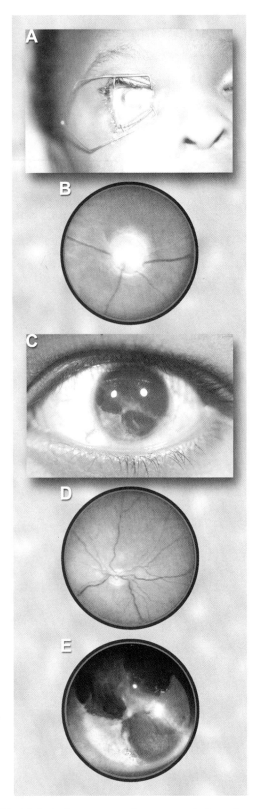

FIGURE 13-1. A: Opaque anterior segment in Peters' anomaly. **B:** Deeply excavated and atrophic optic nerve viewed endoscopically, indicates that further anterior segment surgery would be futile. **C:** A 10-year-old child with a healed corneal laceration and occluded pupil. **D:** Diagnostic endoscopy reveals a normal-appearing disc and retina. **E:** Same eye after sector iridectomy with 20/60 acuity. (A and C courtesy of Norman Medow, MD.)

severe inflammation. Although uncommon, it can create great difficulty for all concerned. Frequent application of steroid drops or ointment is, at the least, a nuisance and often not effective. Systemic steroid administration can be difficult. If the surgeon is wary that this problem may complicate the postoperative course, intraocular injection of dexamethasone (Decadron 0.1 to 1.0 mL) has proved useful in almost ensuring a quiet eye.

Medow and Sauer (12) were among the first to use endoscopy in the management of pediatric ophthalmic disease. While a number of studies are in progress, they have elucidated a few areas in which this approach can be helpful.

Occasionally, one may be confronted with a child of any age who demonstrates an opaque cornea or some other derangement of anterior segment architecture that obstructs a posterior view in association with a normal-appearing ultrasound. Particularly in the setting of glaucoma, diagnostic endoscopy can be of great value. A single incision can permit insertion of the endoscope to evaluate the ocular interior. If an atrophic or extensively excavated disc is observed (or some other major abnormality), further surgical intervention of a more profound nature can be avoided (Fig. 13-1). If, on the other hand, the retina and optic nerve appear to be at least somewhat functional, the surgeon may proceed with more aggressive treatment to salvage what is possible. In the case of the glaucomatous eye, ECP can be performed at that time.

ENDOSCOPIC GONIOTOMY

One of the most significant impediments to successful performance of goniotomy concerns the frequent combination of uncontrolled IOP and opaque cornea. The technique of goniotomy is straightforward as long as the angle can be viewed. It is the inability to visually monitor the progress of surgery that results in inadequate treatment and complications. The endoscope is ideal for this procedure in that it circumvents the need to image from outside of the eye to access the interior.

Endoscopic goniotomy can be performed by a one-handed or a bimanual technique. First, a beveled clear corneal incision is made that is not water tight. This ensures ease of mobility when manipulating the endoscope and other instruments. Children's eyes tend to collapse in the presence of open incisions, so some measures must be taken to maintain the stability and depth of the anterior chamber. This can be achieved with infusion through an anterior chamber maintainer or by filling the anterior chamber with a nondispersive viscoelastic. If a bimanual approach is selected (Fig. 13-2), the endoscope is introduced into the anterior chamber by one of the surgeons or by an assistant. It is held in position in such a way as to monitor the course of surgery despite any corneal opacities. The surgeon then introduces a goniotomy (or other) blade through a second

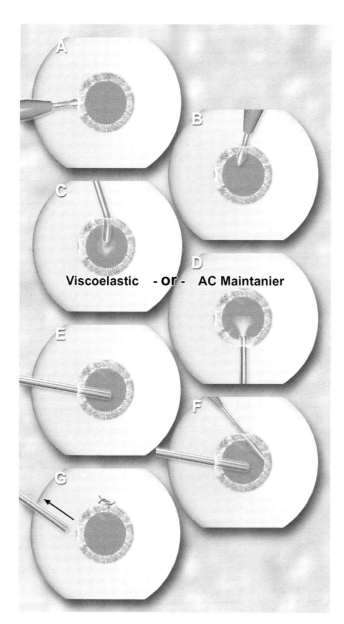

Viscoelastic - or - AC Maintanier

FIGURE 13-2. Endoscopic goniotomy: bimanual technique. **A:** Generous clear corneal incision is fashioned. **B:** A second clear corneal incision is made about 90 degrees from the first. **C:** Viscoelastic fills the anterior chamber. **D:** Alternately, an anterior chamber maintainer is inserted (third incision) to maintain depth. **E:** Surgeon or assistant inserts endoscope and maintains view of potential goniotomy site. **F:** Surgeon inserts blade and, under endoscopic visualization, performs goniotomy. **G:** All instruments are withdrawn and viscoelastic removed. Incisions are sutured.

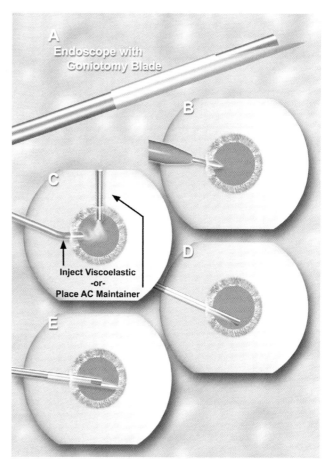

Endoscope with Goniotomy Blade

Inject Viscoelastic -or- Place AC Maintainer

FIGURE 13-3. Endoscopic goniotomy: single-handed technique. **A:** The goniotomy blade slides onto the shaft of the endoscope and is retracted toward the handle so that the blade does not protrude beyond the endoscope tip. **B:** A generous clear corneal bevelled incision is fashioned. **C:** Viscoelastic is injected or an anterior chamber maintainer is placed. **D:** The endoscope with blade is inserted into the anterior chamber and the goniotomy blade is now advanced so that it extends beyond the tip of the endoscope. **E:** The instrument is advanced until the blade engages the target tissue and then the goniotomy is performed under endoscopic visualization.

clear corneal incision that is about 90 degrees from the first entry site. While looking at the video monitor, the surgeon passes the blade into the region of the angle and, under direct visualization, creates the desired incision (Fig. 13-3). The instruments are withdrawn from the eye and the viscoelastic is removed. It is important to suture the incision sites. In an adult eye, this would not be necessary presum-

ably because of the geometry of the incision and the rigidity of the eye. In children, these wounds tend to leak, creating a host of problems that we have tried to avoid all along. Materials for this purpose vary widely, including 10-0 nylon and 10-0 Vicryl.

An alternative is the single-handed approach (Fig. 13-4). In this method, a goniotomy blade is slid over the endoscope and retracted toward the handpiece, so that the blade does not protrude beyond the tip. A clear corneal incision is fashioned and viscoelastic injected or an anterior chamber maintainer placed. The endoscope with blade is introduced into the anterior chamber, and then the goniotomy blade is advanced on the shaft of the endoscope so that it extends beyond the tip. The endoscope is advanced until the blade engages the target tissue. The surgeon's second

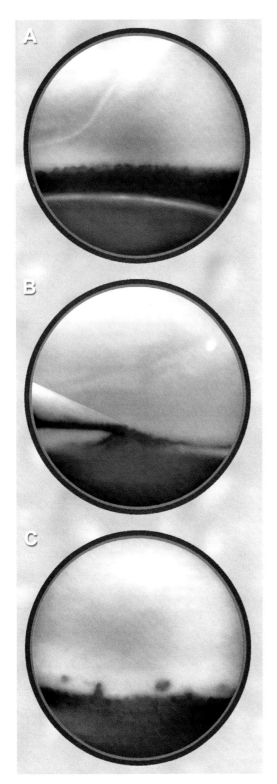

FIGURE 13-4. A: Endoscopic goniotomy. **B:** Blade engages tissue. **C:** Same area after dividing tissue anterior to angle structures.

hand can be used to steady the endoscope. After an adequate goniotomy has been performed, the instruments and any viscoelastic are removed from the eye and the incision or incisions sutured.

This approach can be effective in achieving the physical goal of goniotomy. It may be especially beneficial in the more intractable cases, in which the difficulty may be not so much the potential for the eye to respond to this technique but rather the surgeon's ability to adequately execute it, given the impediments to visualization that these eyes can present. Certainly, additional experience will be required to establish the validity of this approach.

CONCLUSION

In the setting of childhood glaucoma, ECP represents another tool in the arsenal. One may debate where exactly it fits in the scheme of things. Whereas ECP typically achieves IOP control in the range of 90% for adult glaucoma, regardless of the mechanism or severity, the procedure's success in children is only moderate. Few serious complications have been observed, and the reoperation rate is lower than for TSCPC. In addition, the immediate and long-term risks of filtration with or without mitomycin-C and the difficulties associated with tube implantation can all be avoided. The minimally invasive nature of ECP clearly has advantages. Although goniotomy and trabeculotomy are most appropriate for primary congenital glaucoma, it seems absurd to consider TSCPC for refractory patients or those with secondary or aphakic forms of medically uncontrolled disease. Perhaps future experience will make clear whether tube implantation or ECP is the treatment of choice. No matter what order these therapeutic alternatives occupy in the surgeon's management paradigm of pediatric glaucoma, it is invaluable to have a new and significant option, such as ECP, when addressing a disorder that may not respond to *any* treatment modality at all.

Finally, one might conjecture that the combination of an outflow procedure, such as tube implantation, in combination with an inflow-reducing technique, specifically ECP, might prove to be beneficial for the more difficult cases of pediatric glaucoma. After all, resetting the balance between inflow and outflow in a given eye is not a scientifically based titratable maneuver, but rather one that relies on the surgeon's experience and fund of empirical knowledge, as well as some luck. This combined approach might be an important one to study.

REFERENCES

1. deLuise VP, Anderson DR. Primary infantile glaucoma. *Surv Ophthalmol* 1983;28:1–23.

2. McPherson SD Jr. Results of external trabeculotomy. *Am J Ophthalmol* 1973;76:918–922.
3. Freedman SF, McCormick M, Cox TA. Mitomycin-C augmented trabeculectomy in postoperative wound modulation in pediatric glaucoma. *Journal of American Academy of Pediatric Ophthalmolgy & Strabismus* 1999;3:117–124.
4. Mandal AK, Walton DS, John T, Jayagandan A. Mitomycin-C augmented trabeculectomy in refractory congenital glaucoma. *Ophthalmology* 1997;104;996–1001.
5. Susanna R, Oltrogge EW, Carani JCE, et al. Mitomycin as adjunct chemotherapy with trabeculectomy in congenital and developmental glaucomas. *J Glaucoma* 1995;4:15–17.
6. Coleman AL, Smyth RJ, Wilson MR, Tam M. Initial clinical experience with the Ahmed glaucoma valve implant in pediatric patients. *Arch Ophthalmol* 1997;115:186–191.
7. Eid TE, Katz JL, Spaeth GL, Augsburger JJ. Long-term effects of tube-shunt procedures on management of refractory childhood glaucomas. *Ophthalmology* 1997;104:1101–1106.
8. Wallace DK, Plager DA, Snyder SK, et al. Surgical results of secondary glaucomas in childhood. *Ophthalmology* 1998;105:101–111.
9. Uram M. Endoscopic cyclophotocoagulation in glaucoma management. *Curr Opin Ophthalmol* 1995;11:19–29.
10. Chen J, Cohn RA, Lin SC, et al. Endoscopic photocoagulation of the ciliary body for treatment of refractory glaucomas. *Ophthalmology* 1997;124:787–796.
11. Neeley DE, Plager DA. Endocyclophotocoagulation for the management of difficult pediatric glaucomas. *JAAPOS* 2001;5:221–229.
12. Medow NB, Sauer HL. Goniotomy for congenital glaucoma. *J Pediatr Ophthalmol Strabismus* 1997;34:258–259.

ENDOSCOPIC CYCLOPHOTOCOAGULATION FOR POST-PENETRATING KERATOPLASTY GLAUCOMA

Glaucoma may result as a consequence of corneal transplantation for a variety of reasons in the early and late postoperative periods. This problem may ultimately result in profound visual loss either from the effects of markedly elevated intraocular pressure (IOP) or as a consequence of graft rejection. It is therefore important to identify the underlying cause.

ETIOLOGY

If glaucoma develops in the early postoperative period, one must consider the typical causes of this problem that might be seen after any form of intraocular surgery, including transient inflammation, steroid response, pupillary block, and intraocular hemorrhage. Several other mechanisms also have been proposed to account for the IOP rise in these patients, such as compression of the angle structures as a consequence of the surgical technique or collapse or distortion of the trabecular meshwork arising from the loss of structural support following Descemet membrane incision. The overall incidence of this problem has been reported to be 9% to 31%.

On the other hand, a marked and chronic elevation in IOP may develop as a late effect of corneal transplantation, and this form of post-penetrating keratoplasty (post-PK) glaucoma is the focus here.

There are numerous potential causes of post-PK glaucoma, with a reported incidence of 18% to 29% (1–3). Some of these underlying problems are listed in Table 14-1.

By far the most common problem contributing to the development and progression of post-PK glaucoma is the formation of peripheral anterior synechiae (PASs). By physically impeding access to the angle, therapeutic measures directed to facilitating aqueous outflow often fail. If the PASs are newly developed, laser or mechanical lysis can normalize function. If the PASs become longstanding, however, an alternative method of diminishing IOP is necessary.

Typically, surgical intervention is required, the indications being a threatened corneal graft or optic nerve. Trabeculectomy has had low effectiveness in this situation, with very low potential for successful IOP control while posing a substantial risk for chronic graft failure. In addition, the risk of development of an immediate or delayed-onset choroidal hemorrhage is significant.

Tube implantation has fared better, at least as far as controlling the IOP is concerned. In one or more surgeries, success has been achieved in about 70% of patients. Still, this result has come at a high cost, for the incidence of acute graft rejection is 35% to 41% and of chronic rejection in 23% to 42% of eyes. There is also a significant risk for the development of serious complications, reported in up to 30% eyes with tube implants (4–7).

Transscleral cyclophotocoagulation can be performed on multiple occasions to optimize success in controlling IOP. About 50% to 70% of these eyes will ultimately achieve controlled IOP. Nevertheless, the incidence of graft rejection is high, reported in up to 44%; this is accompanied by a host of serious complications, including a 40% to 50% incidence of visual loss and 10% risk of phthisis (2,8–10).

TABLE 14-1. ETIOLOGIC FEATURES OF EARLY AND LATE POST-PENETRATING KERATOPLASTY GLAUCOMA

Early (9%–31%)
- Inflammation
- Steroid response
- Pupillary block
- Hemorrhage
- Compression of angle
- Distortion/collapse of trabecular meshwork

Late (18%–29%)
- Chronic graft rejection
- Steroid response
- Peripheral anterior synechiae
- Pigmentary dispersion
- Aphakic penetrating keratoplasty with intact vitreous face
- Epithelial ingrowth
- Aphakia and preexisting glaucoma
- Combined penetrating keratoplasty and cataract surgery
- Repeat penetrating keratoplasty
- Early choroidal detachment and hypotony (resolves with angle-closure and late glaucoma)

There are clearly no good historical choices for the management of this problem.

TECHNIQUE

Eyes with post-PK glaucoma can be managed with endoscopic cyclophotocoagulation (ECP) through a limbal or pars plana approach, whichever is more efficacious. If there is marked disruption of anterior chamber, iris/lens, or iridocapsular architecture, it is sometimes more effective to perform the entire treatment through the pars plana or to have multiple entry sites, both anterior and posterior (Fig. 14-1).

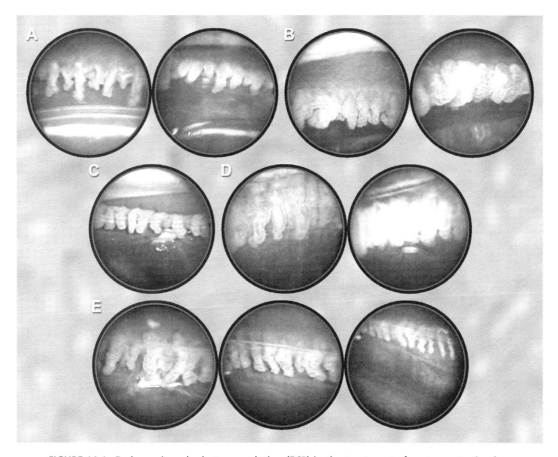

FIGURE 14-1. Endoscopic cyclophotocoagulation (ECP) in the treatment of post-penetrating keratoplasty glaucoma. **A:** Posterior chamber pseudophakia with preoperative IOP of 46 mm Hg on MMT before and after 360-degree ECP. Final IOP was 17 mm Hg. **B:** Posterior chamber pseudophakia with preoperative IOP 33 mm Hg on MMT before and after 300-degree ECP. Final IOP was 20 mm Hg. **C:** Posterior chamber pseudophakia, pars plana approach with preoperative IOP of 40 mm Hg on MMT with 300-degree ECP. Final IOP was 12 mm Hg. **D:** Posterior chamber pseudophakia pars plana approach with preoperative IOP of 29 mm Hg on MMT with 300-degree ECP. Final IOP was 19 mm Hg. **E:** Anterior chamber pseudophakia pars plana approach with preoperative IOP of 37 mm Hg on MMT with 270-degree ECP. Final postoperative IOP was 20 mm Hg.

TABLE 14-2. HISTORICAL DATA COMPARING SURGICAL TREATMENTS, THEIR SUCCESS, AND INCIDENCE OF CHRONIC CORNEAL TRANSPLANT REJECTION

Procedure	Successful IOP Control (%)	Chronic Graft Rejection (%)
Trabeculectomy	25	30
Tube implantation	70	30–42
TSCPC	50–70	44
ECP	90	0

IOP, intraocular pressure; TSCPC, transscleral cyclophotocoagulation; ECP, endoscopic cyclophotocoagulation.

RESULTS

Chen and associates (11) reported on a group of 16 patients with post-PK glaucoma with a mean follow-up of 15.4 ± 6.1 months (range, 7.8 to 25.8 months). This group experienced 90% success in controlling IOP (≤21 mm Hg) with no devastating complications or visual loss. One of the 16 patients (6%) developed signs of acute graft rejection, which resolved within 10 days; remarkably, no patients experienced a chronic rejection event.

Although this relatively small group of ECP patients was not studied in a comparative fashion, the data indicate a very high success rate, minimal complications, and sparing of the corneal graft (Fig. 14.1). Post-PK glaucoma patients require an extensive amount of ECP, 300 to 360 degrees, to achieve a satisfactory result.

A consideration for future study concerns patients in whom retransplantation is contemplated. After their first PK, they were found either to be steroid responders or to develop frank post-PK glaucoma, requiring surgical intervention. Should these patients undergo prophylactic ECP? A pilot study is currently under way to assess the value of this approach.

While the management of post-PK glaucoma requires further study, the data are highly suggestive that ECP may represent the best hope for maximizing the potential for IOP control while achieving one of the cardinal therapeutic goals of the treatment in the first place—saving the corneal graft. This facet represents one area where conventional medical, laser, and surgical therapy have failed (Table 14-2).

REFERENCES

1. Simmons RB, Stern RA, Teekhasaenee C, Kenyon KR. Elevated intraocular pressure following penetrating keratoplasty. *Trans Am Ophthalmol Soc* 1989;87:79–91.
2. Wheatcroft S, Singh A, Casey T, McAllister J. Treatment of glaucoma following penetrating keratoplasty with transscleral YAG cyclophotocoagulation. *Int Ophthalmol* 1992;16:397–400.
3. Foulks GN. Glaucoma associated with penetrating keratoplasty. *Ophthalmology* 1987;94:871–874.
4. Fellenbaum PS, Almeida AR, Minckler DS, et al. Krupin disc implantation for complicated glaucomas. *Ophthalmology* 1994;101:1178–1182.
5. McDonnell PJ, Robin JB, Schanzlin DJ, et al. Molteno implant for control of glaucoma in eyes with penetrating keratoplasty. *Ophthalmology*1988;95:364–369,
6. Sherwood MB, Smith MF, Driebe WT Jr, et al. Drainage tube implants in the treatment of glaucoma following penetrating keratoplasty. *Ophthalmic Surg* 1993;24:185–189.
7. Sidoti PA, Baerveldt G. Glaucoma drainage implants. *Curr Opin Ophthalmol* 1994;11:85–91.
8. Cohen EJ, Schwartz LW, Luskind RD, et al. Neodymium:YAG laser transscleral cyclophotocoagulation for glaucoma after penetrating keratoplasty. *Ophthalmic Surg* 1989;20:713–716.
9. Noureddin BN, Wilson-Holt N, Lavin M, et al. Advanced uncontrolled glaucoma: Nd YAG cyclophotocoagulation or tube surgery. *Ophthalmology*1992;99:430–437.
10. Shields MB, Shields SE. Non-contact transscleral Nd:YAG cyclophotocoagulation: a long-term follow-up of 500 patients. *Trans Am Ophthalmol Soc* 1994;92:271–278.
11. Chen J, Cohn RA, Lin SC, et al. Endoscopic photocoagulation of the ciliary body for treatment of refractory glaucomas. *Ophthalmology* 1997;124:787–796.

ENDOSCOPIC CYCLOPHOTOCOAGULATION FOR KERATOPROSTHESIS GLAUCOMA

KERATOPROSTHESES

The need for keratoprosthesis implantation is, fortunately, quite small. Most of us do not have to attend such patients or deal with their ongoing difficulties. Nevertheless, severe glaucoma often develops in these eyes, and its diagnosis and management can be vexing.

Most eyes requiring this extreme intervention share a few common causes. By far the most frequent problem necessitating keratoprosthetics is alkali- and, to a lesser extent, acid-induced destruction of the external ocular surface. Far less common are patients with cicatricial ocular pemphigoid, Stevens-Johnson syndrome, or trauma, or those whose eyes have irreversibly failed repeated corneal transplants.

There are a variety of keratoprosthetics, the geometry, optical design, and composition of which are the focus of ongoing research. However, there are essentially two basic methods for implantation of these devices: one anchors the prosthetic to the cornea, and the other implants it through permanently fused eyelids. A host of intraoperative and postoperative complications can be experienced with these devices (Table 15-1).

Cornea-Anchored Keratoprostheses

The focus of this discussion will be on the glaucoma associated with these eyes. To begin, one can easily imagine how a corneally anchored keratoprosthetic would permit more opportunities for glaucoma treatment than would those inserted through the eyelids. First, there is access to the external ocular surface. Therapeutic trials of various glaucoma medications may be attempted to improve the situation. Failing this, transscleral cyclophotocoagulation (TSCPC) might theoretically be attempted to address the elevated intraocular pressure (IOP) without having to actually open the eye surgically. However, there seem to be no reports of this in the peer-reviewed world literature. Given that the initial pathology was extreme ocular surface disruption, filtration surgery would be doomed to failure. Tube implantation has been reported with fairly good outcome. One study (1) described 55 keratoprosthetic eyes, of which glaucoma developed in 36 (64%). All underwent tube implantation; IOP was controlled in 81%, with 25% requiring additional medication and 14% ultimately experiencing progressive glaucomatous damage.

Eyelid-Implanted Keratoprostheses

In patients with keratoprostheses implanted through the eyelids, the difficulty of even detecting glaucoma should be apparent. Often the only indication that there is a problem is when the patient experiences diminishing visual function. Assessment of IOP is usually estimated by "finger tension" and optic nerve status determined by viewing with the direct ophthalmoscope through the keratoprosthetic.

From a therapeutic vantage, topical therapy is not possible, nor is filtration surgery, tube implantation, or TSCPC because the ocular surface cannot be approached. Extensive surgery would be required to access a large enough surface

TABLE 15-1. COMPLICATIONS ASSOCIATED WITH KERATOPROSTHESES

Intraoperative expulsive choroidal hemorrhage
Hypotony
Extrusion
Retinal detachment
Retroprosthetic membrane
Reoperation
Vitritis
Eyelid necrosis surrounding optical cylinder
Endophthalmitis
Fistulization with aqueous leak
Eyelid cellulitis
Macular edema
Vitreous hemorrhage
Choroidal effusion
Glaucoma

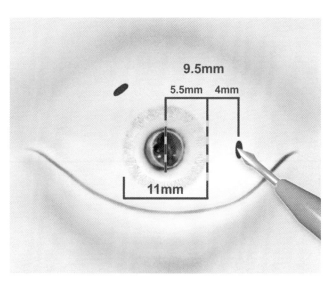

FIGURE 15-1. Estimating incision sites for endoscopic cyclophotocoagulation with eyelid-anchored keratoprostheses.

area to theoretically create a trabeculectomy or implant a seton, but postoperatively, these areas could not be monitored. Essentially, there was no treatment methodology available to address this situation. It would seem that ECP is ideal in that only one or two small sclerotomy incision sites are required to execute the procedure, and monitoring these sites after surgery is not necessary.

A study of six patients with lid-implanted keratoprostheses and uncontrolled glaucoma managed by ECP has been described (2). In all but one case, the precipitating event resulting in anterior segment destruction was alkalai contact; the remaining patient suffered from Stevens-Johnson syndrome.

ENDOSCOPIC CYCLOPHOTOCOAGULATION

Technique

The ECP technique is fairly straightforward, although two assumptions must be made in order to proceed: the keratoprosthesis is presumed to be centered, and the pars plana is expected to be located as it would be in a normal eye.

As implied by these assumptions, it initially seemed that the only possible route into these eyes would be to estimate the location of the pars plana. Assuming keratoprosthesis centration, an 11-mm-diameter cornea, and the desired insertion site 3.5 to 4.5 mm from the theoretical limbus, one would make the incision 9 to 10 mm (corneal radius of 5.5 mm + 3.5 to 4.5 mm) from the center of the keratoprosthesis (Fig. 15-1).

The skin of the eyelid is marked with this distance and then a no. 15 blade (or surgeon's preference) is used to incise the skin down to the sclera. This is easier said than done. Once the sclera is reached, it is best not make the incision but rather to do a bit more dissection, exposing enough sclera so that it can be sutured later. It would be ill advised to leave the sclerotomy open at the completion of

surgery; on the other hand, it is more difficult to expose more sclera for suturing at the conclusion of surgery when the eye is still open.

Once the sclerotomy is fashioned, the laser endoscope is inserted. Because the pars plana is "below" the ciliary processes, it must be tilted "upward" to access the target tissue. If the keratoprosthesis has a long vault, it will extend posteriorly into the vitreous cavity. It is best not to repeatedly bump into it. Some prostheses have a shorter optical vault that does not impede the approach to the ciliary processes. Vitrectomy is typically not required.

Ciliary Body in Keratoprosthesis Glaucoma

In this group, all but one patient experienced destruction of the ocular surface due to alkalai contact (2). When viewing the ciliary processes in these eyes, intraocular damage characterized by pigmentary disruption and gliosis was observed to varying degrees. In addition, the ciliary processes appeared to be "melted," with flattening of their normally convex shape (Fig. 15-2). In effect, the ciliary body appeared much as it does after cyclocryotherapy. A search must be made for "viable"-appearing processes, and the degree to which ciliary body destruction has already taken place should be appreciated before one decides on the extent of ECP to be performed. This may necessitate the creation of a second sclerotomy site with all of its associated difficulties. Alternatively, a curved endoscope can be used to access a broader region through a single incision, assuming that its geometry does not conflict with the positioning of the keratoprosthesis.

Initially, it was thought that eyes with keratoprosthesis glaucoma would respond in a manner that was similar to

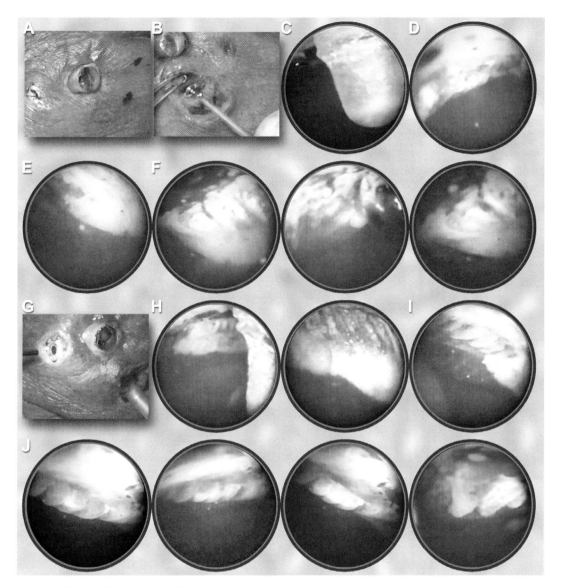

FIGURE 15-2. Images of ciliary processes and pars plana destroyed as a consequence ocular surface alkalai injury. **A:** External view of eyelid anchored prosthesis with marks for three incision sites. **B:** Insertion of laser endoscope through a trocar placed in the sclerotomy site. **C:** View of the long vault of a keratoprosthesis in the posterior chamber. **D:** Images of a "wiped-out" posterior iris-ciliary body region presumably due to the original anterior segment injury and its subsequent inflammatory response. **E:** Extensive destruction of pars plana region that bears a similar appearance to cyclocryotherapy. **F:** Alkalai injury and its inflammatory response have apparently destroyed a large area of ciliary processes. **G:** Because there was so little ciliary process tissue to laser in this hemisphere, the laser endoscope was removed from the first site and replaced with an infusion cannula. This is where using a trocar system can be quite helpful because it would be relatively difficult to suture an infusion cannula in this situation. A second sclerotomy site was created and the laser endoscope is inserted. **H:** Looking around the keratoprosthesis, this panoramic view indicates previous damage to the ciliary body in this hemisphere as well. **I:** Some viable ciliary processes are located, and endoscopic cyclophotocoagulation (ECP) is performed. The border between previously damaged ciliary processes/pars plana and uninvolved tissue is visible. **J:** ECP of viable ciliary process tissue.

those with post-penetrating keratotomy glaucoma, that is, require extensive ECP to achieve an adequate response. This assumption was probably accurate. However, not until the ciliary body in the first keratoprosthesis patient was observed did it become apparent that these eyes might behave more like those with neurovascular glaucoma, being quite sensitive to cyclophotocoagulation, presumably because a portion of the ciliary body was already rendered nonfunctional with diminished baseline aqueous production. In this situation, it is important to determine the extent of destroyed (nonfunctional) ciliary body before initiating treatment. As an example, if a single sclerotomy images 180 degrees and most of the processes are damaged, only a minimal amount of ECP should be performed. In this case, there is most likely extensive involvement of the other half of the ciliary body, so that very little cyclophotocoagulation would be expected to create a considerable effect.

The opposite situation was observed in the Stevens-Johnson syndrome patient. In that case, as one would surmise, the ciliary body was normal in appearance, and so almost 360 degrees of ECP was performed with a good outcome.

Once ECP has been completed, the endoscope is removed from the eye. At this juncture, one can elect to inject an antibiotic, such as vancomycin, 500 to 1000 μm, into the vitreous cavity, as well as 0.1 to 0.3 mL of dexamethasone (Decadron) as a prophylactic measure. Recall that there is no opportunity to use intraocular or topical medications after the completion of surgery. The sclerotomy sites and skin incisions can then be closed.

Results

As far as IOP was concerned, all of the patients experienced at least some decrease in IOP. Indeed, all but one eye was soft. Unfortunately, one of the six eyes developed phthisis. "Successful" IOP control was achieved in 67%. In addition, all but one patient discontinued systemic carbonic anhy-drase inhibitors, which is the only glaucoma medication that these patients can use. There was no perioperative visual field loss.

There were a number of deteriorating features in these patients despite a "good" outcome. Progressive visual field loss, as measured at least 1 year after surgery, was observed in 33%. Apparently, the destructive forces that are active in these eyes can continue despite the successful manipulation of one variable, IOP. Loss of visual acuity was observed in 33% of these patients, presumably for the same reason that progressive field loss occurs. There appeared to be no other findings to explain this observation. Transient vitreous hemorrhage was seen in 50% of patients and was undoubtedly due to the creation of sclerotomy sites or instrument manipulation within the eye. Spontaneous resolution was the rule. Aside from phthisis, there were no other devastating complications. Finally, 33% of these patients required a second surgery to achieve these results (Table 15-2).

In summary, ECP seems to be the only method available for management of keratoprosthesis glaucoma with eyelid-implanted prostheses (Table 15-3). It may also be similarly valuable in eyes with keratoprostheses anchored to the cornea, although these patients have more options (medication, tube implantation). ECP demonstrates far less morbidity and possibly more efficacy than tube implantation in this setting. Finally, there may be some benefit to prophylactic ECP in these keratoprosthesis patients in view of their great propensity to develop blinding glaucoma. Only further experience will tell.

TABLE 15-2. ENDOSCOPIC CYCLOPHOTOCOAGULATION IN THE MANAGEMENT OF KERATOPROSTHESIS GLAUCOMA

	Patient						Successful result (%)
	1	2	3	4	5	6	
Etiology	Alkalai	Alkalai	SJS	Alkalai	Alkalai	Alkalai	
IOP (finger tension)							
Preop	Hard	Hard	Hard	Hard	Hard	Hard	
Last postop	Soft	Soft	Soft	Moderate	Soft-moderate	Phthisis	67
Systemic CAIs							
Preop	Yes	Yes	No	Yes	Yes	Yes	83
Postop	No	No	No	Yes	No	No	17
VF loss							
Periop	No	No	No	No	No	No	0
1-yr postop	No	No	No	Yes	No	Yes	33
Reoperation	No	No	No	Yes	Yes	No	33
VA loss	No	No	No	Yes	No	Yes	33
Minor complications	No	Yes[a]	Yes[a]	No	Yes[a]	No	50
Devastating complications[b]	No	No	No	No	No	No	0

[a]Vitreous hemorrhage.
[b]Except phthisis.
SJS, Stevens-Johnson syndrome; IOP, intraocular pressure; CAIs, carbonic anhydrase inhibitors; VF, visual field; VA, visual acuity.
Data from Uram M. Endoscopic cyclophotocoagulation in the management of keratoprosthesis glaucoma (*in press*).

TABLE 15-3. ADVANTAGES OF ENDOSCOPIC CYCLOPHOTOCOAGULATION IN THE TREATMENT OF KERATOPROSTHESIS GLAUCOMA

- Only option in eyelid-implanted keratoprostheses
- Another treatment option in corneally anchored keratoprostheses
- Far less intraoperative and postoperative complications than tubes
- Potential prophylactic benefit

REFERENCES

1. Netland PA, Terada H, Dohlman CH. Glaucoma associated with keratoprosthesis. *Ophthalmology* 1998;105:751–757.
2. Uram M. Endoscopic cyclophotocoagulation in the management of keratoprosthesis glaucoma (*in press*).

ENDOSCOPIC POSTERIOR VITRECTOMY AND VIEWING TECHNIQUES

BASIC CONCEPTS

Endoscopy and laser delivery for the purpose of endoscopic cyclophotocoagulation (ECP) requires a major paradigm shift in glaucoma treatment. To use this approach, new technology, surgical methodologies, and complication management must be mastered. Although it is not difficult under most circumstances to achieve facility with ECP, the surgeon must undergo a complete transformation in order to perform it. Vitrectomy does not require this adjustment.

Benefits

The value of ophthalmic endoscopy centers on two basic advantages. The first of these is the fact that it allows a posterior view when anterior segment conditions preclude a posterior view. Corneal opacification, flattened or blood-filled anterior chamber, miotic pupil, opacified lens or lens capsule, and cyclitic membrane are but a few of the possible impediments that may be encountered. Recall that the image appearing on the endoscope-assisted video monitor is derived from the tip of the endoscope. A pars plana insertion by definition bypasses these obstacles. As will be discussed shortly, ultimate addressing of these anterior segment conditions may or may not be required.

The second broad area of advantage conferred by endoscopy is generated by its ability to image anatomy not accessible by other means in a given eye. The posterior iris, sulcus, and ciliary body are impossible to see in a particular eye on surgeon demand. The pars plana and peripheral retina can often be a problem as well.

To many vitrectomy surgeons, a significant limitation to accomplishing the surgical goal is loss of image clarity to a sufficient degree that surgery becomes impossible. It is under these circumstances that endoscopy can be most powerful.

When to Use

Some discussion has arisen regarding how often this technique should be used. *In every case* may be the proper answer. First, the surgeon can never know what is being missed if he or she fails to look. A typical example of this is when a "simple" vitrectomy for vitreous hemorrhage is performed through the operating microscope. At the completion of surgery, insertion of the endoscope often reveals a significant amount of residual hemorrhage and vitreous. It may be argued that leaving this material behind is not important to the surgical outcome, and indeed it may not be. But that is not the point. The fact that so much biomaterial remains in the eye illustrates that conventional imaging may not reveal the totality of each eye's anatomic status. In patients with active proliferation, this residual material may become a key feature in eventual failure.

Furthermore, some of the endoscopically monitored vitrectomy skills can be difficult to acquire, and, unless the surgeon is somewhat accomplished in endoscopic imaging, it will be difficult or impossible to achieve the desired goal. For example, endoscopic membranectomy can be challenging because there is no stereopsis. The surgeon must have a good "feel" for where exactly the instrumentation is within the eye. This ability usually cannot be acquired on a casual basis.

As will be discussed, some vitrectomy techniques are actually simpler to perform when imaged endoscopically. Peripheral retinal endophotocoagulation and air-fluid exchange fall into this category. The skill level needed for these maneuvers is not staggering, and many surgeons can perform them on the first try. Using these techniques can save a vast amount of time during surgery as well as minimize frustration when the operating microscope view becomes inadequate.

The tradeoff between stereopsis and panorama was discussed previously but is of greatest importance regarding endoscopic vitrectomy. We have all learned that stereoscopic vision enables most posterior segment surgery and in some disorders, such as macular pucker, this assertion is true. Stereopsis is paramount for successful execution. However, in many other posterior segment disorders this ability is less significant. Three-dimensional vision is not particularly important when removing vitreous with a vitrector, creating retinotomies or retinectomies, peeling membranes from the more peripheral portions of the retina, removing fragments of lens anteriorly and posteriorly, or performing endophotocoagulation or endodiathermy, airfluid exchange, or silicone oil injection, among a host of other maneuvers. Indeed, many situations benefit from the surgeon's ability to see what is happening to the surrounding tissue during an intraocular maneuver, rather than having a smaller field of view with some measure of stereopsis.

Unless a particular vitrectomy procedure is short in duration, the problems of increasing media opacification limits three-dimensional viewing as well. Noncontact, wide-angle imaging systems do not promote a high degree of stereopsis in many situations, and contact, wide-field viewing systems are more difficult and cumbersome to use. For maneuvers adjacent to the retinal periphery, especially during microscope imaging through a middilated or less pupil, there is probably little, if any, three dimensionality to the image. Scleral depression compounds this situation.

There are a few other minor advantages to endoscopy in the context of posterior vitrectomy. Initial sclerotomy sites, especially those for infusion, may be easily inspected. This can be helpful when beginning surgery in an eye with proliferative vitreoretinopathy (PVR) and anterior retinal retraction, choroidal hemorrhage or effusion, or very dense hemorrhage or debris. Before opening the infusion line, the surgeon can ensure that the cannula is not inadvertently placed underneath the retina or choroid (Fig. 16-1).

At the conclusion of surgery, especially in the aphakic or pseudophakic eye, final inspection of the retinal periphery and sclerotomy site can be accomplished in a minute or two without resorting to indirect ophthalmoscopy and scleral depression. In this regard, it is important for the surgeon to remember that retinal breaks and other pathology will be

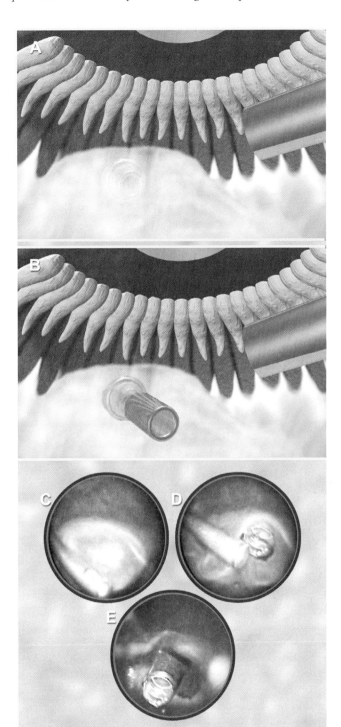

FIGURE 16-1. Infusion cannula inadvertently placed under retina that is retracted anteriorly. **A:** Infusion cannula under retina. **B:** Retinotomy allows cannula to project into vitreous for proper infusion. **C:** Infusion cannula under retina. When infusion begins, detachment of overlying retina is increased. **D:** Retinotomy is fashioned with vitrector. **E:** Cannula is now infusing into vitreous cavity and edges of retinotomy site are photocoagulated.

more apparent in the fluid-filled eye rather than the gasfilled (or, to a lesser extent, oil- or perfluorocarbon liquid–filled) eye.

Finally, endoscopy is not a religion. It is not an either/or decision that the surgeon must make. Rather, it seems absurd not to always combine it with microscope viewing. The endoscopy handpiece is essentially the same size as the typical endoilluminator, yet it can have two or three functions instead of one and, because ophthalmic endoscopy typically demands xenon or metal halide illumination sources, the intraocular lighting is better than with commercially available vitrectomy units. If the surgeon can easily see with the microscope, then the endoscopic image can be ignored, but when the exterior-to-interior viewing becomes more difficult, the surgeon merely shifts attention to the endoscopic image and continues with the procedure unabated.

TEACHING

Endoscopy confers a great advantage on clinicians interested in teaching those around them about vitreoretinal surgical technique. It is interesting to observe the reaction of residents, fellows, nurses, and technicians who may have assisted in many operations yet have seen little of the procedure, even though their operating microscope may be equipped with a video camera. Observing the anatomy, especially of the retinal periphery or region of the ciliary body, can be a novel experience, even for a well-seasoned assistant. Furthermore, once such individuals become accustomed to this method of imaging, they may be better able to assist because they can now monitor the course of the procedure and anticipate the needs of the surgeon.

VIEWING TECHNIQUES

Surgeon Placement

Most of the time, vitrectomy surgeons sit at the head of the operating room table. The video monitor of the endoscopy system is usually within a meter or so of the surgeon to enable good visualization. Exactly where to place it depends on the operator's preference and the location of the other equipment used for the procedure. If the endoscopy system and monitor are too far away, the image detail becomes difficult to appreciate. Small video monitors or LCD displays mounted on the operating microscope are thought by many to be distracting and do not provide the clarity required for surgery, so this option is not much of a solution.

It would be fair to say that most endoscopic vitrectomy surgeons place the instrumentation in a fashion similar to the phacoemulsification-ECP surgeon; that is, the endoscopy unit is situated opposite the usual location of the assistant and machines, but within arm's length of the surgeon and assistant. Although vitrectomy is usually performed from the surgeon's typical position, there may be advantages to temporal seating as well. These will be discussed in the next section.

Sclerotomy Placement

Most surgeons use the three-port technique with superior temporal, inferior temporal, and superior nasal sclerotomy placement. Most of the time this is fine. Depending on the location of certain intraocular pathology, however, variations in this approach can be helpful.

In general, if the pathology is restricted primarily to a specific quadrant or two, placing the endoscope sclerotomy and the vitrector (and other instrument) sclerotomies closer to the area of interest will allow ease of access to the pathology site. It can be beneficial in the phakic eye, when working in the peripheral anterior vitreous, in that trauma to the lens may be avoided.

A good example of this is in a phakic eye with PVR confined largely to the inferior hemisphere. If the "working sclerotomies" are fashioned at the 3 and 9 o'clock positions (or lower), it is often evident endoscopically that the lens can be avoided, while the peripheral retina and pars plana can be easily accessed (Fig. 16-2).

The same holds true for pathology located, for example, in the nasal hemisphere. Temporal placement of the surgeon along with the more directed sclerotomy sites can maximize access to the area with the most serious pathology. It only requires a little flexibility on the part of the surgeon.

As a corollary of this, the number of sclerotomies is also not written in stone. If greater advantage can be gained by changing the direction from which instruments are introduced, this option should be considered. These maneuvers are often performed quickly, especially when using a trocar system for some or all of the sclerotomies.

Image Size And Illumination

An important and simple concept for intraocular endoscopy is that the closer the tip of the instrument is to the target tissue, the larger the image size and the smaller the field of view. Conversely, the further the endoscope is from the area of concern, the smaller the image size and the wider the field of view. Inversely, the closer the endoscope tip to the region of vitrectomy, less illumination is needed, and the farther away from the treatment zone, more illumination is needed (Fig. 16-3).

There is no right or wrong choice in this regard. Some surgeons prefer a larger image whereas others think a more panoramic view is better. Clearly, the best option depends on the circumstances. If a particular area of pathology, such as a gliotic band, needs to be removed, it is usually very simple to move the endoscope closer to the tissue, increasing anatomic detail and facilitating its removal or division. On the other hand, air-fluid exchange is much simpler to perform with a wide field of view, fine anatomic detail not being very helpful.

Imaging

When one is first inserting the endoscope into the vitreous cavity, care must be taken not to advance it very far. Rather, the illumination should be increased and the image oriented so that the iris and lens are at the "top" of the picture and the posterior pole at the "bottom." This approach

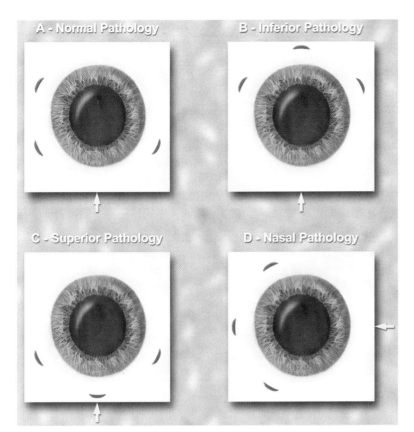

FIGURE 16-2. Eccentric placement of sclerotomy sites can assist in addressing pathology confined to one or two quadrants, especially making the periphery more accessible without traumatizing the lens. Yellow arrow indicates position of surgeon. **A:** "Standard" arrangement. **B:** Inferior pathology. Sclerotomy sites are moved below horizontal meridian. **C:** Superior pathology. Sclerotomies are moved above the horizontal meridian. **D:** Nasal pathology. Surgeon seated temporally and sclerotomies fashioned nasal to vertical meridian. These methods not only bring the instruments closer to the pathology but also diminish the potential for lens contact so that lensectomy may not be necessary in order to dissect membranes from the peripheral retina.

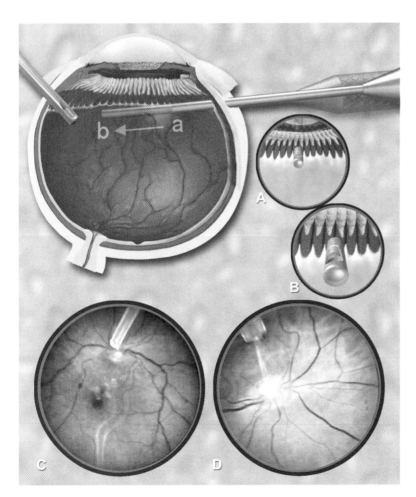

FIGURE 16-3. Magnification, field of view, and illumination requirements vary with distance from the endoscope tip to the target tissue. **A:** Increased distance results in less magnified image, larger field of view, and greater illumination requirements. **B:** Advancing the endoscope toward the target magnifies image size, diminishes the field of view, and lessens the requirement for adequate illumination. **C:** Minified view of aspirating posterior vitreous from disc surface. **D:** Magnified view of same.

makes it simpler to locate instruments introduced through other sclerotomies and to adjust their manipulation within the eye accordingly.

Advancing the endoscope further into the vitreous cavity increases the anatomic detail that can be appreciated. The illumination may need adjustment. Once a satisfactory view and illumination level are obtained, the surgeon holds the endoscope in that position and maneuvers the other instrument as one would if imaging through the microscope. Pathology within the vitreous cavity, such as

hemorrhage or debris, is usually easier to deal with panoramically, whereas maneuvering a pick for removal of a preretinal membrane benefits from a close-up and detailed view.

At first, many of these maneuvers may seem difficult. If so, the endoscope can simply be used as an endoilluminator, with the operating microscope for imaging. One can periodically look at the endoscopy monitor to appreciate what is taking place from that vantage point. By building skill and confidence in this manner, the surgeon will find that the

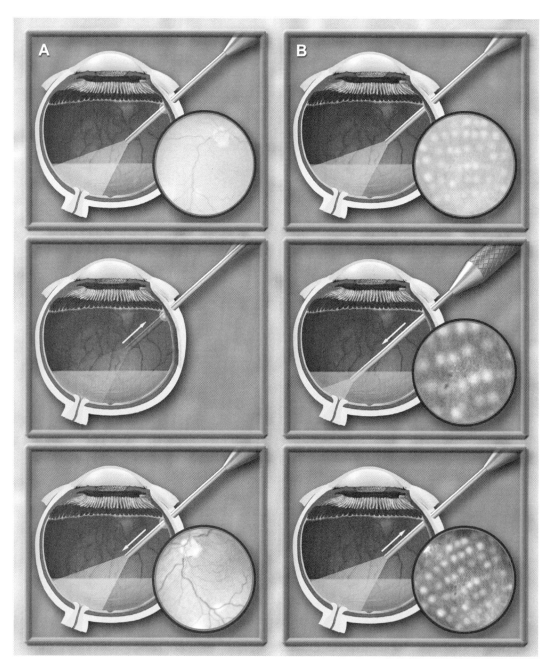

FIGURE 16-4. Methods for clearing fogged images. **A:** Endoscope tip is withdrawn into sclerotomy site, effecting clearing. **B:** Endoscope tip is dipped into residual intraocular fluid, clearing the image.

technique of intravitreal endoscopy soon becomes second nature. Some surgeons have observed that it can replace microscope viewing for most of the procedure even when an adequate image can be obtained through the microscope.

Fogging

A very hazy or foggy image may develop rapidly during the course of endoscopic surgery, but this is simple to reverse. Endoscopy in any body cavity can be plagued by this problem, so ophthalmologists are not alone in this regard.

The most common experience of fogging is during the course of air-fluid exchange. The "warm" balanced saline solution within the eye is being replaced by "cold" room air or gas. Condensation occurs on the tip of the endoscope, just as it can on the posterior aspect of an IOL under the same circumstances. Fogging can also occur in eyes with significant active bleeding or, to a lesser extent, those with dense debris such as that associated with infectious endophthalmitis.

No matter what the cause, there are a few choices available to the surgeon (Fig. 16-4). The most useful and prac-

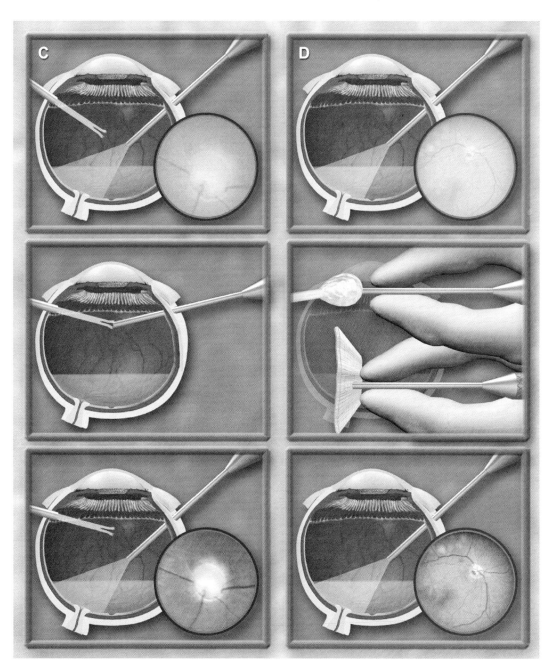

FIGURE 16-4. *(continued)* C: Tip of the endoscope is wiped with a second soft-tipped instrument. **D:** Endoscope is removed from the eye, the tip wiped, and the endoscope reinserted.

tical is to withdraw the tip of the endoscope into its insertion site. Usually a small amount of fluid is present that will spread over the imaging surface, clearing the fog. This maneuver can be repeated several times.

If this proves inadequate, another option is to advance the tip of the endoscope into the remaining intraocular fluid (if there is any), which usually results in immediate clearing of the fog. However, often the image fogs again when the endoscope tip is withdrawn over the fluid meniscus. This procedure can also be repeated as needed.

A third choice presents itself if the other instrument has a soft tip, such as a brush or soft-tipped extrusion cannula. In this scenario, the two instruments are advanced toward each other, and the soft tip is used like a windshield wiper blade to remove the condensation and debris from the imaging system.

Finally, if all of these options fail or cannot be executed, the instrument must be removed from the eye and manually wiped with a dry gauze, a cotton-tipped applicator, or a sponge. However, this is usually unnecessary because the other approaches more than adequately rectify most such situations.

SURGICAL TECHNIQUE

Every surgeon knows that it would be best to examine the internal aspect of all sclerotomy sites at the conclusion of surgery. Equally well known is the fact that this is usually not possible. Most articles in the peer-reviewed literature that address this issue have drawings demonstrating potential problems but no photographs. Clearly, then, one of the great advantages that endoscopy can confer is the ability to examine in intimate detail the status of past and present sclerotomies and provide some solutions for problems associated with their creation.

Incarcerated Vitreous

Incarceration of vitreous is readily apparent in most sclerotomy sites. A V-shaped wedge of vitreous can be observed that is adherent to the site. While some surgeons believe that cutting the vitreous extending from the external surface of the sclerotomy will solve this problem, endoscopy clearly demonstrates that this maneuver is not the solution. Indeed, the internal view of vitreous incarceration does not change as a result of incision of vitreous external to the wound.

The only way to manage this problem is to use a vitrector to mechanically divide and aspirate the vitreous adherent to the internal aspect of the eye wall. This maneuver can be difficult or impossible to achieve. The vitreous base can be very dense and strongly adherent, overpowering the ability of available vitrectors to section and aspirate. Furthermore, the port of the vitrector must be directed to the vit-

reous that needs to be removed, and this often necessitates its approximation to the eye wall. Cutting the vitreous, then, can result in inadvertent laceration of the pars plana, which usually initiates bleeding. If this problem does arise, elevating the IOP, combined with applying direct pressure by the vitrector tip for a few minutes, usually resolves the situation. It is surprising that, even after all this, the vitreous may still adhere to the wound!

Most of the time, this situation does not affect the technical outcome, at least judging by the high level of success associated with vitrectomy. On the other hand, eyes with proliferative disease bear substantial potential for redetachment resulting from proliferation along this vitreous scaffold, anterior contraction, and subsequent detachment of the retina, pars plana, and ciliary body. It is important to preempt the situation by dividing the vitreous incarcerated in the sclerotomy from its more posterior attachment and to the retina. In some situations, a far peripheral retinectomy is required to achieve this goal. It may be surprising to some surgeons that during the course of reoperation for PVR detachment, this anterior retinal retraction to the sclerotomy is partially or completely responsible for the patient's difficulty. This situation is elusive to diagnose and manage through the operating microscope but fortunately is easily detected and remedied by using endoscopy and allied techniques (Fig. 16-5).

Hemorrhage

Occasionally, hemorrhage arises from the internal aspect of the sclerotomy site and persists throughout the procedure. Blindly cauterizing the edge of the wound or raising the IOP may not solve the problem. These areas are easily detected by endoscopy, and direct cauterization, application of direct pressure with an instrument tip, or elevation of the IOP usually suffices to control the situation (Fig. 16-6).

Subretinal Infusion Cannula Placement

As mentioned previously, PVR detachment with anterior traction over the ciliary body or to the posterior iris may make proper infusion cannula insertion difficult. If the cannula ends up being subretinal (even though it is placed properly as measured on the external ocular surface), opening the infusion line will balloon the retina or choroid, exacerbating the situation. Vitrectomy is an unforgiving surgery in the first place, so that ophthalmologists must not sabotage their own potential by initiating this unfortunate chain of events. If there is no place to reasonably insert the endoscope from the pars plana, then it should be introduced from the anterior segment. Before opening the infusion line, the patency of the cannula should be clearly evident. If not, the overlying tissue should be opened with a blade, scissors, or vitrector. Even if a peripheral retinal break

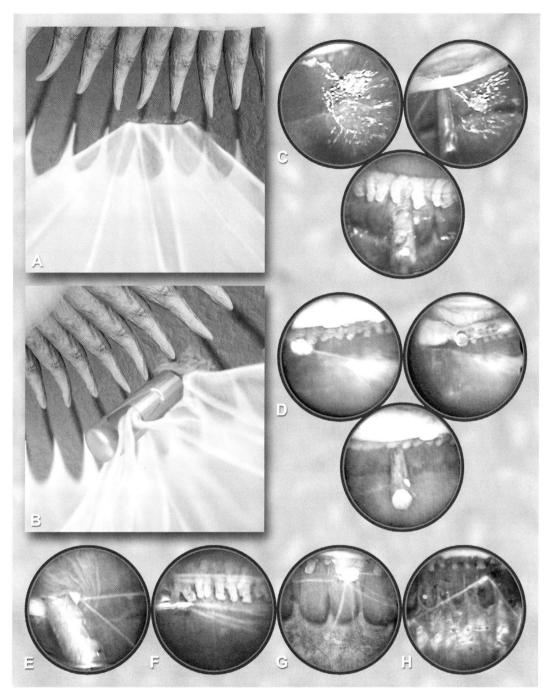

FIGURE 16-5. Vitreous incarceration in sclerotomy site. **A:** Vitreous adherent to internal aspect of sclerotomy and its excision. **B:** Vitrector excising incarcerated vitreous. **C:** Vitreous with asteroid hyalosis adherent to sclerotomy. The vitrector is used to excise this material from the sclerotomy site. **D:** Another instance of this situation. The incarcerated vitreous is removed, releasing tractional elements to the retina and eliminating scaffolding for future proliferation. **E:** Vitreous incarceration in sclerotomy site. Excision may prove to be difficult despite best efforts. **F:** Appearance of residual vitreous incarceration. **G:** Vitreous adhesions emanating from multiple directions are not uncommon after routine vitrectomy. **H:** Appearance of vitreous incarcerated in sclerotomy site from previous vitrectomy in an eye with proliferative diabetic retinopathy. Even though this situation presents a theoretical risk for complications, it has proved to be benign in this instance.

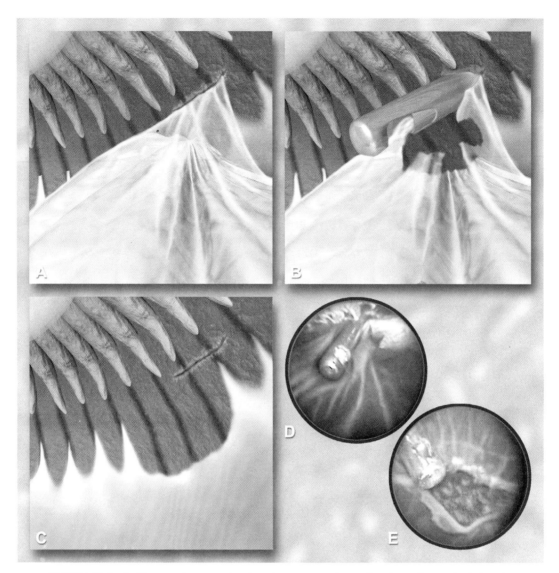

FIGURE 16-6. A: Vitreous incarceration in sclerotomy and associated traction retinal detachment. **B:** Vitrector excises vitreous and retina from this area. **C:** Appearance after this maneuver. **D:** Endoscopic image of vitrectomy/retinectomy from sclerotomy site. **E:** Retina is now freed from its tractional elements and can be easily photocoagulated.

is created at this point, it is most often easily repaired later in the procedure. If these maneuvers do not resolve the problem, the infusion cannula should be removed and placed elsewhere (Fig. 16-7).

Sclerotomy-Induced Retinal Detachment

Occasionally, one performs an uneventful vitrectomy only to have what appears to be a rhegmatogenous retinal detachment develop over the following days or weeks. This problem may be the result of the severing of an anomalous oral tooth during creation of the sclerotomy. This condition is difficult to detect and manage by conventional means. Indeed, scleral depression with indirect ophthalmoscopy tends to obscure the situation. Endoscopy can easily establish the presence of this far peripheral break, and simultaneous endophotocoagulation virtually always resolves the problem (Fig. 16-8).

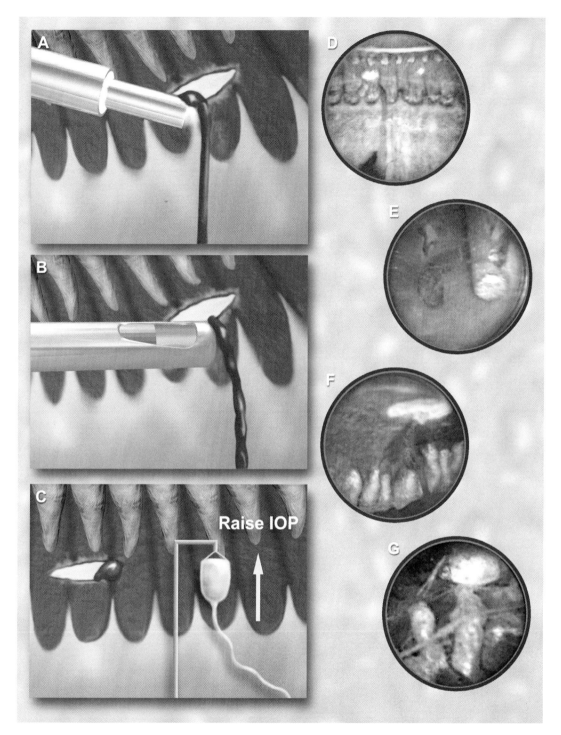

FIGURE 16-7. Bleeding from internal aspect of sclerotomy site. **A:** Treated by cauterization with intraocular wet-field. **B:** Treated by direct pressure with the vitrector. **C:** Treated by raising IOP via increased infusion. **D:** Bleeding from sclerotomy site. **E:** Hemorrhage removed with vitrector as it moves into position for direct pressure. **F:** Bleeding sclerotomy site. **G:** Same area after increasing infusion. Elevated IOP controls the hemorrhage.

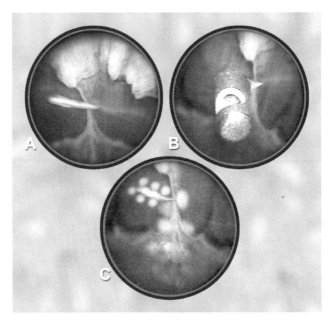

FIGURE 16-8. Anomalous oral tooth inadvertently cut during the creation of a sclerotomy. **A:** Sclerotomy site is well positioned in the mid pars plana, yet the MVR blade severs an elongated insertion of the retina. **B:** Instruments are inserted through this site and manipulated throughout the surgery, enhancing opportunities for subretinal fluid accumulation. **C:** Endoscopic laser retinopexy ensures that this site will not become the origin of a rhegmatogenous detachment.

VITRECTOMY TECHNIQUES AND ENDOSCOPY

SCLERAL DEPRESSION

Vitreoretinal surgeons rely heavily on scleral depression combined with indirect ophthalmoscopy to diagnose and treat a number of retinal disorders. All of the advantages derived from this technique can be applied to endoscopic vitrectomy as well. Scleral depression can elevate the flap of a tear or cause a small retinal operculum to protrude, announcing the presence of significant pathology that must be addressed. This maneuver is especially simple when combined with endoscopy.

Subretinal fluid sometimes remains in an area the surgeon wishes to endophotocoagulate. By applying scleral depression in the target region and displacing the subretinal fluid elsewhere, the laser endoscope can then easily deliver laser energy to the now flattened retina. This maneuver is usually effective (Figs. 17-1 and 17-2).

Occasionally, a particular region of pathology cannot be easily accessed even with endoscopy. This situation might arise as a consequence of anomalous anatomy, less than optimal sclerotomy placement, or a host of other problems. Depressing the area of concentration into view can ease the performance of vitrectomy and limit the time spent struggling with the procedure (Fig 17-3).

There is a down side to scleral depression that can be clearly demonstrated by endoscopy, especially in the management of proliferative vitreoretinopathy (PVR). In this situation, there are often adhesions between the peripheral

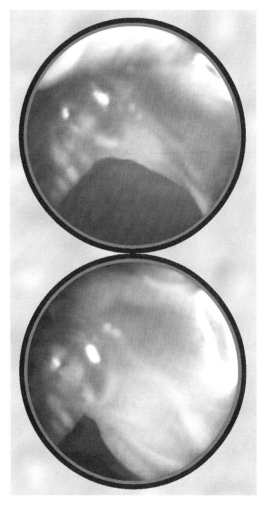

FIGURE 17-1. View of retina with and without scleral depression in the presence of residual subretinal fluid. Scleral depression displaces the fluid so that the area can then be photocoagulated.

retina and the ciliary body, posterior iris, and posterior capsule. Scleral depression releases the traction between these attachments, making them seem to disappear. Even if they could be viewed through the operating microscope, which they most often cannot, the scleral depression would obscure their existence. Intraocular imaging does not require distortion of the existing architecture, whether normal or pathologic, so that the relationship between gliotic tissue and its point of attachment is readily apparent.

Finally, and perhaps most obviously, there are some eyes that should not be subjected to any unnecessary physical stresses, scleral depression being high on the list of maneuvers to avoid. Consider, for example, an eye that is 2 days post phacoemulsification with aggressive endophthalmitis. While vitrectomy would be indicated, the relatively "open" nature of the eye would militate against the use of scleral depression. The same holds true for eyes undergoing vitrectomy for penetrating trauma or intraocular foreign body. Endoscopy usually facilitates a complete evaluation of the intraocular terrain in a relatively atraumatic fashion as well as enabling vitrectomy and allied procedures when the view through the operating microscope is inadequate.

VITRECTOMY

It is essential to master the performance of posterior vitrectomy under endoscopic guidance. The technique can be easily learned but often requires some practice.

The endoscope is inserted with a panoramic view maintained. The vitrector is introduced through the contralateral sclerotomy. With the endoscope held in place, the vitrector is maneuvered into what seems to be the mid-vitreous, and mechanical cutting and aspiration are begun. Every effort should be made not to move the endoscope because maintaining a constant position ensures that the field of view also remains the same. The vitreous will appear white and hazy when illuminated and imaged from within the eye, so what will be experienced is clearing of the view as vitreous is removed.

As the area of vitrectomy enlarges, the cutting/aspiration handpiece is advanced closer to the endoscope, making the image larger. This technique is preferred because it orients the surgeon three-dimensionally. If the surgeon is working in region A and the endoscope tip is in region B, it is not possible to inadvertently traumatize any intervening tissue (Fig. 17-4).

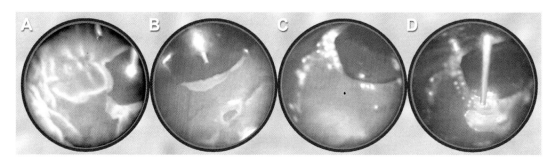

FIGURE 17-2. Displacing subretinal fluid and gas by scleral depression. **A:** Retinal detachment flattening by extrusion of subretinal fluid. **B:** Air-fluid exchange as extrusion continues. **C:** Residual subretinal fluid and gas limit ability to laser and so scleral depression is applied. **D:** Now laser retinopexy can be completed.

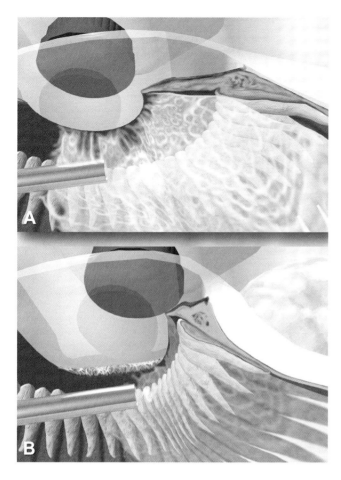

FIGURE 17-3 A,B. Scleral depression can obscure the presence of gliotic attachments by relieving the traction between two points.

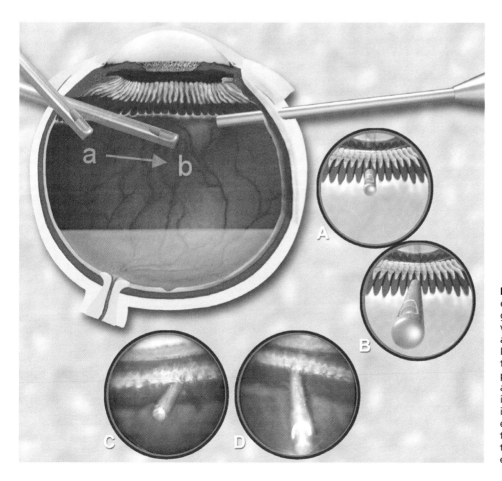

FIGURE 17-4. Relationship between endoscope tip and vitrector. The surgeon should maintain a panoramic view with the endoscope while advancing the vitrector toward it. **A:** Initially, the vitrector is "far" from the endoscope. There is minified and panoramic view. **B:** As the vitrector is advanced toward the endoscope, the image is larger and the field of view is smaller. **C:** Photo of vitrector as it enters the eye and vitrectomy is imitated. **D:** As vitrectomy continues, the vitrector advances toward the endoscope.

This process should be continued until there seems to be no remaining vitreous. The vitrector and endoscope insertion sites should be switched to remove any remaining vitreous that may not have been detectable by imaging through a single entry.

A common experience of the novice is that quite a bit of vitreous remains in the eye after mechanical excision via the operating microscope. Because the whitening effect clearly delineates the presence of vitreous by endoscopy, a more complete removal eliminates this surprise.

When one is first starting, it is best to avoid the phakic eye so as not to inadvertently traumatize the lens. A vitrectomy for an uncomplicated problem, such as chronic vitreous hemorrhage, usually presents the ideal situation.

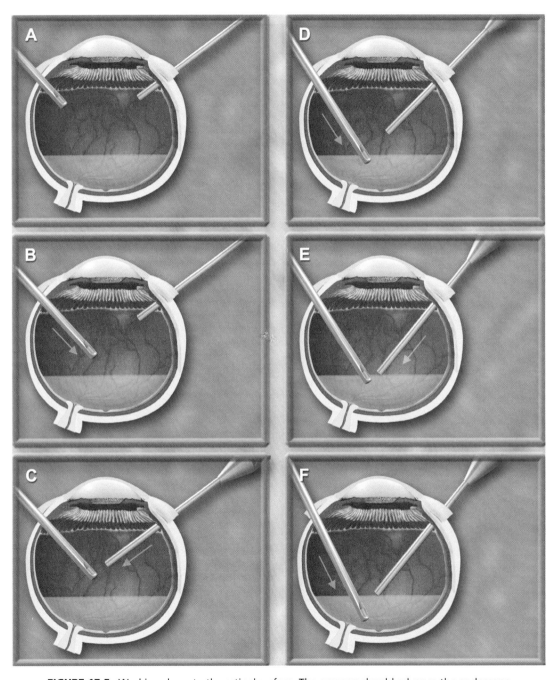

FIGURE 17-5. Working closer to the retinal surface. The surgeon should advance the endoscope tip toward the retina, then move the vitrector to follow. This should be repeated in small steps until the surface is approached safely and the instruments are in proper position for the task. **A:** Both instruments workng anteriorly and peripherally. **B:** The vitrector is advanced while the endoscope remains stationary. **C:** When all of the vitrectors have been removed from this region, the endoscope is advanced. **D:** Then the vitrector is directed more posteriorly creating another panoramic working area. **E & F:** When all the vitreous has been removed from this area, once again the process is repeated by advancing the endoscope and then the vitrector, creating a "new" working space.

When the vitrectomy is being performed closer to the surface of the retina, the endoscope tip is first advanced a bit closer to the target, and then the vitrector tip is moved closer. This should be repeated as frequently as necessary for the surgeon to feel comfortable that the cutter is in the proper position and that the imaging is adequate. In this manner, even fine dissection on the retinal surface can safely and effectively take place (Fig. 17-5).

The same principle of vitrectomy holds true whether one is imaging endoscopically or through the microscope. The closer the vitrector tip is to the surface of the retina, the faster its cut rate should be and the lower its level of aspiration. In this way, control of the tissue can be maximized. If this gross and fine vitrectomy technique can be acquired, almost any other endoscopic intraocular maneuver represents but a minor variation.

Let us reiterate for a moment about the caution that should be exercised in the phakic eye. It is common to become so engrossed in the progress of endoscopic vitrectomy that trauma to the lens might occur, especially during peripheral vitreous excision. Being aware of this potential problem will minimize the risk. Finally, there is no reason that the surgeon cannot confirm the adequacy of vitrectomy at any point during the procedure by viewing through the operating microscope. In most eyes undergoing vitrectomy, the microscope view is adequate to ascertain the position of intraocular instruments and the current intraocular conditions. Only when this view is lost, for the various reasons already discussed, does the true impact of endoscopic vitrectomy become apparent. Then the surgeon may continue with the procedure undeterred and hopefully obtain the desired outcome. If the surgeon has not acquired these endoscopic vitrectomy skills, it is not possible to safely and effectively perform vitrectomy by endoscopic means.

To conclude, the only way to become skillful in endoscopic vitrectomy is to employ the technique frequently and as an adjunct to the operating microscope. When the situation arises that there are no other choices, the surgeon will be competent with this approach and able to effectively execute the procedure.

PRERETINAL MEMBRANECTOMY

Removal of gliotic tissue from the surface of (or beneath) the retina is by far the most demanding of endoscopic procedures. If there is any need for stereopsis, this is where it will be found. Still, two-dimensional imaging by endoscopy can facilitate membranectomy quite well. Perhaps the only relative exception to this is when fine macular dissection is required. Generally, it would be ill advised to perform macular pucker surgery by endoscopic imaging, and such surgery should be avoided. The potential for inadvertent trauma to this area is considerable. Removal of membranes from the surface of the optic nerve or more peripherally, such as in proliferative diabetic retinopathy, is a different matter. The skill that is needed to perform this aspect of vitrectomy has just been discussed. The tip of the instrument (e.g., pick, membrane scratcher, MVR blade) is placed in proximity to the tissue, and the endoscope is advanced toward the area for a close-up view. If an "edge" of the membrane can be imaged, one of the instruments may be manipulated in such a way as to "lift it."

It bears mention that, unlike the view through the operating microscope, the endoscopic image obtained from one insertion site may be more or less advantageous than that from a different sclerotomy, even though the same area of pathology is the focus of attention. The edge of a preretinal membrane may, for example, be much more apparent when the endoscope is inserted nasally than when it is inserted temporally. These types of adjustments are determined at the discretion of the surgeon.

Even though there is no stereopsis, with a little practice it is not difficult to elevate most membranes, especially in the periphery. At first the surgeon should place the tip of the instrument close to the membrane and maneuver it as if it were engaged (Fig. 17-6). In this way, the surgeon can gain

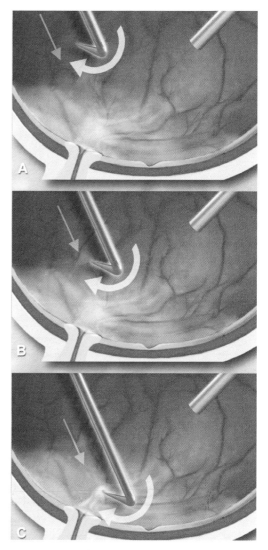

FIGURE 17-6. A-C.: The surgeon should maneuver the tip of the instrument near the edge of the membrane, and repeat as necessary to safely engage it.

a sense of how close to the tissue the instrument actually is. This can be repeated as often as needed to lightly engage the tissue. Then tissue manipulation can proceed as normal.

One of the advantages of endoscopy can be found in the ability to rapidly change the field of view from close-up with high magnification to wide field with low magnification merely by moving the tip of the endoscope away from the target zone. This can be very helpful during membranectomy, when it is important to know precisely what is taking place in the adjacent tissue.

EN BLOC DISSECTION

Consider as an example en bloc dissection of vitreoretinal vascularized membranes in proliferative diabetic retinopathy. The vitreous is left largely intact to provide anterior–posterior traction. It is often straightforward to find a membrane edge posteriorly and insert a fine spatula or blade beneath it. As the edge is gently lifted, its attachments to the underlying retina (pegs) are broken. As long as the retina is not being torn or vessels sheared, this maneuver can be continued. This technique can effect a surprising degree of membrane separation in a brief period.

At the initiation of this maneuver, the endoscope view should be close to the tissue to best define the edge and allow instrument insertion. As the membrane is separated, the wide-field view obtained by withdrawing the endoscope can reveal the extent of traction this maneuver places on adjacent and distant tissues, which can be extremely helpful if the dissection is to continue without reinsertion of the membranectomy instrument (Fig. 17-7).

En bloc dissection is considerably more cumbersome through the operating microscope because both the magnification and the field of view have to be altered. If there is a question regarding continuation of membrane elevation or the need to stop because of strong membrane–retina adhesion, the endoscope can be advanced to inspect the tissue in question in a closer, more magnified view. If the adhesion appears to be significant, delamination, segmentation, or another technique would be required. Usually membranectomy proceeds from anterior to posterior ("outside in"). If it does not, continued elevation of the membrane can proceed. It is this ability to repeatedly shift between close-up/high magnification to wide-field/low magnification that makes the endoscopic image so useful in this situation. Although the operating microscope could also accomplish the same goal given sufficient clarity of the media and pupillary dilation, the process of reimaging and refocusing can add considerably to the time and difficulty of the procedure.

As an added advantage of this approach, if a laser endoscope is used during en bloc dissection or any membranectomy approach and an inadvertent retinal break is created, the laser can be applied at that moment to mark the location for future treatment.

By this approach, most or all of the preretinal gliosis can be elevated from the retina and optic nerve surface and then removed with the vitrector. The difference between the preoperative and postoperative retinal appearance can be astounding. The greatest pitfall with this technique is tearing of the retina or shearing of a vessel by the aggressive tactic of pulling when more stubborn adhesions are detected. Rather, tenacious adhesions are best dealt with focally by delamination or segmentation.

MEMBRANE SEGMENTATION

Unlike en bloc dissection, in which the vitreous is initially left in place to provide anterior–posterior traction, the more typical method used for releasing retinal traction, especially that resulting from densely adherent membranes, involves removing as much vitreous as possible and then dividing or segmenting the preretinal membrane using vertical scissors.

When the posterior pole is involved, the typical approach is to begin vertically, cutting temporally, and then proceed nasally, finally circumnavigating the optic nerve. Once this has been accomplished, cutting of the membrane continues in a more or less radial fashion, from posterior to anterior ("inside out"). Dissection can proceed as a one-handed technique, or it can be assisted by placing a pick-sleeve on the endoscope to assist in tissue elevation and manipulation (Fig. 17-8). Usually, a significant degree of stereopsis is required to perform this feat, it being perhaps the most difficult of endoscopic maneuvers. If this approach becomes the only option, it is best to maximize the image detail by positioning the endoscope tip fairly close to the tissue and then searching for a membrane edge to insert the scissors. Once the scissors are positioned, it is best to withdraw the endoscope, using the more panoramic view, and then segmentation can begin. Hemorrhage is usually controlled by raising the infusion bottle or by endodiathermy.

About one third of these eyes will experience an iatrogenic break as a result of the procedure. The same principles used in other areas of vitreoretinal surgery apply here. All tractional elements should be removed from the area and the break surrounded with endophotocoagulation. If a laser endoscope is being used for the segmentation, then photocoagulation can be performed immediately rather than marking of the area for later treatment. At the conclusion of surgery, retinal tamponade is required.

MEMBRANE DELAMINATION

An alternative method for removing dense, broad-based preretinal membranes requires a bimanual technique using the endoscope with the pick-sleeve for imaging, illumination, membrane edge elevation, and stabilization, along with horizontally cutting scissors.

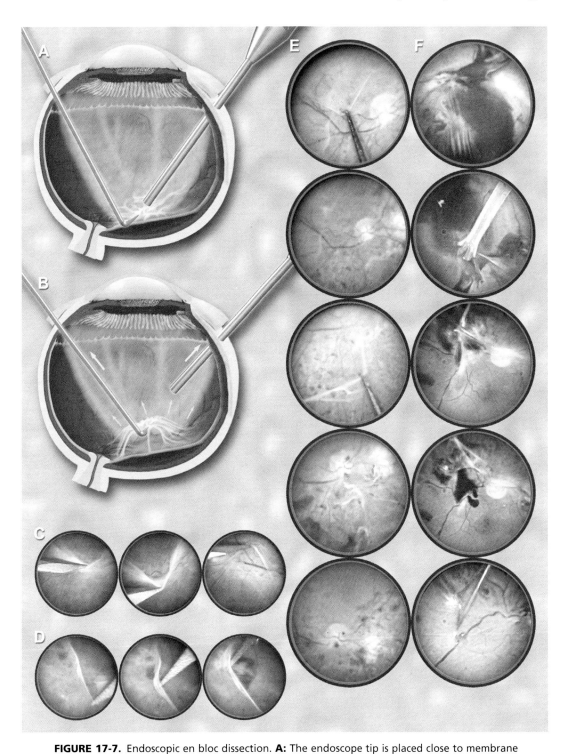

FIGURE 17-7. Endoscopic en bloc dissection. **A:** The endoscope tip is placed close to membrane edge for high-magnification view of vitreoretinal interface and insertion point for instrument, such as a spatula. **B:** Once the membrane edge is being lifted and separated from retina, the endoscope tip is withdrawn to a more panoramic position, enabling dissection to proceed while its effect on adjacent retinal tissue and vitreous is monitored. **C, D:** Clinical example. The membrane edge is engaged while the endoscope tip is close, creating a more magnified view. Once this has been accomplished, the endoscope is withdrawn, allowing a more panoramic image. **E, F:** Some views of endoscopic en bloc dissection.

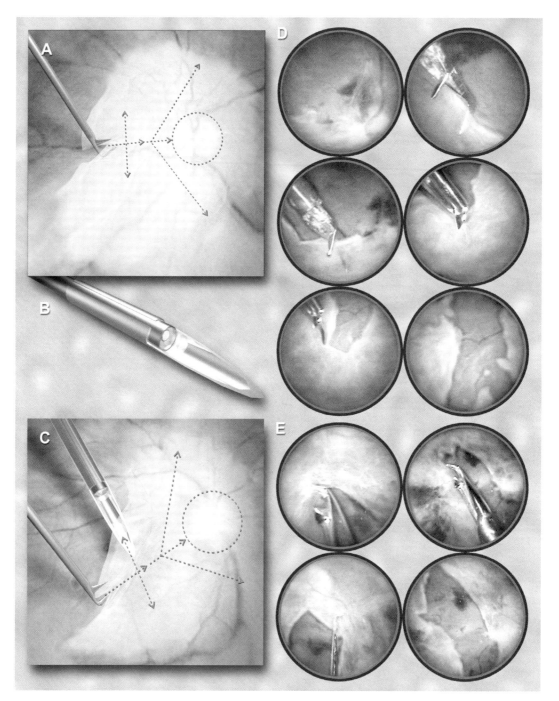

FIGURE 17-8. Endoscopic membrane segmentation. **A:** Typical method of cutting membranes with vertical scissors. **B:** Endoscope pick-sleeve. **C:** View of segmentation assisted by endoscope with pick-sleeve. **D, E:** Views of endoscopic membrane segmentation.

In this approach, most of the vitreous is first removed with the vitrector. Then the surgeon elevates the edge of the membrane by the endoscope with a pick in one hand while cutting the fibrovascular attachments with scissors in the other hand. Once again, it is desirable to start the dissection centrally and continue toward the periphery. Hemorrhage and the creation of iatrogenic breaks are the most significant risks. This maneuver is somewhat more difficult than membrane segmentation in that a panoramic view is not possible because the endoscope pick must remain in proximity to the scissors, serving its function of holding on to the edge of the tissue being divided (Fig. 17-9). Therefore, there is no stereopsis and no trade-off for panorama.

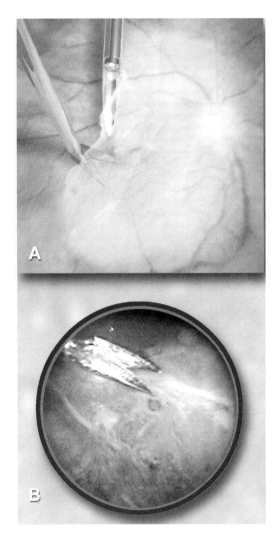

FIGURE 17-9. Endoscopic membrane delamination. **A:** Endoscope pick lifting edge of membrane, allowing horizontal scissors to cut attachments. **B:** Photos of endoscopic delamination.

MEMBRANECTOMY FOR RETINAL STARFOLD

Although just a variation of the previously discussed technique, membranectomy for retinal starfold bears some scrutiny. Several techniques for opening these folds are fairly simple to perform endoscopically (Fig. 17-10). Perhaps the most common technique is to use a bent needle, pick, spatula, or membrane scratcher with one hand while positioning the endoscope with the other hand so as to image from a moderate distance. The instrument tip is passed gently along the surface of the retina to engage any membranes and lift them off. The endoscopic pick-sleeve can also accomplish this task in a similar manner but is used with one hand. Diamond-dusted membrane scratchers, soft-tipped cannulas, and retinal brushes can remove membranes by abrading them from the tissue surface and stretching the retina while progress is monitored endoscop-

ically from a moderately panoramic vantage. Simply grasping the membrane with end-gripping diamond-coated 20-gauge fine forceps and pulling it toward the central vitreous cavity under endoscopic control can be quite effective. Dissection with viscoelastics or perfluorocarbon liquid seems to be less useful.

REMOVAL OF IMMATURE PRERETINAL MEMBRANES

When immature preretinal membranes are present, early PVR changes can be observed consisting of alterations in the appearance of the retinal surface, increasing immobility of the detached retina, and presence of pigment cells on the retinal surface. The instruments typically used to remove or section thick preretinal membranes do not seem to work nearly as well with these immature membranes in that they do not definitively remove the gliotic tissue from the retinal surface; also, for a great deal of effort only a small area of pathology ultimately is addressed. However, with use of a soft-tipped scraping instrument, such as the diamond-dusted membrane scratcher, expansive yet thin areas of immature membranes and pigment cells can be swept from the retinal surface, mobilizing the retina and removing the foundation for progressive and more severe proliferation. This maneuver is easily performed endoscopically and is actually one of the methods that is simpler to execute under endoscopic visualization than through the operating microscope. Usually, mid- to wide-field imaging is best because it enables a complete appraisal of a vast area of retina that can be swept clean of these immature membranes by this method (Fig. 17-11).

SUBRETINAL MEMBRANECTOMY

Typically, subretinal proliferation of gliotic tissue does not require surgical intervention because it is not responsible for retinal detachment. On the other hand, there are situations in which this problem plays a significant role in the cause of retinal detachment; in this scenario, such pathology requires intervention. Although most subretinal proliferation can be seen through the operating microscope, endoscopic imaging and membranectomy guidance is simple. In addition, subretinal endoscopic viewing often reveals the presence of unsuspected proliferation that can then be addressed.

To remove discrete bands, an overlying retinotomy is fashioned and a forceps is used for extraction. If the surgeon has the choice between creating a small posterior retinotomy or a larger peripheral retinotomy to access the subretinal proliferation, the latter is preferable. In the case of more diffuse subretinal proliferation, a larger peripheral retinotomy is usually better, with removal of this tissue

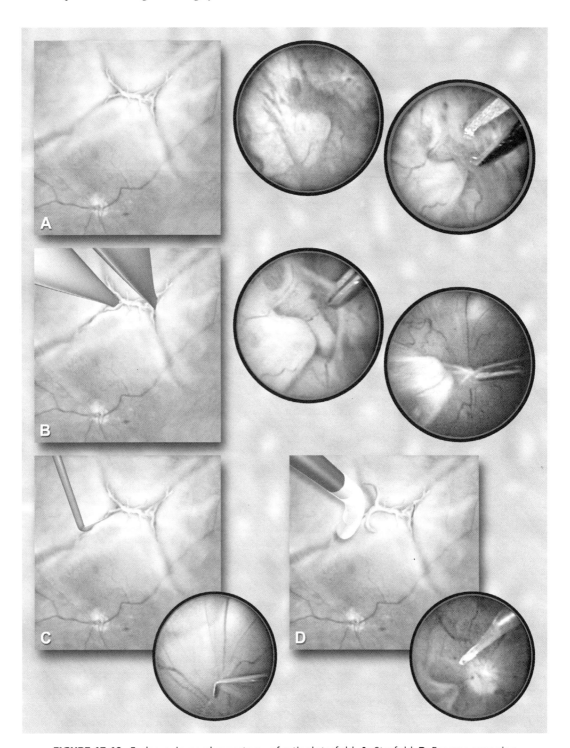

FIGURE 17-10. Endoscopic membranectomy of retinal starfold. **A:** Starfold. **B:** Forceps engaging membrane in center of fold and pilling from retinal surface. **C:** Pick engaging gliotic tissue and pulling from retinal surface. **D:** Diamond-dusted membrane scratcher engaging and removing membranes.

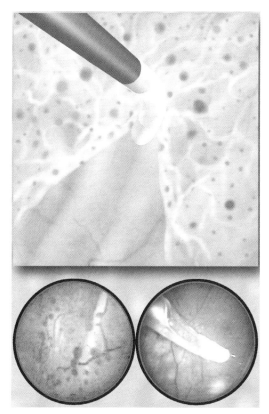

FIGURE 17-11. Endoscopic removal of immature proliferative membranes. Wide-field view monitors diamond-dusted membrane scratcher as it "wipes" immature membranes and pigment cells from vast expanses of retina. Conventional instrumentation and visualization would make this much more difficult or impossible.

undertaken with a membrane scratcher or other scraping-type instrument. Endoscopy has great value in this situation because a clear, magnified, relatively close view of the subretinal proliferation can be obtained that cannot be acquired with the microscope. Essentially, one can image the posterior aspect of the retina from the subretinal space (Fig. 17-12).

AIR-FLUID EXCHANGE

It is not uncommon for the surgeon to be plagued by a poor microscope image near the conclusion of vitrectomy, particularly a lengthy or complicated one. The cornea or lens may lose clarity, the pupil may become miotic, and so forth. Introducing air into the eye changes its optics, and if the patient is phakic or pseudophakic, imaging difficulties can be compounded as a result of the lensing required for an adequate view. Furthermore, condensation can occur on the surfaces of intraocular lenses (IOLs) that can obscure the posterior view yet may not be easily cleared. All of this can be frustrating when experienced near the conclusion of

surgery when everything has gone well, and it can be even more daunting if the course of the procedure has been trying. It is a relief then to be able to execute air-fluid exchange and internal drainage of subretinal fluid despite a deteriorating microscope view, using the endoscopic approach.

After infusion of air has begun, a soft-tipped extrusion cannula or brush is inserted through one of the sclerotomies and aspiration is activated. The endoscope is inserted through the opposite sclerotomy, maintaining a panoramic view and bright illumination. It is simplest to execute this procedure when the "top" and "bottom" anatomy are properly oriented. Air bubbles will be seen entering the eye, and then the meniscus of air and fluid will become visible. The endoscope should be maintained in its current position, but the soft-tipped cannula is advanced below the air-fluid level while it continues to aspirate. This is the point at which fogging of the endoscope tip most often occurs.

Maneuvers to clear the image have been previously examined; however, in general, the most useful technique for rectifying this situation is to retract the endoscope tip into the sclerotomy. Fluid in this area will usually spread over the tip, clearing the image. This method may require several repetitions. As the fluid level becomes lower, the aspirating tip is advanced more posteriorly, "following" the air-fluid level. The endoscope can be advanced as needed, but a wide-field view is preferred. Ultimately, the smallest amount of fluid will puddle over the optic nerve and can be easily aspirated. The soft tip of the extrusion cannula allows the surgeon to gently contact the surface of the optic nerve or retina while aspirating without damaging these structures. Because of their flexibility, these instruments also provide a margin of error in the event that they inadvertently contact these structures while being maneuvered under endoscopic control.

INTERNAL DRAINAGE OF SUBRETINAL FLUID

As a variant of the previous discussion, air-fluid exchange can be combined with active or passive internal drainage of subretinal fluid through a preexisting retinal break or a retinotomy created expressly for the purpose of drainage, all under endoscopic guidance. This simple technique can be profoundly helpful in a number of situations.

First, an air-fluid exchange is performed as completely as possible, as described in the preceding section. If there is subretinal fluid, it will cause the overlying retina to balloon, making their detachment seem more bullous and extensive. This is not cause for concern. The next step is to access a retinal break. If an existing break can be found, the tip of the cannula is directed to its edge and aspiration initiated (while air infusion continues). The subretinal fluid will be seen to stream into the cannula, and the ballooning retina will flatten. Aspiration continues until the retina is com-

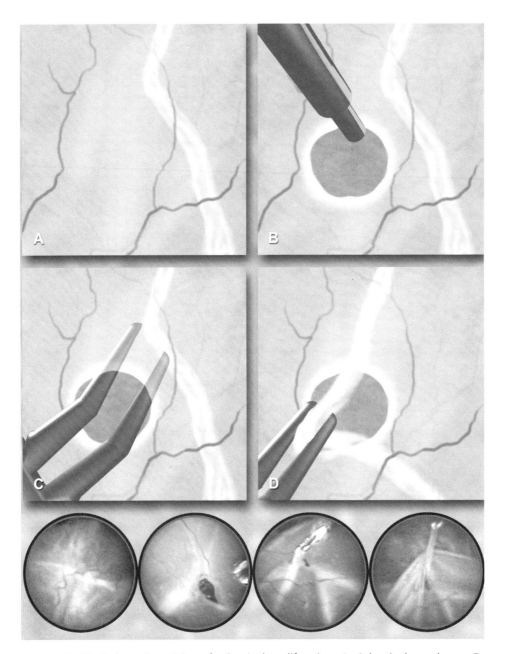

FIGURE 17-12. Endoscopic excision of subretinal proliferation. **A:** Subretinal membrane. **B:** Retinotomy is created by wetfield coagulation overlying gliotic band. **C:** Forceps are inserted through retinotomy into subretinal space. **D:** Band is grasped and pulled into vitreous cavity through retinotomy.

pletely flat. Endophotocoagulation can then be applied. If a preexisting retinal break cannot be found or is difficult to access, a drainage retinotomy can be created in a traction-free area of the retina with the endodiathermy probe and the subretinal fluid then aspirated. The retina should flatten completely. Occasionally, significant pockets of subretinal fluid remain despite the apparent lack of residual membranes or retinal stiffness. A second retinotomy can then be created to permit further internal subretinal drainage and ultimate flattening of the retina.

An impediment to complete drainage may be encountered when one is aspirating through a break overlying or adjacent to a scleral buckle. In this situation, the retina flattens too nicely over or next to the buckle, making it difficult for more distant subretinal fluid to find egress at that site. Should this occur, draining through a different preexisting or iatrogenic retinotomy site will complete the maneuver (Fig 17-13).

One of the great advantages of endoscopy is evident in this situation. Merely by a slight movement of the hand holding the endoscope, the image in a partially or com-

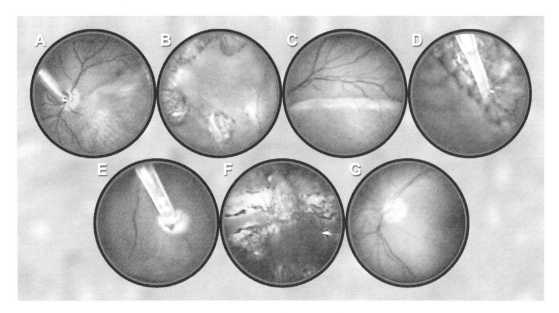

FIGURE 17-13. Endoscopic internal drainage of subretinal fluid. **A:** View of retinal detachment extending into macula. **B:** Peripheral retinal break. **C:** Fold at edge of macular detachment. **D:** After air-fluid exchange, a soft-tipped cannula is inserted through a preexisting retinal break or a drainage retinotomy, and aspiration is performed. The ballooning retina will flatten. **E:** This maneuver in the presence of a scleral buckle can be a problem. If the retina flattens on the buckle, precluding further internal drainage, a more posterior retinotomy must be fashioned for completion. **F:** Now the peripheral retinal break is flat on the scleral buckle and its edge seems to disappear **G:** Following complete drainage of subretinal fluid, the macula is reattached.

pletely air-filled eye can shift from anterior to posterior view, from a panoramic minified wide-field mode to a close-up magnified view—on surgeon demand, despite deteriorating anterior segment conditions, and all without an assistant. This would certainly not be possible while imaging through the operating microscope except under ideal conditions. The significance of this advance will become evident in the discussion of pseudophakic retinal detachment and PVR management.

RETINECTOMY

There may come a time during the course of vitrectomy for complicated retinal detachment when removal of membranes does not mobilize the retina sufficiently to permit its flattening. Dense but focal areas of membrane proliferation that are too stubborn to remove in an efficient manner, as seen with some perforating injuries, may also fall into this category. Under these circumstances, it may be more productive for the surgeon to excise them than try to mobilize them through extensive dissection. Although the indications for this technique will be discussed, attention here will be focused on the technique itself.

A few surgical principles are involved in the performance of retinectomy (Table 17-1). First, circumferential orientation is often helpful in releasing tractional elements, and the

more peripherally this is performed the better. Hemostasis should first be attained through the creation of one or more rows of endodiathermy. Then the vitrector or scissors can be used to cut the retina. The retinectomy should be somewhat more extensive than the area of traction. The more peripheral apron of retina should then be completely excised with the vitrector. Some form of tamponade should be used, such as gas or silicone oil injection, and the edge of the retina photocoagulated. This technique can be helpful in the management of PVR and diabetic traction detachment. Typically, the endoscope is used to give a panoramic view of the situation. Often, the moment traction is released, the retina is seen to flatten. Because many retinectomies are extensive and peripheral in nature, the microscope does not usually present a sufficient peripheral field of

TABLE 17-1. CONSIDERATIONS IN RETINECTOMY

- Removal of as much surface membrane as possible
- Endodiathermy of the extent of retinectomy and more
- Circumferential orientation
- Peripheral better than posterior
- Excise peripheral retinal apron
- Air–fluid exchange
- Internal drainage of subretinal fluid
- Endophotocoagulation
- Gas or silicone oil tamponade

view to accomplish this task with ease. All of the maneuvers in this technique—such as endodiathermy, vitrectomy, air-fluid exchange, silicone oil injection, and endophotocoagulation—are relatively simple to perform under endoscopic control and do not require stereopsis.

A variation of this approach is the more circumscribed retinectomy, which can be performed for more focally intense gliosis, as seen in penetrating trauma. The basic components and endoscopic imaging are the same. First, to maintain hemostasis, endodiathermy is applied to the area to be cut. Then scissors or a vitrector is used to cut the retina. The freed retina flattens with air-fluid exchange, but the relatively immobile dense gliosis does not. This area can then be excised. The cut edge of the retina is then photocoagulated and gas or silicone oil tamponade applied (Fig.17-14).

There are a few more guidelines that the surgeon should appreciate when considering retinectomy. Usually, the more posterior the retinectomy site, the more difficult it is to manage—a factor that should be taken into consideration. Residual surface membranes may add to the difficulty of the procedure by making retinectomy sites gape open and enlarge. Clearly, this is not helpful for reattaching the retina. Care should be taken to remove as much of the pre-retinal membranes as possible when one is considering retinectomy. Peripheral retinal stiffness may aid in more posterior dissection by contributing to anterior–posterior traction. If a retinectomy is fashioned peripherally early in the procedure, this advantage is lost. It is better to reserve this technique for the later stages of surgery. Finally, radial retinectomies are a problem in that they tend to extend posteriorly beyond their original intention and do not seem to be particularly helpful in their role of permitting retinal reattachment. It is best to avoid them.

ENDOPHOTOCOAGULATION

Certainly one of the great advances in vitreoretinal surgery was the ability to deliver laser energy to intraocular structures through an endoprobe. Given that retinopexy and retinal ablation are among the most commonly required services of the retinal surgeon, being able to perform them without a slit-lamp delivery system was quite a step. Here specific applications of this modality are discussed and variations of the technique examined.

When imaging through the operating microscope, the surgeon is typically required to hold the endophotocoagulation probe in one hand while illuminating with the other. Combining laser and illumination in a single probe can be advantageous but still has its limitations. When the field of

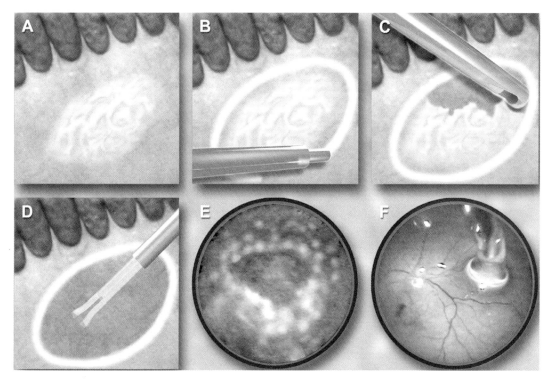

FIGURE 17-14. Endoscopic retinectomy. **A:** An area of dense retinal gliosis is identified. **B:** Using a more panoramic endoscope view, endodiathermy is initiated to an area greater than that of the planned retinectomy. **C:** The retina is then excised with the vitrector. **D:** Air-fluid exchange and internal drainage of subretinal fluid is performed. **E:** Endoscopic endophotocoagulation surrounds the retinectomy site. **F:** Gas or silicone oil tamponade is required.

view is adequate and the treatment directed more posteriorly, this standard technique is acceptable. As the area of interest moves more anteriorly, however, the bimanual approach to endophotocoagulation becomes more difficult.

This is well demonstrated by the near impossibility of bimanual endophotocoagulation of the ciliary body. As noted in the previous discussions about technique, an adequate microscope view is a prerequisite for executing any maneuver and when the image is lost, so is the surgeon. Performing endophotocoagulation typically requires both of the surgeon's hands, media that is clear enough to allow imaging and lasing, and the skill to align the microscope's optics so as to sufficiently view the target zone. At the same time, the surgeon should be able to view the endophotocoagulation probe and maneuver the endoilluminator into a position such that it adequately lights the field. Endoscopic laser delivery is not bound by these limitations. It would be fair to say that "pointing" the laser endoscope at the target zone enables all three functions—imaging, illumination, and laser delivery—simultaneously. The advantages of this configuration, especially when operating under less than ideal circumstances, should be evident.

Basic Considerations

Wavelength

Any wavelength that can be delivered by fiber can be used for endophotocoagulation through the laser endoscope. As a practical matter, however, the green (532-nm) and near-infrared (810-nm) wavelengths emitted by the semiconductor diode laser are ubiquitous. While the physics varies significantly from one to the other, in the context of endophotocoagulation, their tissue effects are fairly similar.

The advantage that the 810-nm laser has over the 532-nm laser for endoscopic cylcophotocoagulation (ECP) has already been discussed, but the distinction is less important when considering retinal photocoagulation. There are several reasons for this. One of the unique and powerful aspects of ECP is in its incorporation of an invisible-wavelength laser that employs very long-duration applications of relatively low power, which can be used to achieve the desired tissue effect while the surgeon can visibly monitor the course of this change. This capability limits overtreatment and undertreatment as well as collateral damage to non-aqueous-producing tissue and prosthetic material. All of this results in specific ablation of the target tissue, accounting for the extraordinary rate of success while minimizing potential complications. This would not be possible using a visible-wavelength laser. The laser flash would obscure the surgeon's view of the tissue effect, and the ciliary body's absorption characteristics of this wavelength would no doubt differ as well.

As far as the retina is concerned, these features are far less important. Indeed, it may be argued that the green wave-

length is slightly more desirable in this context because of its absorption characteristics by the various retinal structures. Still, it is a small point to argue that, for instance, the infrared laser is inferior to the green laser for the management of macular microaneurysms. While this may be true when treating a patient at the slit-lamp specifically for this problem, and even though this pathology can be addressed during the course of vitrectomy with either modality, the main indications for endophotocoagulation are retinal ablation and retinopexy, where the distinction between the two is less apparent. Infrared laser applied through a slit lamp to the posterior segment is usually painful, requiring some type of anesthesia, whereas there is no pain with the green laser. During the course of vitrectomy, when anesthesia has already been applied, this difference becomes moot. As a practical matter, then, there is little difference between these wavelengths, either being perfectly acceptable.

Spot Size

Unlike using the slit lamp for laser delivery, where the spot size can be selected within a certain range, there are substantial limitations to this component of the laser power density equation when one is applying endophotocoagulation. The primary determinant of spot size in this context is the diameter and numerical aperture of the laser fiber used through the endoscope. Most standard endophotocoagulation probes are about 200 μm in diameter, with a numerical aperture of 0.22 or smaller. What this means is that pretty much the smallest lesion that can be created using this fiber is 200 μm in diameter.

A few variables can alter this size. The green laser presents a relatively coherent beam, and so distance from probe tip to target tissue does not play much of a role with regard to spot size. In contrast, the infrared laser has a somewhat divergent beam, so the further away the fiber is from the target, the larger the spot. Another method of enlarging the spot size is to deliver a higher powered laser application with or without a longer duration. The initial laser spot size will be seen to enlarge. The infrared laser seems to spread more than the green under these circumstances. The down side of this approach is that a focal overtreatment may induce tissue explosion characterized by a popping sound and a palpable shock wave. Any intraocular tissue is capable of exploding under these circumstances, especially the retina or ciliary body, so that great care should be taken to ensure that this does not occur.

It is possible to create a smaller lesion than 200 μm with this instrumentation (e.g., to laser a macular microaneurysm). The tip of the laser endoscope should be held relatively close to the target, limiting the potential for beam divergence. Then a relatively short-duration spot is applied. Essentially, only a portion of the laser spot is actually being delivered. With a little practice, the surgeon can create 50- or 100-μm lesions in this manner.

Tissue Effect

By balancing the issues of laser wavelength, power, duration, and distance between the laser endoscope tip and the target tissue, one can create the desired lesion with regard to size and intensity. This latter characteristic varies, depending on the pathology being treated and the wavelength used. In general, the green laser makes a more "superficial" retinal burn and is often white in appearance. Typically, a short duration is used. Because of beam coherence and other factors, the spot size tends to remain more or less constant from lesion to lesion. Infrared laser applications, in contrast, demonstrate more variability in appearance from laser spot to spot, take a bit longer to produce, and may expand to a significantly larger size than the diameter of the laser fiber, depending on the absorption characteristics of the tissue, duration of application, and other features. None of these factors seems to cause as much variability with green laser application under similar circumstances. Finally, the retinal lesions resulting from infrared application are grayish with low power, creamy yellow with moderate power, and white with higher intensity.

Tissue Painting

Understanding the variables that combine to elicit the desired appearance of each laser application, the surgeon now has the option of using an alternate photocoagulation technique on the ciliary body or retina. This approach is referred to as "painting," and it is essentially the continuous delivery of laser energy to the tissue rather than by the staccato pulses with which we are all acquainted. The painting approach is difficult with the green laser, presumably because of the relatively superficial absorption of this wavelength by the tissue. More importantly, as the visible laser is being emitted, it obscures our view of the tissue effect until the application has been completed. It is not a very useful technique with this wavelength. On the other hand, the infrared laser is ideally suited for this purpose because its application is invisible to the surgeon's eye. Furthermore, the barrier filter in the operating microscope or in some endoscopy systems is clear and does not obscure or change the tissue characteristics that we perceive. These features enable the surgeon to continuously apply laser energy to the tissue and visually monitor its effect. In retinopexy, for example, the edge of a retinal tear can be approached by placing several rows of photocoagulation spots around it or by making a ring of confluent and continuous laser applications in the continuous-wave mode (Fig 17-15).

Intraocular Media

Endophotocoagulation may be needed at various times during the course of vitrectomy and for a host of reasons. These eyes can be filled with balanced saline solution (BSS), gas,

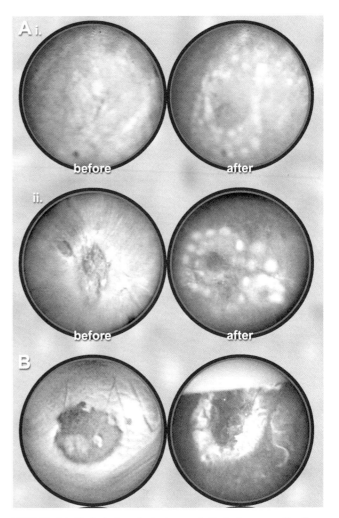

FIGURE 17-15. Painting technique of diode laser application. **A(i & ii):** Retinal break surrounded by several rows of discrete laser applications. **B:** Retinal break treated with continuous application of laser in an uninterrupted fashion.

perfluorocarbon liquid, or silicone oil, and some adjustments to laser power, duration, and treatment distance may be required depending on the intraocular media. Typically, decreasing laser power density is required with gas, and increasing power density with silicone oil. These adjustments are easily made and are not much of a challenge.

On the other hand, there is a situation commonly encountered during the course of vitrectomy in the phakic or pseudophakic eye that can be quite vexing. Specifically, after air-fluid exchange has been performed, the optics of the eye change and must be addressed by alterations in the contact lens used with the operating microscope. Even when using a noncontact, wide-field imaging system and the microscope, optical adjustments must be made. If the delays associated with these adjustments were routinely rewarded with a clear image of adequate magnification, field of view, and stereopsis, it would be satisfactory, but often this is not the case. Typically, the view becomes "minified," with decreased stereopsis and image clarity. If the pupil becomes a bit more miotic, or if there is condensation on the lens surfaces, or if corneal decompensation with epithelial edema or Descemet folds evolves, the view can be diminished or lost entirely. It can be frustrating when these problems arise, prohibiting endophotocoagulation and limiting the potential for successful surgery.

Endoscopic endophotocoagulation circumvents these problems. The surgeon can rely on this technology to execute laser delivery at the appropriate time and not be hampered by these physical impediments. Indeed, many believe that the endoscopic approach to endophotocoagulation is simpler and more efficacious even when a clear operating microscope view is available.

Finally, the surgeon can alternate the focus of attention between posterior and anterior locations within the gas-filled eye with great ease and without loss of image clarity. Magnification and field of view can also be adjusted by small alterations in the position of the endoscope within the eye. None of this is possible when the operating microscope is used for viewing. These features prove to be quite helpful in the execution of the various maneuvers required to surgically manage vitreoretinal diseases.

Endophotocoagulation Techniques

Focal Endophotocoagulation

The management of a number of retinal disorders by laser treatment rests on the focal ablation of some tissue. In this situation, the area of pathology is identified and laser applied, first surrounding the lesion and then directly to it. The power required varies in each situation, but treatment is usually initiated with mild to moderately intense lesions. The ultimate goal is to create a field of confluent burns that incorporates the entire lesion.

Often, the pathology encountered during the course of vitrectomy that demands this approach is vascular in nature (e.g., vitrectomy performed for vitreous hemorrhage that appears intraoperatively to be due to retinal arterial macroaneurysm). The surgeon must be careful not to be overzealous, delivering intensive burns that cause vessel rupture or occlusion. To the contrary, complete coverage of the macroaneurysm with mild to moderately intense burns is the goal. Ultimately, the intensity and extent of treatment are based largely on the surgeon's estimate of how extensive the treatment zone should be rather than following a predetermined "recipe" of parameters.

As far as endoscopic focal endophotocoagulation is concerned, and especially when an infrared laser is being used, the closer the tip of the instrument is to the tissue, the more compact the lesion. The endoscopic image will be relatively magnified, with a small field of view. With use of lower laser power settings with longer duration, more controlled ablation of the target tissue can be achieved. Varying the dis-

tance from the tip of the laser endoscope to the target may also enhance control of the tissue effect. Manipulation of these variables with the green laser is usually not possible, mostly because of the lack of laser beam divergence and the retinal absorption characteristics of this wavelength. In this situation, adjusting the laser power and duration more precisely on the laser console is required.

Laser Retinopexy

There are basically two techniques for laser retinopexy, and both are easily facilitated by endoscopic imaging. Indeed, many surgeons believe that it is simpler to perform these maneuvers by endoscopy even when a clear microscope view is available. The laser applications made in both techniques are typically delivered from close to moderate range but usually not panoramically. As with endophotocoagulation performed through the operating microscope, these techniques can be applied in the BSS-, gas-, perfluorocarbon liquid–, or silicone oil–filled eye.

The first and most common approach is to surround the retinal break or localized area of retinal detachment or lattice degeneration with several rows of moderately intense laser burns spaced fairly close together. Barring the presence of extraordinary tractional forces, such as those seen in PVR, it is surprising how little retinopexy is required to stabilize this pathology.

An alternative approach is to paint a ring of photocoagulation around the retinal break, lattice degeneration, or localized detachment (Fig. 17-16). This technique is more difficult with visible-wavelength lasers for reasons previously discussed. The infrared laser is quite efficacious for this purpose. The laser duration is set on continuous wave, and once the threshold for laser reaction is established by adjustment of the laser power and of the distance of the tip of the laser endoscope from the retina, the treatment can proceed. A large area can be rapidly and effectively addressed by this technique.

Macular Grid Photocoagulation

Not uncommonly, vitrectomy for vitreous hemorrhage is performed only for the surgeon to discover that at least a portion of the underlying pathology is some macular disease, such as branch retinal vein occlusion with macular edema and peripheral retinal neovascularization. It is entirely reasonable to address the macular pathology at the time of surgery by photocoagulating a grid pattern (Fig 17-17), similar to treatment applied at the slit lamp. More precise laser delivery would be desirable in the macula, compared with other areas of the retina, and so endoscopic endophotocoagulation should be effected at relatively close range. This will provide the most detailed view of the tissue as well as the most compact laser spot. Typically, photocoagulation is applied in a "loose" to moderately "tight" pat-

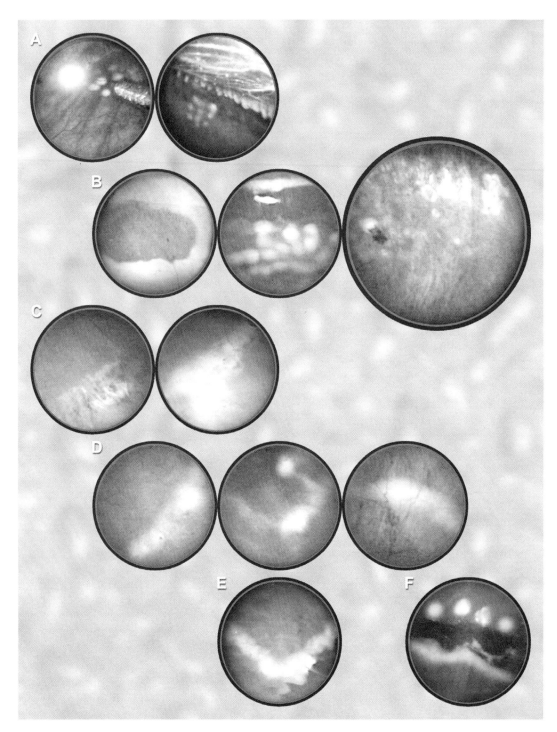

FIGURE 17-16. Endoscopic laser retinopexy. **A:** Scatter pattern of rings placed around pathology. **B:** Continuously applied diode laser retinopexy creating a confluent ring of laser application. **C:** Continuously applied laser to lattice degeneration. Before *(left)* and after *(right)* treatment. **D:** Continuous application laser retinopexy. **E:** Continuous laser application to the cut edge of a retinectomy. **F:** Combination of scatter and continuous application laser retinopexy.

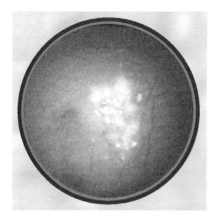

FIGURE 17-17. Endoscopic macular grid pattern of endophotocoagulation after treatment to area of retinal venous obstruction. Note moderately intense lesions scattered in a moderately tight pattern.

tern to areas of edema and hemorrhage, avoiding the fovea by at least 500 μm. The intensity of the lesions created should be mild to moderate; intense applications should be avoided.

Segmental Photocoagulation

The indications for segmental laser application typically relate to the ablation of a quadrant or hemisphere of retina for ischemic disease arising from a multitude of causes. It can also be used for its retinopexy function in the management of certain complex retinal detachments. This is another situation in which endoscopic laser delivery is thought by many to be simpler than viewing through the operating microscope, especially in the gas-filled eye.

Typically, a pattern of moderate-intensity lesions is created in the sector of pathology. The surgeon can elect for a scatter of photocoagulation that varies varying from light to dense, depending on the particular circumstances. Usually, the endophotocoagulation is applied with the tip of the laser endoscope placed a moderate distance from the target (Fig. 17-18). A more panoramic view at the time of laser delivery, especially when one is using the more divergent diode laser, produces larger retinal lesions. This may not be a negative feature considering that often the goal is ischemic retinal ablation. Understanding this, the choice of endoscopic working distance is at the surgeon's discretion.

Panretinal Endophotocoagulation

The technique of panretinal photocoagulation (PRP) is well known to most ophthalmologists, and its indications are numerous. Ablation of ischemic retina or the creation of extensive retinopexy is the most common goal with this technique. Endoscopic performance of PRP is so simple that most retinal surgeons are able to execute this procedure

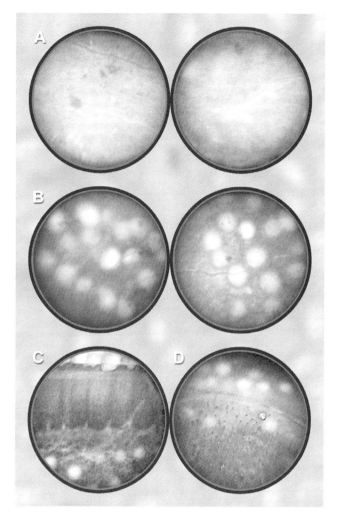

FIGURE 17-18. Endoscopic segmental retinal endophotocoagulation. A quadrant or hemisphere of retina undergoes moderate intensity light to dense scatter of laser applications for the management of ischemic disease. This is best accomplished with tip of endoscope at a moderate distance from the retina, especially when using 810-nm diode laser with its more divergent beam. **A:** Ischemic quadrant of retina in branch retinal vein occlusion. Note the white vessels. **B:** Same areas after segmental photocoagulation. **C:** Ablation carried to the ora if possible. **D:** Peripheral retinal ablation. Note healed laser lesions posteriorly and new laser spots anteriorly that are addressing the schemia of the more peripheral aspects of the retina.

almost immediately. Typically, lesions of mild to moderate intensity are created in a scatter pattern that can vary from light to dense, depending on the clinical situation (Fig 17-19). Hundreds or even thousands of applications can be made. Usually the tip of the laser endoscope is held at a moderate distance from the target tissue, although this option is certainly at the discretion of the surgeon. One of the great advantages of executing this technique endoscopically is that complete treatment of the retinal periphery or even pars plana is possible with relative ease despite deteriorating anterior segment conditions or the presence of

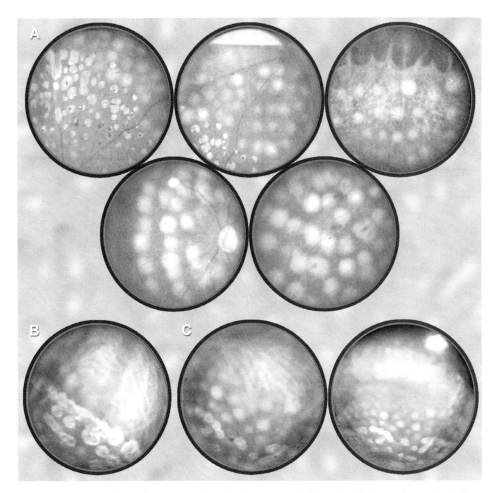

FIGURE 17-19. Endoscopic panretinal endophotocoagulation. **A:** Moderate-intensity lesions with light to dense scatter. **B:** Peripheral retina has previously been left untreated. **C:** This area is now "filled in."

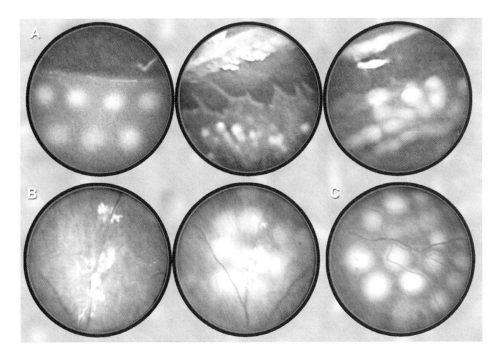

FIGURE 17-20. Endoscopic peripheral retinal endophotocoagulation and ablation. **A:** Define boundary of perfused and nonperfused retina initiate scatter photocoagulation two rows proximal to this region in healthy retina, and then proceed more peripherally in light to dense scatter pattern. **B:** Peripheral retinal neovascularization in Eales' disease. Before *(left)* and after *(right)* treatment. **C:** Peripheral retinal neovascularization in sickle disease after retinal ablation.

intraocular gas. In ischemic eyes, this ability can give the surgeon confidence that complete retinal ablation will be possible intraoperatively, limiting the potential for iris neovascularization and its postoperative complications. In eyes requiring extensive retinopexy, one again can rely on the ability of this approach to effect the planned treatment rather than succumb to conditions beyond the surgeon's control. Finally, in highly ischemic eyes, painting the most involved retinal areas may result in more effective retinal ablation.

Peripheral Retinal Endophotocoagulation and Ablation

Certain disorders result in the development of peripheral retinal schemia. This pathology may be confined to a focal area or may be present in a wide ring involving the mid- to far peripheral retina for 360 degrees. This pathologic state can induce peripheral fibrovascular proliferation that ultimately can lead to vitreous hemorrhage and retinal detachment, necessitating vitrectomy.

The endoscopic photocoagulation principles are the same as in segmental retinal laser ablation. Because fibrovascular proliferation usually begins at the border of perfused and nonperfused retina, treatment is initiated by starting about two laser "rows" proximal to the areas of proliferation and proceeding in a light to dense pattern into the periphery (Fig. 17-20). In some of the disorders underlying this pathology, the retina is ischemic for 360 degrees and so a peripheral ring of endophotocoagulation is applied. In other situations, the area of peripheral schemia may be confined to a hemisphere or more focally, so that less extensive treatment is indicated.

MANAGEMENT OF A FORESHORTENED RETINA

The purpose of membranectomy is to effect increased retinal mobility so that the retina can flatten against the eye wall. Theoretically, removal of all preretinal and subretinal proliferation should result in this outcome. Nevertheless, there are situations in which successful membranectomy has been executed and an air-fluid exchange performed, only to result in the accumulation of subretinal air. The infusion of air should be discontinued immediately and the area of accumulation inspected for residual membranes that might account for this predicament. If they cannot be detected, one can presume that the cause of this difficulty is contraction of the retina itself, rendering it too short and inflexible to reapproximate against the eye wall. In this scenario, a retinotomy must be performed to "relax" the retina and allow its proper placement against the eye wall. Endoscopy is quite helpful for the diagnosis and management of this problem. During the course of air-fluid exchange, a wide-field endoscopic view of

the retinal periphery is easily established. Early in the progress of subretinal air accumulation then, the problem will become evident to the surgeon. Effecting adequate retinotomy is usually done more easily under endoscopic guidance than with use of the microscope because the extent of the treatment area required is usually well beyond that available through the microscope, even with a wide-field imaging system, whereas a panoramic endoscopic view often incorporates the entire treatment zone as well as some surrounding tissue.

The creation of a retinotomy for this purpose is quite simple (Fig. 17-21). Once the subretinal air is observed, the intraocular diathermy is introduced. One or two rows of confluent application are made in a circumferential fashion and as peripherally as possible along the entire extent of the foreshortened retina and then a bit more on each side of the pathologic tissue. The purpose of this maneuver is to effect hemostasis. Then, with use of a vitrector or vertical scissors,

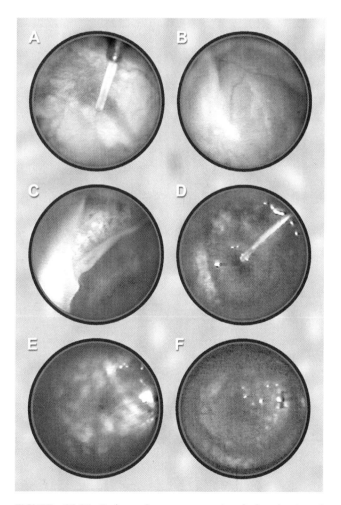

FIGURE 17-21. Endoscopic management of foreshortened retina. **A:** Wide-field view discloses intrinsically stiffened retina. **B:** Close-up view. **C:** Vitrector retinectomy performed with excision of peripheral retinal apron. **D:** Air-fluid exchange and internal drainage of subretinal fluid performed with flattening of retina. **E:** Endoscopic endophotocoagulation to cut edge and margin is applied. **F:** Wide-field view of attached retina.

the diathermized retina is cut. Often, when a sufficient retinotomy is created, the retina flattens spontaneously. The peripheral "apron" of retina should then be excised with the vitrector. Photocoagulation can then be applied to the edge. Ultimately, gas or silicone oil tamponade is required.

PARS PLANA LENSECTOMY

Being able to rapidly shift imaging from the posterior iris region to the macula and back again with a small hand movement is an asset of endoscopy. The anterior segment progress of lensectomy can be monitored through the operating microscope, and the posterior location of nuclear and cortical fragments as well as lens capsule can be monitored endoscopically. In this manner, it would be difficult to miss any lens material that might otherwise be left in the eye if microscope imaging alone were used. Typically, a wide-field view is used to assess the situation posteriorly and to locate scattered lens fragments. Then, the surgeon can advance the phacoemulsification tip toward the fragment and initiate aspiration. Once the fragments are lifted from the retinal surface, further aspiration or fragmentation can begin. This step is repeated as many times as necessary to complete the task. If large fragments are present, it is often best simply to break them into smaller pieces before phacoemulsification is initiated.

In an eye with dislocated lens material, large fragments in the anterior or posterior chamber often are readily apparent. Endoscopic inspection frequently reveals many small lens fragments scattered about the posterior segment, especially in the region of the ciliary sulcus and vitreous base, that are not so obvious. Missing them at the time of surgery may not be very important because the eye may simply heal well following removal of the larger pieces. Still, it is quite disturbing to operate on such a patient only to have these residual fragments rear their heads in some form, such as by elevated intraocular pressure, inflammation, or frank obscuring of the patient's vision. Under these circumstances, additional surgery would be required. Endoscopic imaging combined with fragmentation and vitrectomy can prevent this situation from developing because it enables imaging of all lens fragments. In this situation, the surgeon can then judge whether the fragment must be removed or, alternatively, left in the eye.

Some caution is required for the extraction of lens fragments on the macular surface. Usually, the endoscope is held at a moderate to close distance from the surface and the phacoemulsification tip is brought into proximity, with care taken not to contact the retina. Then, only aspiration is initiated and the fragments are vacuumed into the phacoemulsification tip port. The endoscope can then be withdrawn further from the retina and followed by the phacoemulsification tip. The surgeon can elect to continue with aspiration alone or to proceed with phacoemulsifica-

tion. In any event, the fragment will have been safely removed from the retinal surface, and its disposal can take place in mid-vitreous cavity, away from any structures of importance.

The panoramic retinal view makes it possible to monitor the status of the retina while chasing around the lens fragments. This view is also useful to detect iatrogenic breaks during the evaluation of the retina after lens removal. If breaks are found, endophotocoagulation can be applied immediately.

LENS CAPSULECTOMY

Depending on the underlying pathology, the surgeon may elect to remove the remaining lens capsule. Although this can be done partially or completely using a vitrector, perhaps the ideal method is to grab the edge of the lens capsule with end-gripping forceps and gently pull the capsule from the eye under endoscopic control (Fig. 17-22). This endoscopic capsulectomy can be easily and rapidly performed, resulting in total removal of the capsule so that a scaffold for potential proliferation will not remain in the eye.

There may be other situations in which, despite previous cataract surgery, all or some of the capsule remains in the eye, impeding access to the ciliary body or serving as an unwanted scaffold for proliferation. As described previously, this tissue can be removed from the eye with end-gripping forceps and/or the vitrector under endoscopic control. Usually a moderate or wide-field view is used for this purpose. This tissue is typically undetectable, let alone treatable, by conventional microscope imaging.

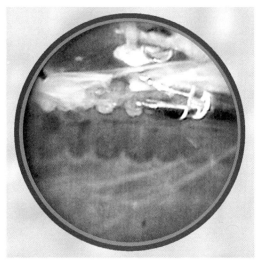

FIGURE 17-22. Endoscopic capsulectomy. End-gripping forceps are used to grab the capsule and literally pull it from the eye in its entirety.

SILICONE OIL INJECTION

Although silicone oil injection is not the most difficult of procedures under most circumstances, it is quite easy to inject silicone oil under endoscopic visualization. Usually, the endoscope is used to present a wide field of view in an air-filled eye. The silicone oil cannula can be visualized within the eye and, when injection begins, the oil can be seen to drip posteriorly onto the optic nerve and macula, gradually filling the eye (Fig 17-23).

This approach presents two advantages over microscope-controlled injection. The first is that the extent of the oil fill can be completely ascertained endoscopically but not microscopically. Once the oil level has passed the midperipheral portion of the retina, the operating microscope cannot be relied on to provide a good view of the far periphery and posterior iris region, at least without other surgical maneuvers. The extent of further oil injection can only be estimated. The endoscope can clearly delineate the air–oil interface anywhere in the eye and the amount injected more precisely controlled.

The second advantage of endoscopy in this situation is realized if silicone oil begins to enter the subretinal space. This feature is especially helpful if the problem can be detected early on. It is difficult and time consuming to remove subretinal oil, especially if it is not detected until a substantial amount of this material has already been misplaced. It is much simpler to completely observe the course of injection from its entry into the eye through the cannula to completion of an adequate fill by endoscopic means.

Silicone oil does not degrade the endoscopic image at all and only mildly attenuates laser delivery. Therefore, all maneuvers that can be performed in the fluid-filled eye can be performed in the silicone oil–filled eye.

PERFLUOROCARBON LIQUID INJECTION

As in air-fluid exchange or silicone oil injection, endoscopy can be useful in monitoring the injection of perfluorocarbon liquid. Typically, this substance is injected into a fluid-filled eye and, because it is "heavier," the perfluorocarbon liquid "sinks" to the posterior pole, creating a clear delineation between itself and the BSS. As more perfluorocarbon liquid is injected, subretinal fluid is pushed peripherally and through retinal breaks, ultimately flattening the retina, as long as there is no significant traction (Fig. 17-24). On the other hand, if strong tractional elements remain, the retina will clearly be unresponsive, so attention may be focused on that particular area. One of the great advantages of endoscopy in this situation is that its wild field of view allows continuous monitoring of the retina as it flattens so that areas with persistent traction or gliosis are readily apparent.

Endoscopy can also be useful in the removal of perfluorocarbon liquid from the eye. Some of this material may inadvertently be left behind because it becomes sequestered in areas that are not visible through the operating microscope, such as the ciliary sulcus or posterior to the iris. Since it can be somewhat of a chore to remove perfluorocarbon liquid postoperatively, its complete aspiration under endoscopic guidance is most helpful.

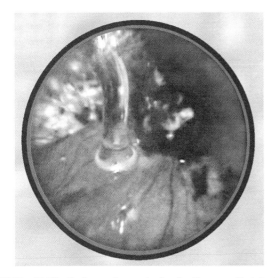

FIGURE 17-23. Endoscopic control of silicone oil injection. Panoramic view is used to follow the course of silicone injection into air-filled eye. Silicone oil drips onto posterior pole and then fills the eye.

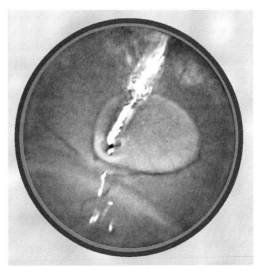

FIGURE 17-24. Endoscopic control of perfluorocarbon liquid injection. Perfluorocarbon liquid injected into water-filled eye over the disc pushes subretinal fluid peripherally while flattening the retina. The basic salt solution–perfluorocarbon liquid interface is easily detected.

ANTERIOR SEGMENT VISUAL OBSTRUCTIONS

Every vitreoretinal surgeon has encountered eyes with obstructions to visualization that are located in the anterior chamber or at the level of the iris, ciliary sulcus, ciliary body, or anterior vitreous. These are usually membranous structures that have arisen as a result of inflammation, residual lens material following cataract surgery, proliferative gliotic tissue, or trauma, or that are congenital. No matter what the cause, they may sometimes be addressed by the creation of a shock wave produced by the neodymium:yttrium-argon-garnet (Nd:YAG) laser that ruptures the structure, creating an opening that will, it is hoped, suffice to improve visual function. However, if this is not the case, then surgical excision is required. Typically, these membranes can be punctured with an MVR blade either from the anterior or posterior segment, and then a vitrector, with or without infusion, can be used to partially or completely excise the structure. Often a subtotal excision is sufficient for most cases, with the creation of a central opening being the goal. In some situations (e.g., adult retinopathy of prematurity after cataract surgery), however, these structures can recur. In these situations, total excision is required to limit the potential for recurrence. Endoscopic imaging can be helpful because a view of the membranous structure and its attachments can be obtained from the anterior and posterior aspects (Fig 17-25). This is not the case with the

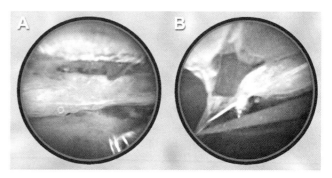

FIGURE 17-25. Endoscopic evaluation and management of anterior segment membrane obstructing a posterior view. **A:** Cyclitic membrane adherent to peripheral retina, ciliary body, and posterior iris with a broad iridomembrane adhesion. **B:** Same area being dissected with MVR blade.

operating microscope. This ability permits total excision of the pathology and limits the potential for the creation of iatrogenic complications, such as retinal detachment.

At times, many of these eyes present with no posterior view, a poor historian for a patient, and no previous medical records. At the time of surgery, assessment of more posterior structures, such as the optic nerve, by endoscope may indicate that the patient has a viable eye or, to the contrary, that optic atrophy is already present and would limit the patient's visual potential even with an outstanding surgical result (Fig 17-26).

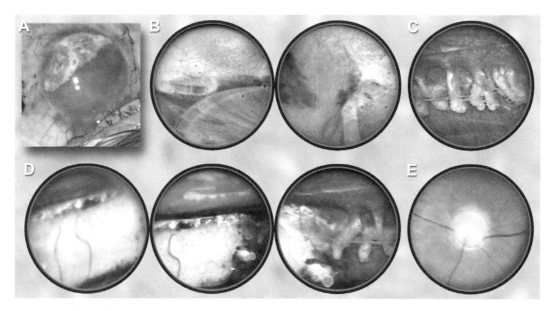

FIGURE 17-26. Assessment of intraocular status despite anterior segment opacities obscuring a posterior view. **A:** Opaque cornea. **B:** Anterior chamber intraocular lens with haptics piercing iris. **C:** Posterior view of haptics piercing iris. **D:** Old cyclocryotherapy. **E:** Advanced cavernous optic atrophy.

ENDOSCOPIC VITRECTOMY FOR DIABETIC RETINOPATHY

Retinal schemia drives the development of fibrovascular proliferation within the eye, and the natural history of this chain of events ultimately creates retinal detachment, vitreous hemorrhage, glaucoma, and blindness. All ophthalmologists understand that there is a lengthy list of underlying disorders that initiate this chain of events, but no matter the cause, there are only a few guiding principles that must be kept in mind in their management. The key to controlling these disorders is to effect sufficient retinal ablation so as to effect regression of the proliferative process. To achieve this goal technically and to rehabilitate the eye maximally, the media must be clear and the retina largely attached.

The surgical option presents itself when retinal ablation is not possible because of impedance from these opacities or retinal detachment. Our surgical goals, then, are to remove media opacification, reattach the retina, and initiate retinal ablation.

The consequences of ocular proliferation in proliferative diabetic retinopathy (PDR) are numerous, presenting a handful of indications for surgery, including vitreous hemorrhage, premacular hemorrhage, severe proliferative retinopathy unresponsive to panretinal photocoagulation (PRP), traction macular detachment, combined traction and rhegmatogenous retinal detachment, anterior hyaloidal fibrovascular proliferation, and iris neovascularization associated with opaque media. Their management options will now be explored.

DIABETIC VITREOUS HEMORRHAGE

The Diabetic Retinopathy Vitrectomy Study (DRVS) (1) has indicated that in type I diabetics, a vitrectomy performed within the first 6 months for dense vitreous hemorrhage enhanced the potential for improvement in anatomic and functional outcomes. Visual recovery was earlier and better in patients who underwent successful surgery. The techniques of vitrectomy, active or passive extrusion, air-fluid exchange, and endophotocoagulation are most commonly used in this situation, and all can be enhanced with endoscopy. More complete removal of vitreous and blood can often be effected. This limits the potential for complications, some of which center on residual hemorrhage or opacified vitreous in the eye that may limit the patient's ultimate visual result or that are associated with hemolytic glaucoma or that mask the presence of retinal breaks. Vitrectomy performed under these circumstances can be expected to improve visual acuity in about 80% of the treatment group, with as many as 35% attaining an acuity of 20/40 or better (Fig. 18-1).

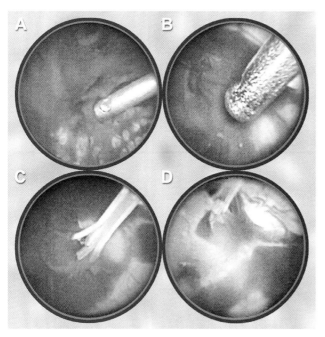

FIGURE 18-1. A-D. Endoscopic vitrectomy for vitreous hemorrhage in PDR.

PREMACULAR HEMORRHAGE

Proliferative diabetic retinopathy is often associated with intraocular hemorrhage, presumably arising from rupture of neovascular vessels. One of the sites where this might occur is the posterior pole. Neovascularization of the disc or retina may bleed, with entrapment of the hemorrhage between the posterior hyaloid and the retinal surface, obscuring the macula and diminishing vision. As with hemorrhage elsewhere in the eye that arises from this condition, spontaneous resolution is common. On the other hand, a number of these patients do not benefit from a conservative approach, ultimately experiencing nonclearing hemorrhage, macular detachment, or premacular fibrosis. Although the data about this are less than definitive, many retinal surgeons believe that large, nonclearing hemorrhages should be treated. The DRVS has addressed this issue and its conclusions are pending.

The surgical approach is straightforward. A complete or partial vitrectomy is performed. This latter approach may be interpreted as a simplified variation of en bloc dissection in that it uses the inherent anterior–posterior (AP) vitreous traction to help elevate the posterior hyaloid. An MVR blade or other sharp instrument is used to incise the posterior hyaloid, usually over a dense area of subhyaloid hemorrhage. This protects the underlying retina from inadvertent laceration. The surgeon can then continue elevating the

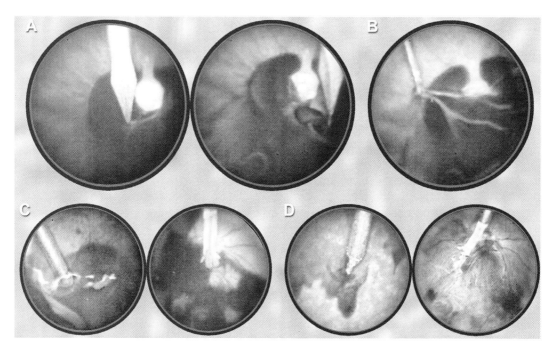

FIGURE 18-2. Endoscopic vitrectomy for preretinal hemorrhage. **A:** Posterior hyaloid over thickest portion of hemorrhage is incised while viewing with high magnification and small field of view. **B:** With the endoscope shifted to a more panoramic view, the membrane is opened more fully and removed. **C:** A vitrector or extrusion cannula is then used to aspirate the hemorrhage. **D:** Air-fluid exchange, endodiathermy, and endophotocoagulation are applied as needed.

posterior hyaloid with the blade or a pick, spatula, or forceps until it is removed from overlying at least the macular region and perhaps even more extensively. This tissue can be removed from the eye with the vitrector. Preretinal hemorrhage is then easily removed by aspirating into the vitrector or by extrusion. An alternative approach is to puncture the posterior hyaloid over the densest area of hemorrhage and to insert the aspirating port of the vitrector or an extrusion cannula into the subhyaloid space. The subhyaloid blood is easily aspirated. Following this, the residual posterior hyaloid membrane can be removed as previously described.

Although the endoscopic approach to each of the techniques has been described, it is important to note that this entire procedure is easily performed by endoscopy alone. Usually, the hyaloid incision should be executed under higher magnification and smaller field of view, with the surgeon then shifting to wide-field imaging for elevation and excision of the posterior hyaloid as well as hemorrhage aspiration (Fig. 18-2). Not infrequently, these eyes require endodiathermy for oozing neovascularization, as well as air-fluid exchange and endophotocoagulation. Although not statistically valid, personal experience has indicated that most patients with this problem who are approached before chronic retinal changes evolve do well, with substantial visual recovery and long-term stabilization of their retinal status.

SEVERE PROLIFERATIVE DIABETIC RETINOPATHY DESPITE ADEQUATE PANRETINAL PHOTOCOAGULATION

Occasionally, patients present with severe proliferation characterized by advancing neovascularization and fibrosis even though they have had extensive PRP. For a time, these patients often have good visual acuity despite progression of their disease. The DRVS demonstrated that eyes in this situation did poorly with photocoagulation alone yet seemed to benefit from removing the vitreoretinal interface. Specifically, 44% of eyes treated by vitrectomy attained 10/20 acuity or better while only 28% of those treated conventionally did as well over a 4-year follow-up period (1). Treatment was thought to be most useful in those patients with severe fibrous and neovascular proliferation.

From a technical viewpoint, vitrectomy and various membranectomy techniques are applied in this situation, with special attention to hemostasis. Many of these patients have lush neovascularization, and so endodiathermy and increasing infusion pressure are critical components of this intervention, perhaps being even more important than when one is performing vitrectomy for the more common situation of traction detachment. While en bloc dissection can be useful in this situation, the surgeon must clearly understand the higher risk of hemorrhage.

One asset of endoscopy lies in its ability to help locate sites of bleeding hidden from the microscope view by a preretinal membrane that has not yet been excised. In the event that bleeding does occur and its source cannot be controlled with endodiathermy or even located, air-fluid exchange can be helpful. Endoscopic imaging under these circumstances is superior to alternatives because it does not require a change in lensing or instrumentation and can be performed most rapidly. In some eyes, several cycles of air-fluid exchange are required during the course of vitrectomy to manage this problem.

Endoscopic endophotocoagulation of the far retinal periphery can assist in diminishing the ischemic drive experienced by these eyes. This procedure can usually be expeditiously performed by this approach in the fluid- or gas-filled eye, again without a change in instrumentation or lensing, which is required by other techniques (Fig. 18-3).

Finally, at the conclusion of surgery, the surgeon may note persistent oozing of blood from one or multiple sites that does not completely respond to conventional techniques. Many of these patients seem to do well with silicone oil injection, limiting their potential for problems in the early postoperative period. Despite the possible need for its removal at a later date, silicone oil can help stabilize the retinal status, especially when the course of surgery has not been smooth.

DIABETIC TRACTION MACULAR DETACHMENT

As fibrovascular tissue proliferates about the disc and macular vasculature, it most often "grows" along the posterior hyaloid face. Subsequent contraction may result in detachment of the macula on a tractional basis. A variation of this problem may be observed when frank detachment is not present but ectopia of the fovea with its associated visual loss evolves. Under these circumstances, vitrectomy is required, primarily to relieve this traction and reestablish more normal macular architecture, with the ultimate hope that technically successful surgery will restore the patient's visual function.

There is no clear agreement among the gurus of vitrectomy as to the best technique for the management of this difficult problem, and so tailoring the approach to a given eye and patient by considering a menu of these techniques might be appropriate.

In PDR, the retina is often thin and prone to tearing, unlike some other forms of traction retinal detachment. Techniques that rely on tissue "pulling" can be effective in the elevation and removal of membranes but at the price of risking break formation or significant hemorrhage. If the retina does not seem to be atrophic, a more vigorous approach may indeed be most useful.

Perhaps the safest approach is to first remove all of the vitreous, relieving AP traction. Sometimes the macula will be

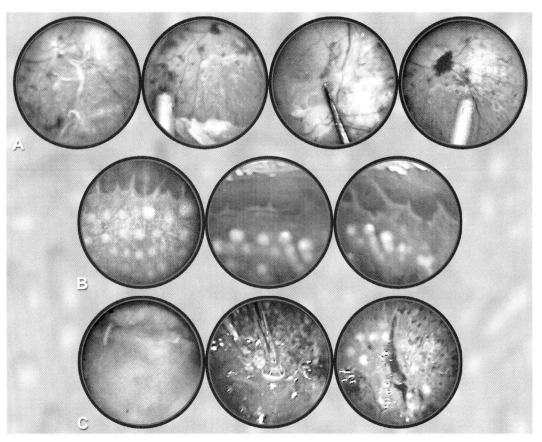

FIGURE 18-3. Endoscopic vitrectomy for severe proliferative diabetic retinopathy (PDR) unresponsive to laser therapy. **A:** Endoscopic views of vitrectomy and membranectomy techniques in this situation. **B:** Endoscopic endophotocoagulation of far retinal periphery effect more complete ablation of ischemic retina, theoretically diminishing the stimulus for persistent and further neovascularization. **C:** Persistent oozing of blood from active neovascularization or damaged retinal vessels despite typical maneuvers to control. Benefit obtained from silicone oil tamponade.

seen to flatten even though fibrovascular proliferation around the disc and macular vessels remains. One of the surgeon's options is to fill in any untreated areas of retina with PRP, then declare victory by terminating the procedure. The rationale here is that the purpose of the procedure was to normalize macular architecture, and that is what has been achieved. On the other hand, some surgeons would argue that the residual fibrous or vascular tissue could serve as a focus for reproliferation in the future. They would advocate membranectomy by segmentation, delamination, or en bloc dissection (Fig. 18-4). While it is true that these approaches would result in a more "complete" management of the patient's retinal disease, they have the potential for creating complications that might ultimately lead to failure. To add to the potential for confusion, some surgeons who strongly advocate membrane segmentation proceeding from posterior to anterior ("inside-out"), whereas others use only en bloc dissection with membranectomy proceeding from anterior to posterior ("outside-in").

The same argument holds true with regard to the instrumentation used for these techniques. Some favor only scissors or vitrector dissection, admonishing those surgeons who use instruments such as picks, blades, needles, or membrane scratchers. When these types of controversies arise, it is clear that there is no one right answer. To be sure, many patients who experience flattening of the macula by removing AP traction do well despite thick accumulations of residual membrane along the vascular arcades. Some macular distortion resulting from further membrane contraction may develop in some of these eyes over the long run. On the other hand, if adequate retinal ablation has been effected to eradicate active neovascularization, this simplified treatment can be extremely effective with relatively little risk to the patient. This approach can be especially helpful in eyes that cannot wait for visual recovery over a lengthy period, which might be necessary with a more aggressive approach.

Suppose that a different scenario develops. Consider that after the AP traction has been removed, the macula or significant amounts of peripheral retina remain with traction detachment. Under this circumstance, it is clear that membranectomy is required. One may be faced with the same

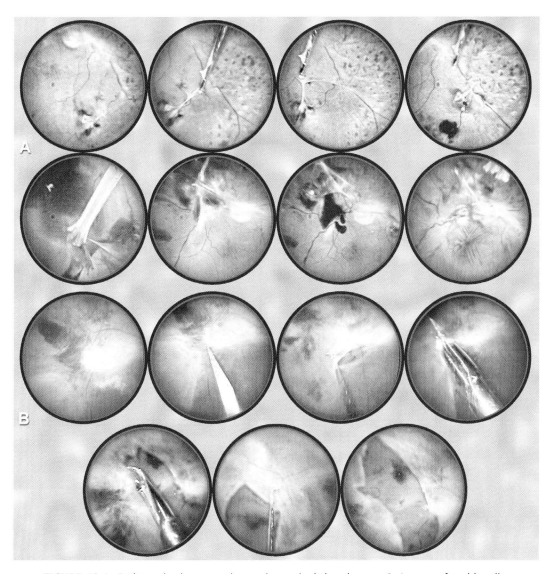

FIGURE 18-4. Endoscopic vitrectomy in traction retinal detachment. **A:** Images of en bloc dissection. **B:** Images of membrane segmentation.

questions as alluded to previously. Should membranectomy proceed with segmentation from posterior to anterior? Should en bloc dissection with anterior to posterior progress have been selected? What instruments should be used? How much fibrovascular membrane should be removed? The answer to all of these questions depends entirely on the surgeon's skill and experience as well as the condition of the eye, but suffice to say that the surgeon should be experienced in all of these methods and their instrumentation to address the wide array of each eye's particular anatomic variables. Choosing one method or set of instrumentation while discounting the others severely limits the surgeon's options when the need arises. Opinions about the perhaps more philosophical issue of how much membranectomy should be performed vary among practitioners.

On a personal note, I typically begin these vitrectomies with the intention of performing an en bloc dissection. If all is going well, I continue as planned. If the procedure is not progressing as smoothly as anticipated or if the adhesion between posterior hyaloid and retina is so strong that extensive delamination becomes necessary, I shift over to completing removal of the AP traction with the vitrector and observing the behavior of the macula. If it flattens, the surgery is concluded. If it does not, I undertake segmentation with vertical scissors until the macular traction is released. The last location considered for membranectomy is nasal to the disc. It seems incautious to be aggressive with membranectomy in this region unless there is extensive retinal detachment because iatrogenic posterior break just nasal to the disc can ultimately be the undoing of an otherwise successful surgery, even though it does not contribute to the patient's ultimate visual function even if all membranes are successfully excised.

It has also been my experience that if the macula is flattened and considerable retinal ablation is performed, even substantial amounts of residual extramacular fibrovascular membranes do not threaten long-term stability. However, I suspect that many knowledgeable and experienced vitrectomy surgeons would disagree.

The value of endoscopy in this situation perhaps may be found when complications arise. Any method of instrumentation used for membranectomy may tear the retina or shear a retinal vessel. Both of these problems must be addressed adequately or surgery will fail.

As far as iatrogenic breaks are concerned, the endoscope can be exceedingly helpful in detecting their presence, particularly when they are hidden beneath a partially cut membrane (Fig. 18-5). This pathology may not be detected by microscope viewing, but relatively close-up endoscopic imaging can easily reveal the nature of this event. The treatment principles are quite straightforward, but their execution may be considerably more problematic. Essentially, all the tractional elements from the region must be removed; then the break can easily be flattened by air-fluid exchange and its edges photocoagulated. Unfortunately, some of these breaks occur adjacent to stubborn or very large membranes with which the surgeon is struggling in the first place. What may ultimately be required is a circumscribed

retinectomy to achieve the goal of flattened retinal break edges that can be lasered. If the location of the break does not permit this, the only other alternative is to densely circumscribe the area with almost confluent or painted laser applications to confine the localized detachment. Gas or silicone oil tamponade at the conclusion of surgery can sometimes be effective in ultimately flattening the area.

Shearing a blood vessel at the time of membranectomy is all too common, and again endoscopy can be useful in locating the exact site of hemorrhage, particularly when it is concealed beneath the edge of a membrane. Once found, this site can be treated by elevating the balanced saline solution infusion pressure, performing air-fluid exchange, and controlling the IOP in that manner, or by direct pressure from an intraocular instrument, endodiathermy, endophotocoagulation, adding thrombin to the infusion, or any combination of these maneuvers (Fig. 18-6).

Finally, there may be an area of retina that seems to have had all of the vitreous and membranes removed and that does not appear to be foreshortened yet does not flatten with air-fluid exchange. Recalling that endoscopy gives a different perspective to the appearance of vitreous than the microscope, a search for adherent vitreous fibers should be made. Often a few long "strands" can be found on the retinal surface, restricting its mobility. Once removed, the retina can be observed to flatten and then can be treated with photocoagulation or other modality.

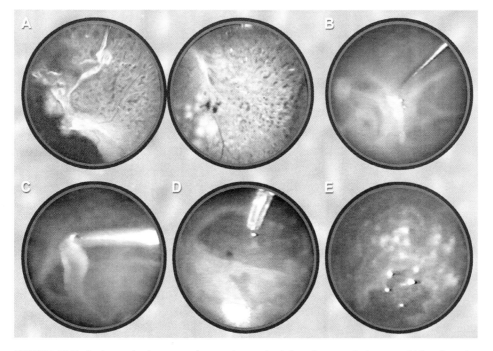

FIGURE 18-5. Endoscopic vitrectomy in traction retinal detachment. **A:** Image of bleeding site hidden by partially cut membrane. **B:** Circumscribed excision of retina for dense proliferation that cannot be dissected. **C:** Vitrector excises retina. **D:** Internal drainage of subretinal fluid with flattening of retina. **E:** View after gas and silicone oil tamponade.

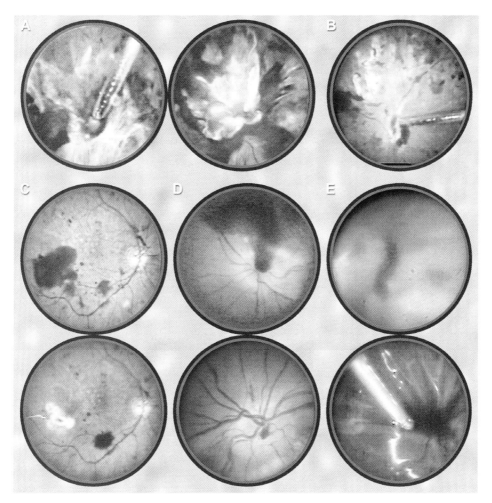

FIGURE 18-6. Hemorrhage from shearing a retinal vessel during membranectomy. **A:** Appearance during *(left)* and after *(right)* application of direct pressure with an instrument—in this case, a vitrector. Bleeding before *(top)* and after *(bottom)*. **B:** Endodiathermy. **C:** Endophotocoagulation. **D:** Raising balanced salt solution infusion pressure: bleeding before *(top)* and after *(bottom)*. **E:** Air-fluid exchange.

Ultimately, about 80% of these traction macular detachments achieve a good anatomic result, with 5/200 vision or better being attained in about 70% of the eyes.

COMBINED TRACTION AND RHEGMATOGENOUS RETINAL DETACHMENT

At times, the contracting vitreous causes so much traction on the retinal surface, particularly adjacent to the epicenters of fibrovascular proliferation, that a hole in the retina develops, ultimately producing a rhegmatogenous component to what otherwise seemed to be a tractional retinal detachment. This rhegmatogenous portion can be localized or it can be extensive, spreading into the retinal periphery.

To avoid any confusion, it should be clear that in traction and rhegmatogenous retinal detachment, surgery is indicated whether or not the macula is involved. Certainly

the prognosis would be better if successful surgery were to be performed prior to any macular detachment, as in purely rhegmatogenous retinal detachment.

One way to look at this situation is to treat it as if it were a tractional retinal detachment with associated iatrogenic break. All vitreous should be removed and, most importantly, any membrane in the region of the break must be completely excised to achieve a relatively free and mobile retinal break and adjacent retina. In this situation then, en bloc dissection or delamination is usually indicated. Segmentation of the membrane adjacent to the break may or may not be successful in permitting hole closure because it might allow residual traction to impinge on the site. Still if the adjacent membrane can be sufficiently segmented so that subsequent air-fluid exchange and endophotocoagulation can be performed, this approach would be acceptable.

Endoscopy can be useful in the detection of the offending retinal breaks. They are often small and round, and

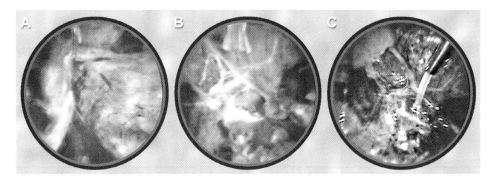

FIGURE 18-7. Endoscopic vitrectomy in traction and rhegmatogenous retinal detachment. **A:** Breaks are often small and located near membrane epicenter. **B:** All adjacent fibrovascular tissue is removed by any suitable membranectomy technique. **C:** Gas or silicone oil tamponade and laser retinopexy.

although we know they are frequently adjacent to the membrane epicenter, they may be hiding beneath the edge of a membrane, making them difficult to detect with the microscope. Close- or medium-range endoscopic imaging can easily detect this pathology, streamlining treatment.

Once the offending membrane and breaks have been addressed, the principles of vitrectomy for traction detachment that have already been discussed apply (Fig. 18-7).

Scleral buckling may be a consideration in rhegmatogenous detachment but is rarely necessary. Once the area of the retinal breaks has been freed of the vitreous and membrane attachments, gas tamponade and photocoagulation suffice to flatten the retina and create permanent adhesion.

ANTERIOR HYALOIDAL FIBROVASCULAR PROLIFERATION

Aside from the cumbersome name, this uncommon event is usually devastating. Neovascularization with fibrous prolif-

eration is thought to be initiated in the retinal periphery and extend anteriorly, along the ciliary body, to ultimately involve posterior iris or lens capsule. This entity is seen most often in highly ischemic eyes that have undergone previous vitrectomy (usually for traction retinal detachment) and may have exhibited uncontrolled neovascularization unresponsive to PRP in the past. Cases have been reported in which previous vitrectomy was not performed. On a personal note, I have evaluated several patients in whom this severe problem developed on the heels of successful cataract/intraocular lens surgery. The earliest clinical manifestation of this problem is far peripheral neovascularization with vessels that may be seen to spread onto the anterior vitreous face or posterior lens capsule by slit-lamp biomicroscopy. As the condition advances, anterior vitreous hemorrhage evolves or a more fibrous component to the proliferation becomes evident anteriorly, which will ultimately result in anterior retinal and ciliary body detachment. These anterior changes obscure a posterior view, but advanced cases demonstrate a posterior spreading of this

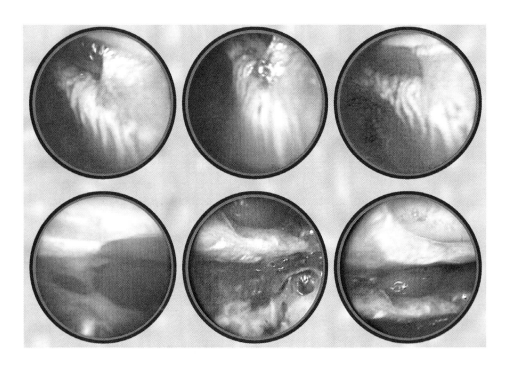

FIGURE 18-8. Endoscopic views of anterior hyaloidal fibrovascular proliferation.

proliferation, so that ultimately the entire interior of the eye is lined by a lush fibrovascular membrane.

Early intervention might be helpful and consists of complete vitrectomy, removal of anterior fibrovascular membranes, and extensive PRP involving the entire retinal periphery. Endoscopy is useful in these situations because often the anterior segment does not permit an adequate posterior view with the microscope, so that much pathology can be missed (Fig. 18-8). In addition, the key to treatment is extensive and peripheral endophotocoagulation, for which laser endoscopy is ideal. Overall, the prognosis is grim, with surgery often being an act of desperation.

IRIS NEOVASCULARIZATION ASSOCIATED WITH OPAQUE MEDIA

As discussed previously, iris neovascularization is a serious problem and one that screams for the ophthalmologist's attention; it is not to be taken lightly. To develop the first few twigs of fine iris or angle vessels requires a massive amount of ocular schemia. Immediate and unrelenting attention is required to thrash these vessels into submission (Table 18-1).

Once they have been detected, dense PRP is required. This treatment often proves to be effective in preventing the development of neovascular glaucoma and its complications. But what if the patient has a dense cataract, opacified cornea, hyphema, or some anterior segment condition that does not permit adequate visualization and laser delivery by the usual means? What if there is a poor or moderate view of the retina due to vitreous hemorrhage?

TABLE 18-1. BEST METHODS FOR DETECTING EARLY IRIS NEOVASCULARIZATION

- Be suspicious and go out of your way to look for it.
- Examine the pupillary border with extreme care; that is usually where iris neovascularization starts.
- Use high magnification and bright illumination on slit-lamp examination.
- If at first glance you don't see any neovascularization, concentrate on the pupillary border or angle for longer than you might during an otherwise routine examination.

The choice is clear. These patients require vitrectomy for the purpose of enabling PRP. Endoscopy can be a superior method in this situation for a few reasons. First, lensectomy in such an eye would be ill advised, since it may catalyze a progression, rather than regression, of iris neovascularization. The microscope view may be inadequate, with any significant anterior segment opacification making endophotocoagulation impossible. On the other hand, even in the presence of an opaque lens or totally opacified cornea, the laser endoscope may easily effect complete and dense PRP from posterior to anterior retina. The same holds true for vitreous hemorrhage. Endoscopic vitrectomy followed by endoscopic PRP can effectively control the situation (Fig. 18-9). Often, there exists a combination of these problems that makes it impossible to achieve adequate retinal ablation by ordinary means.

Finally, if neovascular glaucoma is already present, after completion of posterior treatment, endoscopic cyclophotocoagulation can be undertaken in any eye, no matter what

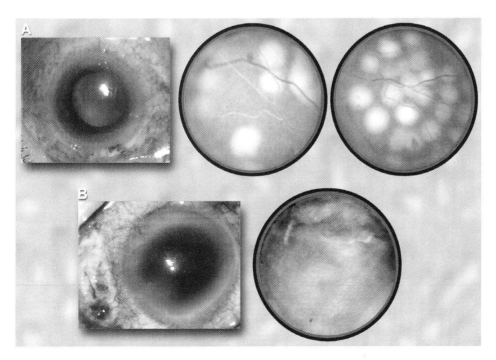

FIGURE 18-9. Endoscopic vitrectomy and endophotocoagulation for iris neovascularization. **A:** Panretinal photocoagulation in the presence of dense cataract. Lens has been spared to maintain anterior–posterior barrier to diffusion of angiogenic substances. **B:** Hyphema, cataract, and vitreous hemorrhage prevented routine retinal ablation. Endoscopic vitrectomy and endophotocoagulation circumvent these impediments.

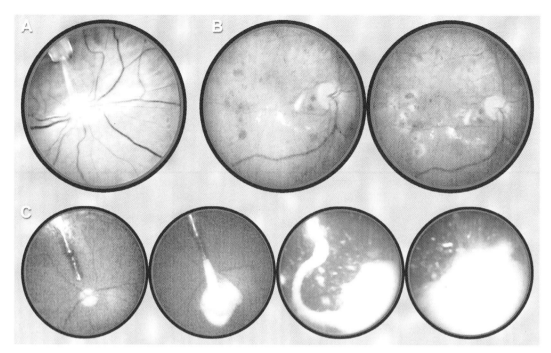

FIGURE 18-10. Endoscopic removal of posterior hyaloid for intractable macular edema. **A:** Endoscopic monitoring of posterior hyaloid removal. **B:** Endoscopic endophotocoagulation. **C:** Intraocular injection of triamcinolone.

the patient's lens status, on the surgeon's demand. These techniques have already been discussed extensively. Combining endoscopic cyclophotocoagulation with endoscopic PRP in this situation is superior to any other treatment in terms of safety and efficacy. Surgeons who are skilled in these techniques will not require more brutal and destructive procedures, such as panretinal cryotherapy or cyclocryotherapy, or the more involved and potentially more devastating tube implantation that would, in any event, require an additional surgery.

DIABETIC EXUDATIVE MACULOPATHY ASSOCIATED WITH TRACTION

Some patients with diabetic exudative maculopathy demonstrate a thickened and taut appearance to the posterior hyaloid associated with profound visual loss but do not respond well to focal photocoagulation. Documentation may be difficult but can be demonstrated at times by ocular coherence tomography. These eyes may seem to have run out of therapeutic options. In this situation, vitrectomy

with removal of the posterior hyaloid can sometimes effect significant resolution of edema and exudation. This anatomic change is often associated with significant visual improvement. The technique is simple, typically consisting of vitrectomy followed by stripping of the posterior hyaloid with a pick or forceps. Perhaps the biggest risk to the patient is that, despite surgery, no benefit is gained. Endoscopy can be helpful in identifying membrane edges and residual vitreous in the eye that may not be apparent through the operating microscope. Focal photocoagulation may also be applied through the endoscope to the macula and paramacular region to any areas of leakage. Intraocular injection of triamcinalone has been associated with some remarkable instances of resolving edema and improved visual function (Fig. 18-10).

REFERENCE

1. Diabetic Retinopathy Vitrectomy Study. Research Group Early virectomy for severe vitreous hemorrhage in diabetic retinopathy. Diabetic Retinopathy Vitrectomy Study Report 2. *Arch Ophthalnology* 1985;103:1644–51.

ENDOSCOPIC VITRECTOMY FOR OTHER RETINOPATHIES

PROLIFERATIVE RETINOPATHY OF BRANCH RETINAL VEIN OCCLUSION

Not uncommonly, vitrectomy is performed for vitreous hemorrhage, the etiology of which is unknown preoperatively. Once the blood is cleared, it becomes apparent that the underlying cause was retinal fibrovascular proliferation from branch retinal vein occlusion (BRVO). The pathogenesis of the neovascularization is identical to that seen in diabetic retinopathy—that is, capillary nonperfusion—although it is usually sectoral in nature rather than being more global, as in the diabetic eye.

The management principles are the same. After removal of the vitreous hemorrhage with the vitrector, a search is made for the focus of neovascularization, which may well have a tractional component. Typically, these areas will be found toward the periphery in the involved quadrant or hemisphere. Endoscopy facilitates their identification because it is easy to follow the course of a vessel from the posterior pole to the ora serrata without changing lensing or other mechanical issues, as would be required with the microscope. Once detected, the vitrector may be used to remove any anterior–posterior (AP) tractional elements. Usually, an involved membranectomy is not required. The key to permanent resolution of this problem is to effect segmental retinal ablation, which can often be completed intraoperatively. Recalling that retinal neovascularization usually begins at the border of perfused and nonperfused retina, a segmental pattern of panretinal photocoagulation is made. Usually this begins two "rows" of laser applications proximal to the area of neovascular-

ization and proceeds more distally, to the ora serrata if possible (Fig. 19-1).

As an example, suppose that an inferior temporal BRVO with retinal neovascularization is diagnosed after a vitreous hemorrhage is removed. This fibrovascular membrane is observed in the midperiphery. Photocoagulation of the sector begins several rows proximal to the membrane and proceeds peripherally as far as possible. It is not important to ablate more proximally nor is it necessary to address other quadrants of the retina. This technique is highly effective in managing this disorder, with complete regression of neovascularization being the rule.

Furthermore, unlike many of the ischemic retinal disorders that result in the development of neovascularization and require dense retinal ablation to effect regression of the pathologic process, BRVO seems to be more sensitive to laser treatment. Light- to moderate-density applications usually prove sufficient for the purpose at hand. In the end, if endophotocoagulation is inadequate, further treatment can easily be applied at the slit lamp. Many of these BRVO patients do well, not only demonstrating resolution of their pathology but, in the end, showing considerable improvement in visual function, which remains stabilized without further treatment.

The benefit that endoscopy confers in this situation is in detection of the more peripheral sites of neovascularization that may not be apparent through the microscope, as well as the capacity of endoscopic endophotocoagulation to easily complete the necessary retinal ablation into the far periphery. These are key features in the relatively simple and efficacious management of this problem if the proper diagnosis is made.

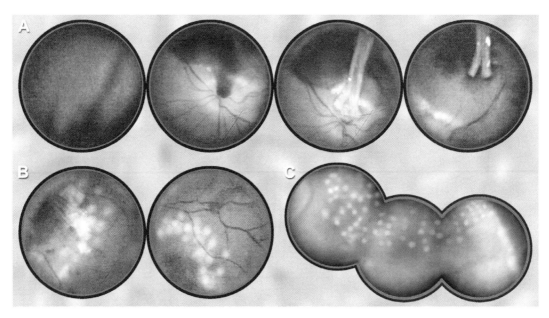

FIGURE 19-1. Endoscopic vitrectomy in branch retinal vein occlusion. **A:** Vitreous hemorrhage cleared by vitrectomy. **B:** Retinal neovascularization in mid periphery detected by endoscopy. Photocoagulation is applied. **C:** Another case. After all tractional components are removed, segmental panretinal photocoagulation is applied.

PERIPHERAL PROLIFERATIVE RETINOPATHIES

A number of disorders eventually create a sufficient amount of nonperfused ischemic retina to drive the development of fibrovascular proliferation and its attendant complications. Among the most common are sickling retinopathies, Eales' disease, and peripheral proliferative retinopathy as a variant of diabetic ophthalmopathy. The ischemia arising from these disorders may be more localized in nature, and so their treatment may also be less expansive than in diabetic retinopathy, although the principles are the same. Indeed, management is much the same as in BRVO. Vitrectomy removes hemorrhage and AP traction. Areas of fibrovascular proliferation are detected, and peripheral retinal endoscopic endophotocoagulation is applied to the ischemic region, be it in a 360-degree ring around the periphery or more focally (Fig. 19-2). Endoscopy proves to be most valuable in the detection of peripheral areas of neovascularization that may not be as evident through the microscope as well as in streamlining laser delivery, a key component in effecting resolution and long-term stability in these diseases. Indeed, even though many of these disorders cause blindness if left to their natural history, they are often easily remedied by this approach, with the added potential of recovering excellent acuity.

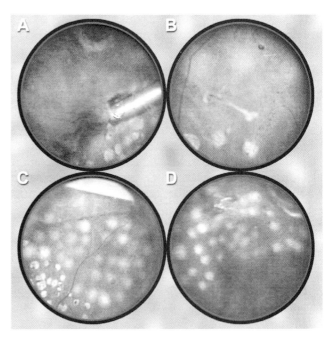

FIGURE 19-2. Endoscopic vitrectomy in peripheral proliferative retinopathy. **A:** Principles are identical to branch retinal vein occlusion. In this instance of Eales' disease, vitrectomy removes hemorrhage and anterior–posterior traction. **B:** Endoscope follows course of major arcades from posterior to anterior to identify sites of proliferation. **C:** Scatter peripheral laser ablation performed endoscopically in peripheral ring. **D:** Peripheral ring of panretinal photocoagulation in sickle retinopathy.

EXUDATIVE MACULOPATHIES

Occasionally, at the time of vitrectomy for some other problem, the surgeon may be surprised to find a disorder of the macula characterized by focal or diffuse exudation. A therapeutic opportunity exists here that one perhaps should not disregard. We are all well acquainted with the methods of slit lamp–delivered laser for the management of these problems, and so they are easily applied in the context of this situation. As an example, consider the eye undergoing vitrectomy for diabetic vitreous hemorrhage or traction detachment. Once the media have been cleared or the retina flattened, the presence of active maculopathy with edema and exudation becomes apparent. Focal endophotocoagulation, as described previously, can be quite helpful in resolving the problem and possibly improving the potential for visual recovery.

In the diabetic eye especially, it is well known that macular edema and exudation cause permanent profound visual loss more frequently than proliferative disease. One might argue that treatment of the macula can be performed postoperatively, so that the surgeon need not pursue this avenue intraoperatively. To the contrary, just as in the case of endophotocoagulation for proliferative disease, eyes fare better when treated during surgery because circumstances may evolve that prevent timely postoperative intervention. In our diabetic vitrectomy example, if the surgeon elects to treat the maculopathy later but postoperative vitreous hemorrhage occurs, then proper management of the maculopathy cannot be achieved. There could be many variations on this theme, but the point is that if active macular leakage is evident at the time of vitrectomy, the surgeon should consider treatment (Fig. 19-3).

The endoscope can be especially useful in this situation because when many of these instruments are held 1 to 2 mm from the retinal surface, high magnification with good resolution of microaneurysms or other pathology, along with simultaneous laser delivery, is possible. This cannot be achieved by conventional means (Fig. 19-4).

There has been much interest in injection of triamcinolone into the vitreous for the purpose of diminishing macular edema arising from a host of disorders, including

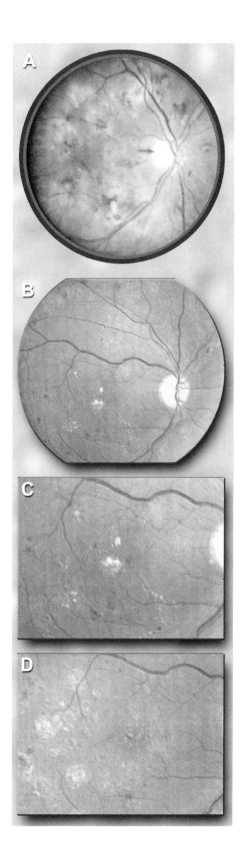

FIGURE 19-3. Focal endoscopic endophotocoagulation for diabetic macular edema. **A:** Patient demonstrated chronic macular exudation and subsequently developed a vitreous hemorrhage and extramacular traction retinal detachment. At vitrectomy for these latter problems, focal treatment to the macula was applied. **B:** Vitrectomy was performed to remove subsequent vitreous hemorrhage and repair tractional detachment. **C:** Macular laser was applied intraoperatively. **D:** Three months after treatment, the foveal region was dry and most of the lipid exudation had resolved.

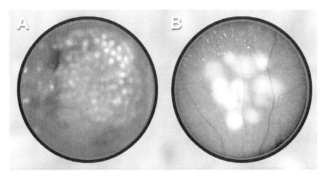

FIGURE 19-4. Focal endoscopic endophotocoagulation. **A:** Underlying macular edema from branch retinal vein occlusion (BRVO) discovered at vitrectomy. A grid pattern of photocoagulation is applied intraoperatively. **B:** Small area of retinal neovascularization in BRVO managed by focal ablation.

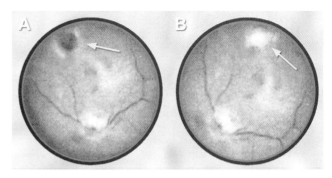

FIGURE 19-6. A: Retinal arterial macroaneurysm discovered at vitrectomy. **B:** Focal treatment was applied intraoperatively.

diabetic retinopathy, branch and central vein occlusion, and macular degeneration (1–5). The long-term outcome of this maneuver is yet to be determined, although it is quite simple to perform and seems to result in marked visual recovery in some patients (Fig. 19-5).

Nondiabetic vitreous hemorrhage undergoing vitrectomy may reveal the presence of a number of underlying disorders that can be addressed at the time of surgery. Perhaps the most common of these is BRVO. Management of the proliferative aspects of this disorder has been discussed, but what of the exudative manifestations? For the same reasons described for diabetic maculopathy, grid or focal endoscopic endophotocoagulation can be executed during vitrectomy. While the patient is recovering from surgery, the macular disease will simultaneously be on its potential course for resolution.

Ruptured retinal arterial macroaneurysm occasionally causes nonclearing vitreous hemorrhage requiring surgery. Discovering the location of the macroaneurysm permits the laser endoscope to effect treatment precisely and with high image magnification and resolution (Fig. 19-6). It is impor-

tant to surround these lesions with a ring of laser spots. Following this, mild laser applications should be made to the surface of the macroaneurysm, with care taken to ensure that the spot size is larger than the lesion. Inadvertent rupture by an overly intense "small" spot would be unfortunate. Overzealous treatment can also result in arterial occlusion distal to the retinal arterial macroaneurysm, so that care must be taken to avoid this situation as well.

Submacular hemorrhage with breakthrough into the vitreous cavity not uncommonly arises from a subretinal neovascular membrane. Often the patient presents with a vitreous hemorrhage of unknown cause only to have this unfortunate event reveal itself after clearing of the blood. Some of these lesions may still appear to be actively bleeding, and so intraoperative photocoagulation may be helpful in limiting the disease process. Moderate-intensity confluent lesions directed to the entire extent of the subretinal membrane are the desired tissue effect.

Certainly, many other macular exudative processes that one could stumble onto during the course of vitrectomy have not yet been described. Reporting of their management and outcomes might benefit all of us.

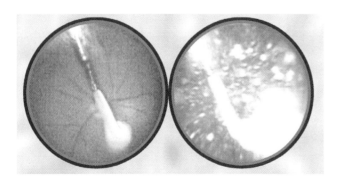

FIGURE 19-5. Intravitreal injection of triamcinolone for the management of macular edema.

REFERENCES

1. Branch Retinal Vein Occlusion Study Group. Argon laser scatter photocoagulation for prevention of neovascularization and vitreous hemorrhage in branch vein occlusion. *Arch Ophthalmol* 1986;104:34–41.
2. Jonas JB, Sofker A. Intraocular injection of crystalline cortisone as adjunctive treatment of diabetic macular edema. *Am J Ophthalmol* 2001;132:425–427.
3. Danis RP, Ciulla TA, Pratt LM, Anliker W. Intravitreal triamcinolone acetonide in exudative age-related macular degeneration. *Retina* 2000;20:244–250.
4. Ip MS, Kumar KS. Intravitreous triamcinolone acetonide as treatment for macular edema from central retinal vein occlusion. *Arch Ophthalmol* 2002;120:1217–1219.
5. Martidis A, Duker JS, Greenberg PB, et al. Intravitreal triamcinolone for refractory diabetic macular edema. *Ophthalmology* 2002;109:920–927.

ENDOSCOPIC VITRECTOMY IN RETINAL DETACHMENT SURGERY

RHEGMATOGENOUS RETINAL DETACHMENT

One of the interesting applications of ophthalmic endoscopy is in the management of rhegmatogenous retinal detachment (RRD). Although certainly the mainstay of treatment is scleral buckling, there are situations in which vitrectomy may be preferred, and it is here that endoscopy can be valuable.

Vitrectomy for complicated retinal detachment has taught us that release of vitreoretinal traction, laser or cryoretinopexy, and gas tamponade can achieve retinal reattachment. In the past, the lack of technology and surgical expertise negated the value of this approach. This is no longer the case. The surgeon may choose between these two approaches, especially in the pseudophakic eye.

Endoscopy simplifies vitrectomy for RRD in several ways (Figs. 20-1 to 20-3). First, removal of vitreous with hemorrhage, debris, and opacification may ultimately result in clearer vision for the patient, assuming that reattachment has been successful and the retina attains a good measure of function. Second, it simplifies the search for retinal breaks, obviating the need for indirect ophthalmoscopy. This feature can be especially helpful in the presence of an opacified posterior capsule that obscures a view of the retinal periphery. Even tiny retinal holes at the far periphery can be easily detected by endoscopy and often simultaneously photocoagulated at the point of their discovery. Third, air-fluid exchange with internal drainage of subretinal fluid can be performed simply and rapidly under endoscopic guidance,

almost always resulting in a flattened retina. This is clearly a safer, more controllable, and often more compete maneuver than external drainage. Fourth, as just alluded to, endoscopic endophotocoagulation in the air-filled eye with a flattened retina is quite simple and effective. It is less traumatic than transscleral cryopexy and perhaps diminishes the risk of inciting proliferative vitreoretinopathy (PVR). It can also be effected without a change of instrumentation. Fifth, postoperatively, patients have a minimum of discomfort when compared with scleral buckling, especially of the encircling type. Finally, it can simplify reoperations for retinal detachment with less trauma to the eye than a repeated scleral buckle procedure.

GIANT RETINAL TEAR AND DETACHMENT

Formerly a difficult task, management of this problem has been greatly simplified by the introduction of perfluorocarbon liquid (PFCL). To begin, vitrectomy is performed, with special attention paid to the edge of the retinal tear (Fig. 20-4). It must be freed from all of its tractional attachments. Endoscopy can be helpful, especially when the tear is very large, because the panoramic view enables the surgeon to visualize the impact of surgery on the entire tear as the vitrectomy proceeds. This method of imaging clearly indicates the presence of even a small amount of residual traction on the tear edge, which might not be apparent when the operating microscope is in use. Furthermore, because these tears

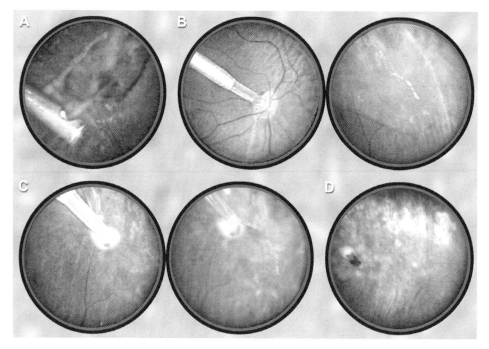

FIGURE 20-1. Endoscopic vitrectomy in rhegmatogenous retinal detachment. **A:** Removal of vitreous. **B:** Identification of breaks. **C:** Air-fluid exchange with ballooning retina *(left)* and internal drainage of subretinal fluid through preexisting break or retinotomy *(right)*. **D:**Endoscopic endophotocoagulation.

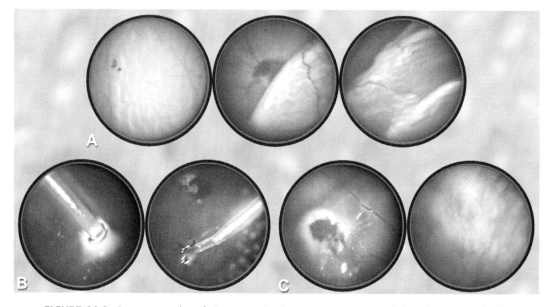

FIGURE 20-2. Some examples of vitrectomy in rhegmatogenous retinal detachment. **A:** *(left)* Phakic eye *(center)* two breaks *(right)* breaks flat on buckle. **B:** *(left)* Laser around break and ciliary processes; *(right)* lens, attached retina, and laser. **C:** *(left)* Flat retina *(right)*. start of laser

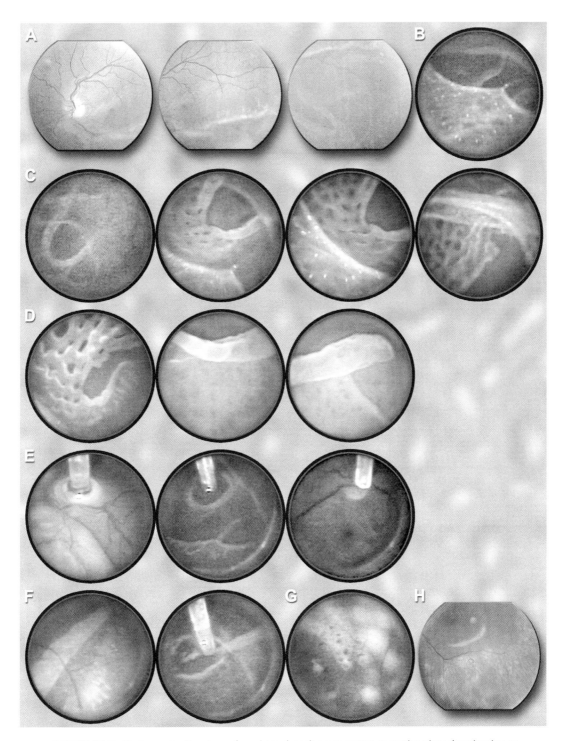

FIGURE 20-3. Endoscopic vitrectomy for schisis detachment. **A:** Preoperative view showing inner and outer wall breaks. **B:** Intraoperative view after vitrectomy. Note horizontally oriented inner wall break with dots of subretinal precipitates, overlying more vertically oriented outer wall break. **C:** As the endoscope is advanced, greater anatomic detail can be appreciated. In this instance, the moth-eaten appearance of the outer wall with its rolled-over edge can be appreciated. **D:** As the endoscope is passed through the inner wall, details of the outer wall and its rolled edge can be seen. **E:** Air-fluid exchange is performed with internal drainage of subretinal fluid through the full-thickness break created by the inner and outer wall break. The macula is now flattened. **F:** The rolled edge of the outer wall break remains even after removal of the subretinal fluid. Although it is probably not very important to the long-term success of this surgery, the soft-tipped extrusion cannula is directed through the inner wall break and is used to unroll the outer wall break edge. **G:** After endophotocoagulation. **H:** Appearance of the retina postoperatively.

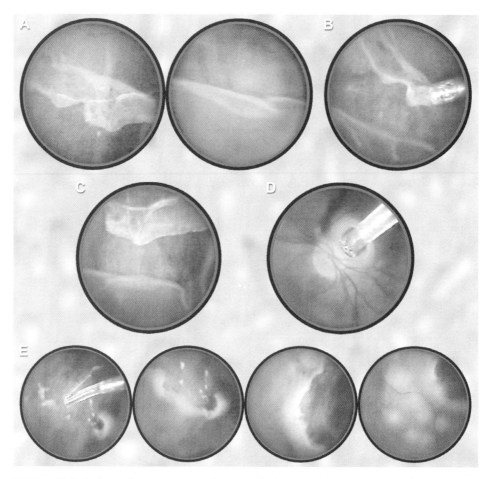

FIGURE 20-4. Endoscopic management of giant retinal tear and detachment. **A:** Giant tear with rolled edge. **B:** Vitrectomy frees edge of traction. **C:** The anterior and posterior edges are now highly mobile. **D:** Perfluorocarbon liquid is injected through a soft-tipped cannula to force subretinal fluid anteriorly, flattening the retina. **E:** The retina adjacent to the giant tear is now flat and endoscopic laser retinopexy is performed in an "interrupted" and "painted" fashion.

are usually anterior in their placement, they may be difficult to view through the operating microscope but are easily accessed endoscopically.

After the vitreous has been removed, the edge of the tear is rolled over; if it is less flexible, this indicates that an element of PVR has begun. Membranectomy using a pick, spatula, or diamond-dusted membrane scratcher may be effective at freeing the edge. If, however, it cannot be completely mobilized, it is better to excise the stiffened edge completely so that it is once again mobile. Hemorrhage can be controlled with endodiathermy.

At this point, the PFCL is introduced over the optic nerve, and the posterior retina will be seen to flatten as subretinal fluid is pushed peripherally. This injection is continued until the edge of the giant tear is flattened. Care should be taken not to allow PFCL to enter the subretinal space. Once the edge is apposed to the eye wall, the laser endoscope can be used to apply several rows of laser application to the complete extent of the tear as well as perhaps an extra clock hour or two on each end of the break. This latter

detail can help to prevent postoperative extension of the break. Painting the edge of the tear with a laser is also an acceptable alternative.

Once completed, an air-PFCL exchange is made. Care should be taken so that posterior slippage of the retina does not occur at this time. If it does, the retina can often be massaged back into position with a soft-tipped cannula or brush. Then, long-acting gas or silicone oil is injected.

There are three additional issues to be examined. First, a scleral buckle is not necessary in this procedure; in fact, the architectural distortion it creates can contribute to posterior slippage. If all the vitreoretinal attachments are removed and the edge of the break is free (which must be accomplished), gas or oil tamponade following laser retinopexy will be sufficient. Second, many of these eyes have a relatively clear lens preoperatively, and the question of whether to perform lensectomy may arise. Lens removal is not necessarily required to effect repair of this problem, and the lens often is not traumatized during this procedure. On the other hand, much of the work is performed in the anterior vitreous cavity, so lens trauma would certainly not be a surprise. This is an issue that must be considered on an individual basis. The point, however, is that lensectomy is not strictly required to resolve this problem. Finally, no matter how elegant the surgery has become, these eyes are at high risk for the development of PVR, and this should be emphasized to the patient. Although these steps may appear to be complex, the procedure is actually a great improvement over what has been used in the past. An experienced vitrectomy surgeon who is nevertheless a novice in endoscopy may be able to execute the entire course of surgery under endoscopic guidance.

PROLIFERATIVE VITREORETINOPATHY

Proliferative vitreoretinopathy is one of those troubling disorders that often affront us despite our best efforts and following our most elegant surgery. It can be disheartening for all despite a stunning performance on the part of the surgeon and excellent cooperation by the patient. The reason that a well-executed procedure does not lead to the anticipated outcome is that vitrectomy, under the best of circumstances, can address only the pathologic anatomy that is present at the time of surgery and cannot prevent further proliferation, retinal atrophy and break formation, or perhaps, ultimately, retinal cell death.

Because of this great uncertainty, patient selection is crucial. Certainly, when PVR develops in the better eye, strong consideration should be given to intervention. More of a problem is the patient with a good fellow eye. In this situation, it is important to have a frank discussion concerning the possible benefits and problems that can arise from PVR surgery as well as the considerable potential for reoperation, anatomic, and functional failure despite extreme efforts.

The classification of the various stages of PVR is well known and will not be reviewed here. Rather, consideration of the various technical approaches to the management of this problem will be explored. The surgical principles involved in the management of this disorder are generally well agreed on, although authorities vary in the details. I myself think that the management of PVR is challenging and that each eye presents a set of variables that differ from other eyes sufficiently so as to defy having a "routine" for treating all cases.

Consider that the postoperative reattachment is dependent on having a free and mobile retina, without residual traction, a well-functioning RPE pump, and good mechanical tamponade. The intraoperative goal, then, is to satisfy these parameters.

Scleral Buckling

Most authorities agree that an encircling scleral buckle is helpful but differ on the reason for its placement, the type of buckle used, and when during the procedure it is applied. Some experts believe that a wide, moderate-height buckle can support the retina, assist in relief of residual traction, and close many of the retinal breaks that might be encountered during the course of surgery. Others think that a moderate-width or even narrow band is sufficient, its primary purpose being to elevate the vitreous base, presenting it to the surgeon for easier dissection. If, on the one hand, the surgeon subscribes to the latter philosophy, the buckle should be placed prior to vitrectomy. If, on the other hand, the surgeon intends the buckle to have a more long-term function, it can be placed either before or after the vitrectomy. As usual, there is no clear answer.

Still, this minor controversy points to an undeniable fact: if the peripheral vitreous is not removed, the patient and surgeon will most likely pay for it later, as the vitreous ring contracts and results in redetachment and failure. All of this contraction does not necessarily have to proceed in a posterior direction. To the contrary, anterior forces may develop, causing detachment of the ciliary body and leading to hypotony or phthisis. Endoscopy can be supremely helpful in the complete excision of the anterior vitreous and any of its anterior or posterior attachments. This ability can negate the value of a scleral buckle altogether, at least for those who place it for the purpose of better vitreous base access.

Lensectomy and Intraocular Lens Explantation

This portion of the surgery is also controversial. Some think that lensectomy is required in all PVR cases, even if the lens is clear, because it will hinder access to the vitreous base, it will undoubtedly be traumatized during surgery and therefore demonstrate progressive opacification, and gas or silicone oil tamponade will likely cause cataract formation in and of itself. If this occurs, it would be difficult to follow the patients postoperatively, or, in the case of an otherwise successful outcome, it would require another surgery to rehabilitate the patient's vision. This aspect of PVR surgery again seems to merit individual determination rather than proceeding as if rules were in effect. Some eyes can tolerate PVR vitrectomy well and maintain a clear lens postoperatively; this is potentiated by endoscopy in that it permits a panoramic and complete view of the vitreous base when imaging may be difficult through the microscope.

Some surgeons believe that all intraocular lenses (IOLs) and capsular material should be removed, presumably eliminating them as scaffolding for future proliferation. Although a controlled study has not addressed this assertion, its validity seems to be questionable. Opacified capsule surely limits the microscope view of the retinal periphery and more anterior structures, even with scleral depression. Removing the IOL and capsule can reestablish the view. Endoscopy completely circumvents this issue by permitting a view of this region despite IOL or capsular limitations. The endoscopic vitrectomy surgeon will rarely need to explant a lens unless it is unstable or has some other intrinsic problem.

Pupil Stretching and Iridectomy

When confronted with the PVR patient who has a miotic pupil from underlying pathology or in whom this situation develops during the course of surgery, microscope imaging becomes difficult or impossible. To move ahead with the operation, the surgeon must either stretch the pupil in some way or perform an iridectomy. The endoscopic surgeon is not hampered by this situation because the anterior segment status is not important as far as posterior imaging is concerned. Surgery can proceed under endoscopic guidance, but it should be clear that PVR surgery is challenging under any circumstances and the degree of difficulty increases when the surgery is performed solely by endoscopic imaging.

Opaque Cornea

Some eyes demonstrate an opaque cornea in concert with a PVR detachment. In this situation, some recommend removal of the cornea with placement of a keratoprosthesis. Following the vitrectomy, corneal transplantation is required. Endoscopy eliminates the need for this approach, again because anterior segment opacification is irrelevant as far as posterior endoscopic imaging is concerned. The down side is that the surgeon needs to be experienced in endoscopically guided vitrectomy and associated techniques in order to be successful in this situation.

Reviewing for a moment, the capable endoscopic vitrectomy surgeon can eliminate scleral buckling, lensectomy, IOL explantation or capsulectomy, pupillary stretching or iridectomy, keratoprosthesis, and corneal transplantation procedures (or any combination of these) in PVR surgery. Certainly, this diminishes operative time and patient morbidity as well as allowing the surgeon to concentrate on the task at hand, that is, removing vitreoretinal traction, membranectomy, retinal tamponade, and photocoagulation.

Surgical Technique

In PVR, the vitreous is detached, shrunken, and retracted in an anterior direction. Circular contraction of the vitreous base, which is strongly adherent to the underlying retina, results in the radial folds that are seen in this condition. To make matters worse, newly developed membranes on the surface of the retina or vitreous may contract, exacerbating this radial folding. When the vitreous base shrinks toward the center point of the vitreous cavity, the retina is pulled forward, referred to as anterior loop traction. Then there are membranes on the retinal surface that contract tangentially,

resulting in starfolds. Finally, subretinal proliferation of these membranes may at times contribute to detachment. The first order of business is to remove as much of the vitreous as possible with the vitrector. Endoscopy will often reveal the presence of vitreous that may not be seen through the microscope because of the characteristics of internally illuminating and viewing this structure rather than imaging from the outside of the eye to the inside. Still, this task is usually accomplished without much difficulty.

When to address the vitreous base during the course of the procedure is a different issue. Some believe that posterior dissection of membranes should be the next step because it may afford more opportunities to find a membrane edge. Furthermore, and perhaps more importantly, the tension on the retina arising from contraction of the vitreous base can assist in posterior dissection. If this advantage is lost, particularly when exacerbated by the iatrogenic creation of a significant retinal break, the posterior membranectomy becomes more difficult. Some surgeons place PFCL posteriorly at this point and carry on the posterior-to-anterior dissection using the tension it creates to assist in membranectomy. Others feel that vitreous base removal should be performed after core vitrectomy. In so doing, an important pathologic feature of PVR, anterior loop traction, is completely eliminated as well as some element of the circular traction. It probably makes no difference as to which approach is selected, depending more on the pathologic geometry of the retina in question.

Let us assume, for the sake of this discussion, that the posterior membranes and hyaloid will be addressed first (Fig. 20-5). Very often a pick or spatula is used to elevate an edge. If the edge is highly adherent, an MVR blade may be needed to start the process. Once the edge is delineated, it can be grasped by a forceps and stripped from the retinal surface. This process is repeated until all of the membranes that can be grasped in this manner are removed. These membranes and hyaloid should be stripped to the vitreous base, where they can be removed with the vitrector.

Large fixed retinal folds may now be evident (Fig. 20-6). With bent needle, spatula, or pick the surgeon can gently scrape along the retinal surface in the recess of the fold to engage any membranes. Once an edge is elevated in this manner, its dissection can continue with the same instrument or a forceps can be introduced to complete the task. Very adherent membranes may require sharp dissection with the MVR blade. On the other hand, immature membranes are not very cohesive, so that usually no matter what instrument is applied in their removal, fragmentation will occur. I find the diamond-dusted membrane scratcher to be helpful in this situation because it can remove sheets of these immature membranes and pigment cells rapidly and completely and without causing trauma. In tougher membranes that are nevertheless diffuse, a metal membrane scratcher may be used. Care must be taken with this instrument not to tear the retina because so doing will render it

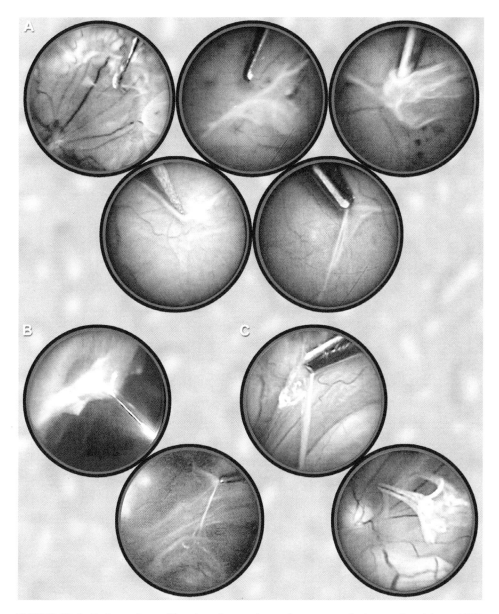

FIGURE 20-5. Endoscopic proliferative vitreoretinopathy surgery. **A:** A spatula, pick, or MVR blade is used to elevate edge of membrane posteriorly. **B:** A spatula is used to elevate and separate membranes in an anterior direction. **C:** End-gripping forceps is used to strip membrane anteriorly to vitreous base.

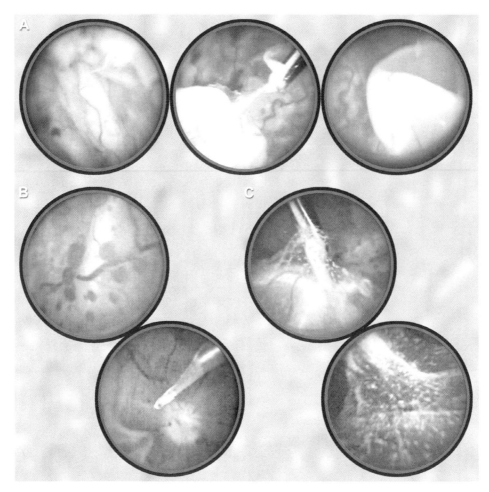

FIGURE 20-6. A: Large fixed folds are addressed with spatula, pick, MVR blade, bent needle, or forceps to engage membrane in recess. **B:** Immature diffuse membranes are managed with a diamond-dusted membrane scratcher. **C:** More dense and diffuse membranes are removed with metal membrane scratcher.

more mobile, impeding the remainder of the membranectomy. This process is continued, with removal of as much of these membranes as possible with this instrument.

Now more tangential traction, if present, can be addressed (Fig. 20-7). Starfolds can be opened in a similar manner to the larger folds, by passing a bent needle, spatula, or pick in a recess, "fishing" for a membrane, and then elevating it for forceps or vitrector removal. Some assert that an alternative method is the only way to proceed in this situation. In it, an end-gripping forceps is used to grasp the membrane and pull it off the retinal surface. This technique works quite well but not universally. Whichever approach seems to get the job done is probably the correct one to use.

Iatrogenic breaks frequently, if not always, develop during the course of membranectomy, and the surgeon should not despair. The alternative, leaving the membrane, often results in reproliferation and detachment. Release of all tractional elements is the goal, and any break with a free perimeter is easily managed.

There may be a small or extensive amount of residual retinal stiffness due to foreshortening, preretinal membranes that cannot be removed for one of several reasons, or subretinal membranes that contribute to retinal detachments (most do not). Thus, the situation may not look good. Ignore these areas for now.

If all or most of the hyaloid and membranes has been removed, the retina can be mobile to the point of interfering with vitreous base dissection. Posterior placement of PFCL can help to flatten and stabilize the posterior retina, as well as to potentially indicate areas of the retina thought to be free but in fact are not free.

Vitreous Base Dissection

No matter when in the course of vitrectomy the surgeon addresses this region, complete vitreous base excision and membranectomy in the posterior iris and ciliary body region is essential for a successful outcome in PVR.

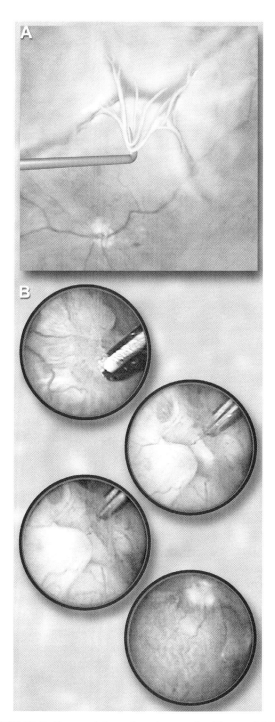

FIGURE 20-7. Tangential traction characterized by starfolds. **A:** Offending membrane can be removed as in larger fixed folds with spatula, pick, MVR blade, or bent needle. **B:** End-gripping forceps grab membrane in center of fold and pull off retina.

Endoscopy can be supremely helpful in this area because its dissection is a crucial part of the procedure, yet this is the most difficult anatomic site to access even under the best of circumstances. For surgeons who initiate PVR surgery with scleral buckling and lensectomy, the microscope view can

be extremely poor at this point in the procedure. Endoscopy can clearly delineate that pathologic anatomy and its effect on the surrounding structures. Scleral depression is often used to bring areas of interest into the microscope view. The endoscopic approach does not require this. In fact, scleral depression can relieve points of vitreous adhesion to the peripheral retina, pars plana, ciliary body, lens, or posterior iris, obscuring their presence, whereas the endoscopic view clearly indicates their existence.

Contraction and anterior retraction of the vitreous can drag the retina centrally and anteriorly in PVR, affecting various points of adhesion that must be excised (Fig. 20-8) This anterior retraction can create a retinal trough at the pars plana. More extreme changes can draw the retina to a sclerotomy site, ciliary body, iris near the sulcus, lens capsule, or posterior iris at the pupil. Typically, an MVR blade or scissors is used to divide these adhesions and separate the structures. This action can relieve some or all of the posterior radiating folds. These problems can be detected and addressed with relative ease endoscopically, whereas they can be difficult or impossible to manage by more conventional means.

Freeing the retina from its most extreme anterior attachments (if present) will permit access to the vitreous base for its removal. There are a few variations on the microscope-guided technique for completing this portion of the operation, but, basically, the peripheral retina is scleral depressed into view and the vitrector is used to "shave" the vitreous as close to the retinal surface as possible for 360 degrees. The endoscopic approach is usually simpler because scleral depression usually is not needed. Furthermore, the visualization difficulties that can be present with microscope imaging are irrelevant with endoscopic guidance.

At times, it is not possible to remove enough of the vitreous base to relieve all of the traction and relax the posterior radial folds. In this situation, the surgeon can make vertical incisions with the MVR blade through the vitreous base every few millimeters until the desired amount of retinal relaxation is obtained (Fig. 20-9).

Testing Retinal Mobility

Let's assume that the surgeon now believes that all tractional elements are removed and the retina will reattach. This may be the moment of truth. To test the true mobility of the retina, the infusion pressure of the balanced saline solution is raised and a soft-tipped extrusion cannula is used to aspirate subretinal fluid through a preexisting retinal break or a retinotomy site. If the retina seems to be flattening in all quadrants, congratulations are exchanged and gas or silicone oil tamponade is completed with any indicated endophotocoagulation, and the procedure is finished. Large retinal breaks or retinotomies invalidate this test.

If, on the other hand, the retina does not respond as one might wish, further investigation is required as to the cause

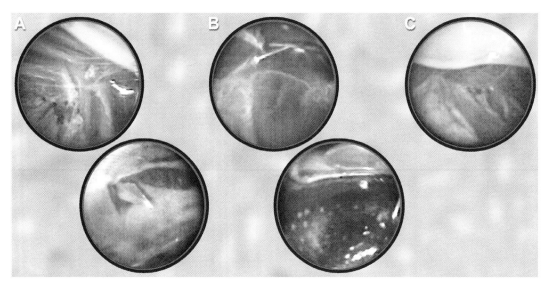

FIGURE 20-8. Anterior retinal retraction to sclerotomies, ciliary body, lens, or posterior iris. **A:** An MVR blade is helpful in dividing these adhesions and freeing the retina from the tractional elements. **B:** Ciliary body detachment can by repaired by dividing the adhesion with a vitrector. **C:** View of detached retina adherent to crystalline lens.

of immobility. The first suspect would be residual epiretinal membranes and vitreous remnants. These, if detected, must be removed as previously discussed.

The next most likely root of persistent detachment is subretinal proliferation. Once detected, a small retinotomy is made overlying any bands and a forceps is inserted subretinally to grasp and remove them.

If these problems are not present or have been addressed without benefit, the only other consideration is that the retina is foreshortened and most likely will never be able to be sufficiently mobilized to allow reattachment. Before contemplating retinectomy, one might consider massaging the shortened retina with a soft-tipped instrument to stretch it from its contracted state to one that would allow more mobility (Fig 20-10). Sometimes, 10 or 15 minutes of this activity, proceeding in a posterior to anterior direction, proves useful in achieving this goal.

Retinectomy

At times, perhaps often, we have executed all of these steps—vitrectomy and membranectomy of the posterior, equatorial, and peripheral retina and vitreous base—yet have not been rewarded with a mobile retina. In addition, one may encounter extensive or simply very dense membranes that are not effectively addressed by these membranectomy techniques. In considering the option of retinectomy, the surgeon may rely on a few guidelines. Usually, it is unknown preoperatively whether a retinectomy will be required. It is only after executing all of these other maneuvers that this option should be considered.

Caution should be exercised the more posteriorly one elects to perform retinectomy. Good hemostasis and removal of all debris is important in helping to prevent future proliferation. This includes the more peripheral side

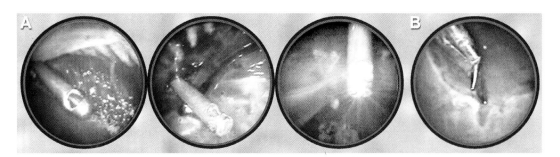

FIGURE 20-9. A: Excising vitreous base with vitrector by endoscopy. **B:** Radial cuts every few millimeters in vitreous base relax the radial fold if complete excision is too difficult.

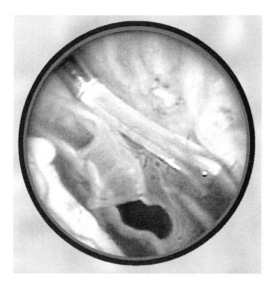

FIGURE 20-10. Endoscopic view of massaging foreshortened retina with soft-tipped cannula or brush in posterior to anterior direction. Doing this for 10 to 15 minutes can increase elasticity.

of a retinectomy site, which is or will become avital and therefore should be excised. If the retina is densely adherent to a particular area (e.g., a perforation site), circumcised retinectomy is the method of choice. The same holds true when the retina becomes adherent to a sclerotomy site and maneuvers such as vitrectomy, air-fluid exchange, or massage cannot effect release. It is simple and necessary to use the vitrector to excise this portion of the retina so that the

remainder may flatten. Finally, limbus parallel retinectomies are preferred, with little or no utility ascribed to radial ones.

Endoscopy can greatly facilitate the execution of retinectomy, especially after surgery has been under way for some time, because there may be a loss of anterior segment clarity, confounding the microscope view. Usually, a moderate-to wide-field view is chosen to monitor the effect retinectomy is having on the surrounding retina (Fig. 20-11). Once an adequate retinectomy has been performed, endoscopic imaging often instantly reveals relaxation of the surrounding retina, which may not be apparent with the hazier or smaller field of view through the microscope. Sites of even subtle bleeding can also be easily detected and treated endoscopically.

Air-Fluid Exchange and Endophotocoagulation

Let's continue to assume that we have been amazingly successful and the retina is now mobilized (Fig. 20-12). Next, air-fluid exchange is performed with internal drainage of subretinal fluid. The retina should flatten nicely. Once achieved, laser retinopexy can be executed, although the extent of its application varies among surgeons. Surely, any areas of retinal break formation, retinotomies, or retinectomies should be treated. Many retinal surgeons also apply the laser to the periphery for 360 degrees and extend treatment, at least to some degree, posteriorly as well. Overly intensive applications focally or extensive treatment

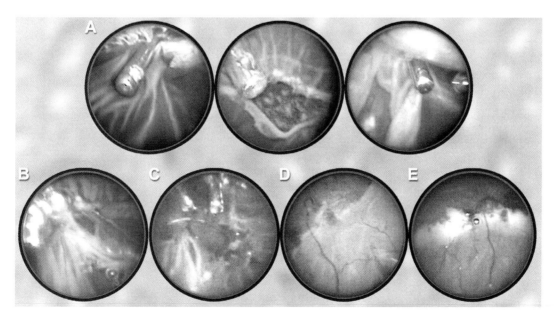

FIGURE 20-11. Endoscopic retinectomy. **A:** View of retinal excision from sclerotomy site. **B:** Foreshortened retina adherent to sclerotomy site. Note ciliary processes. **C:** Retinectomy is performed, freeing attachment and some elements of traction. **D:** The edges of the retina are now flattened as air-fluid exchange is performed. **E:** The flat edge is then photocoagulated in a continuous fashion.

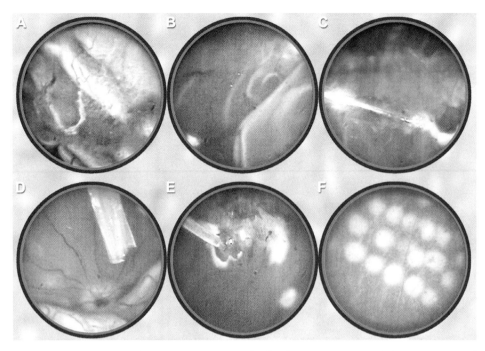

FIGURE 20-12. The proliferative vitreoretinopathy (PVR) retina is now mobile. **A:** PVR retinal detachment with some vascularized membranes and hemorrhage. **B:** The retina is mobilized after membranectomy. Note retinal break. **C:** The edge of the retinal break is demarcated with wet-field coagulation. **D:** Air-fluid exchange is performed using extrusion through a silicone brush. **E:** Extrusion through the retinal break. The mobile retina is now fixed almost flat. **F:** Peripheral laser retinopexy.

throughout the retina can incite postoperative inflammation. This negative feature must be kept in mind when one is considering how much of the retina to incorporate into the treatment zone. There is no standard amount and so one must exercise judgment in each individual case.

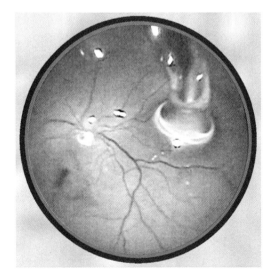

FIGURE 20-13. Endoscopic view of air–silicone oil meniscus ensuring adequate fill without overfilling or underfilling.

Long-Term Retinal Tamponade

The PVR eyes that experience intraoperative reattachment must have some form of retinal tamponade, either with perfluorocarbon gas or silicone oil. The difference in outcome between these two options is not significant. Still, many surgeons use silicone oil liberally, whereas others have never employed this material. There are certainly no clear indications for using one over the other. I prefer to use silicone oil in the eyes of patients with significant retinectomies who have failed vitrectomy with gas tamponade or who cannot cooperate with postoperative positioning. I have no proof, however, that my indications have provided the patients with an enhanced opportunity for success.

The simplest method of achieving a complete fill is to perform an air-silicone oil exchange. Endoscopic imaging can be useful because the air-oil meniscus can be clearly defined as the exchange is taking place. This feature is helpful in preventing underfilling or overfilling (Fig. 20-13). Inadvertent subretinal injection of silicone oil is a major problem because it usually occurs near the conclusion of surgery (to everyone's dismay) and must be addressed by removing it from the eye and either refilling or identifying why the oil bubble surface tension has been broken, permitting this event to occur. This problem can be difficult to detect through the operating microscope until the oil migrates posteriorly because it often begins peripherally, where the view can be limited.

Surgery Under Silicone Oil

As an aside for those surgeons who use silicone oil, it is not an uncommon experience to have a patient with reproliferation of PVR or failure attributable to some other cause who comes to further vitrectomy. It is feasible to perform the various membranectomy tasks in the silicone-filled eye. This material helps to stabilize the retina during dissection as well as to maintain an excellent level of media clarity. Endoscopic imaging is enhanced by this characteristic of silicone oil so that these membranectomies usually proceed with relative ease.

The same features assist endoscopic endophotocoagulation in the silicone oil–filled eye. The vitreous cavity is usually very clear, and silicone oil does not attenuate laser delivery to a significant degree.

At the conclusion of these maneuvers, it is still often necessary to remove the oil from the eye and either use gas or replace the oil for long-term tamponade.

Table 20-1 summarizes the approach to endoscopic management of PVR.

Anticipated Outcomes

In a number of major studies, PVR reattachment rates have been as high as 60% to 70%. These reports included a mix of grade C and D PVR detachments of both the anterior and posterior forms. Final anatomic success rates included patients who underwent multiple surgical interventions. A report of endoscopic vitrectomy for PVR included only the most severe grade of PVR detachment managed with a single procedure and without silicone oil. Anatomic success was achieved in 60% of these eyes, which was comparable to other studies that mixed the theoretically less severe (and therefore presumably easier to repair) stages, using multiple procedures as required, with or without silicone oil tamponade. One might speculate that 30% to 40% of patients treated for severe PVR ultimately experience failure as a

TABLE 20-1. SUMMARY OF ENDOSCOPIC MANAGEMENT OF PROLIFERATIVE VITREORETINOPATHY

1. Remove the core vitreous.
2. Remove posterior, equatorial, and peripheral vitreous remnants and membranes.
   a. Elevate membrane edge posteriorly with blade, pick, or spatula.
   b. Strip membranes posterior to anterior with forceps.
   c. Remove membranes starting in between large fixed folds with blade, pick, or spatula.
   d. Strip these membranes with forceps posterior to anterior.
   e. Remove tangential traction and starfolds with forceps, pick, spatula, or blade.
3. Dissect the vitreous base.
4. Remove all very anterior tractional elements to iris, ciliary body, and pars plana.
5. Remove subretinal membranes that keep the retina elevated.
6. Test retinal mobility.
7. Perform retinectomy for densely adherent membranes or foreshortened retina that prevent retinal reattachment.
8. Perform air–fluid exchange with subretinal fluid drainage.
9. Perform endophotocoagulation of retinal breaks, retinotomies, retinectomies, and the retinal periphery.
10. Establish long-term retinal tamponade with gas or silicone oil.

As another option, the surgeon may consider placing or revising a scleral buckle or performing a lensectomy.

result of reproliferation of gliotic tissue, whereas 60% to 70% can have successful reattachment if all tractional forces are released and scaffolding for future proliferation is eliminated, albeit with one or multiple procedures.

The former may represent our ability to effectively manage this problem, and future pharmacologic or mechanical innovations will be required to achieve any greater success. On the other hand, by using endoscopy and adapting our current vitreoretinal surgical techniques, more complete tissue dissection and photocoagulation at the time of initial PVR surgery are possible. This may minimize the need for repeated intervention in patients whose failure is not due to reproliferation.

ENDOSCOPIC VITRECTOMY FOR POSTERIORLY DISLOCATED LENS MATERIAL

One of the most common duties of the modern vitreoretinal surgeon is to perform a posterior vitrectomy and remove dislocated lens material. Phacoemulsification has markedly increased the need for this service, so that most retinal surgeons are now skilled in managing this problem. Endoscopy can greatly enhance our ability to remove posterior lens material not only by assisting in the removal of cortical or nuclear fragments that can be seen through the microscope but also by identifying scattered pieces that are otherwise not apparent (Figs. 21-1 to 21-8).

Novice endoscopists when first dealing with this problem may be surprised to observe how much lens material retained in the posterior iris, sulcus, and peripheral anterior vitreous regions is missed by microscope imaging. One might argue that these remnants are not very important in that they will ultimately disappear or be sequestered within the eye, without clinical sequelae. This may be true. Nevertheless, how often have we removed cortical remnants only to be rewarded within days by seeing residual material of a significant degree in the eye? As discussed earlier in the section on cataract surgery, a surprising amount of lens material can be found in many eyes that have undergone phacoemulsification, and this is especially true when intraoperative complications have developed.

Removal of cortical material by endoscopic means is usually simple. A complete vitrectomy must first be performed so that all of the lens material is freely floating. Small pieces scattered throughout the vitreous are often removed simultaneously. Once mobile, the cortical fragments can be easily aspirated into the port of the vitrector or phacofragmentation needle. Using a wide-field endoscopic view is helpful, primarily because it reveals the totality of the situation, allowing the surgeon to clearly define the scope of the procedure required to correct the problem. Stereopsis is not necessary to accomplish this task, and frequently even lens pieces that are somewhat distant from the aspirating handpiece will "fly" into its port because there is no vitreous to impede their movement.

Larger fragments require a bit more caution, especially if they are close to the retinal surface. Advancing the endo-scope so that a medium to high magnification view can be helpful in attaining finer visualization and control in this situation. Still, most of these lens pieces can be aspirated alone or cut and aspirated with the vitrector, without requiring phacofragmentation.

Once the vitreous is removed and residual cortical material excised from the anterior vitreous and region of the sulcus, small fragments will often be found on the macula. They are usually removed easily by aspiration alone, but care must be taken not to traumatize the retina. Usually, the endoscope is advanced to within 3 or 4 mm of the retinal surface so that a higher magnification image is obtained. Then the tip of the vitrector, fragmentation needle, or extrusion needle is carefully advanced so that it just overlies the fragments. They can then be aspirated into the instrument's port. Excessive suction should be avoided so that the macula does not follow these fragments. The surgeon should be especially careful if the retina is already detached. Usually, low suction is required for this task if the vitreous has been completely removed from the posterior pole. Nuclear fragments present a measure of increased difficulty. Unless they are quite small, usually it is not possible to remove these fragments with the vitrector, and fragmentation is required. The same endoscopic principles previously mentioned apply in this situation as well. A wide-field view is used to locate the fragment after complete vitrectomy. Then aspiration is applied to draw it into the port of the fragmentation needle. If it must be removed from the macular surface, the surgeon must shift to a higher magnification image, which is achieved by moving the endoscope tip closer to the fragment. Then the phacoemulsification needle is carefully advanced toward the nuclear material, ultimately aspirating it into its port. The needle is retracted into the mid- or anterior vitreous cavity while the aspiration continues, and at the same time the endoscope is withdrawn again to create a more panoramic view. At this point, fragmentation can be safely added to the aspiration function. Usually a small to moderate amount of nuclear material can be removed in this fashion, and the remaining piece will break off and float posteriorly. This process can be

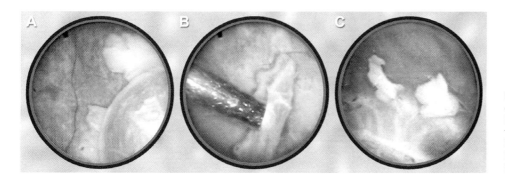

FIGURE 21-1. Endoscopic image of dislocated lens material. **A:** Nucleus and cortex on retinal surface. **B:** Removal of this material by posterior fragmentation. **C:** Retained nuclear fragments causing glaucoma and inflammation.

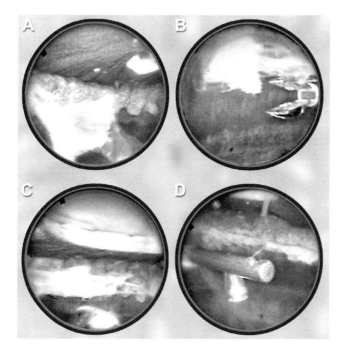

FIGURE 21-2. Retained cortex. **A:** Image of this material overlying ciliary body. **B:** Removal with forceps. **C:** Close-up view. **D:** Removal with a vitrector.

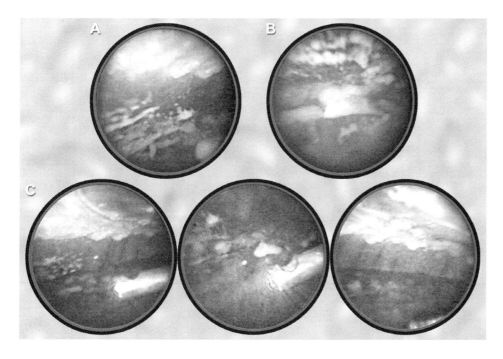

FIGURE 21-3. Lens fragments. **A:** Cortex scattered over pars plana. **B:** Cortex scattered over peripheral retina. **C:** Removal with vitrector.

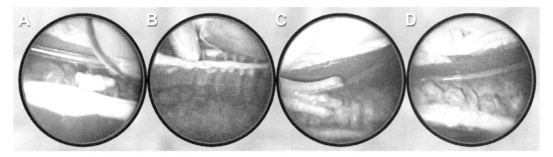

FIGURE 21-4. Case of recurrent inflammation and intraocular pressure elevation of indeterminate etiology. **A:** Diagnostic endoscopy reveals lens fragment overlying ciliary processes. **B:** Attempt to remove by suction through vitrector was unsuccessful. **C:** Extrusion brush was maneuvered into proper position. **D:** Lens fragment is no longer present.

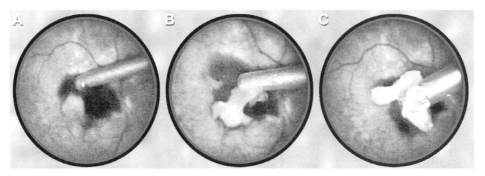

FIGURE 21-5. One day after complicated phacoemulsification. **A:** Lens fragments and hemorrhage on macular surface. **B:** Fragments are carefully aspirated from retinal surface. **C:** Vitrector and aspirated lens fragments are brought into mid vitreous cavity, where removal is completed.

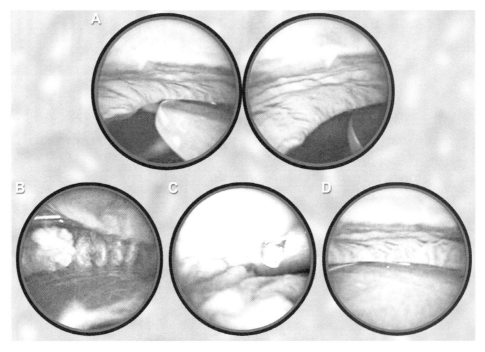

FIGURE 21-6. Uncontrolled intraocular pressure elevation following complicated phacoemulsification. **A:** Posterior chamber intraocular lens is slightly decentered and tilted with lens fragment evident in angle. **B:** Residual fragment overlying ciliary body. **C:** Vitrector used to aspirate lens fragments (iris at bottom of image). **D:** All fragments are now removed and the lens is repositioned.

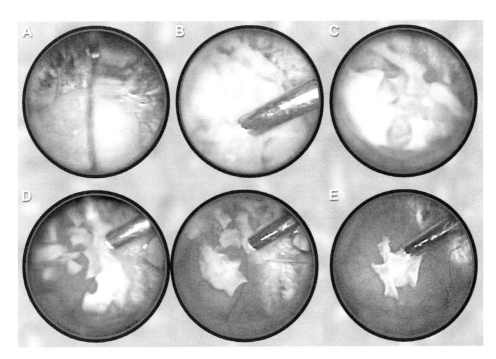

FIGURE 21-7. Eye with previous extensive laser treatment for proliferative diabetic retinopathy undergoing phacoemulsification. Most of the lens falls posteriorly. **A:** A large nuclear fragment on retina surface. **B:** The endoscope is advanced so that a close-up view permits gentle aspiration of the large fragment into the port of the fragmentation needle. **C:** The fragment is then elevated into the mid-vitreous cavity, where phacoemulsification can then be applied. Typically, the fragment will break off and fall posteriorly again. **D:** This process is repeated, breaking the large fragment into smaller and smaller pieces. **E:** Removal of the last fragment.

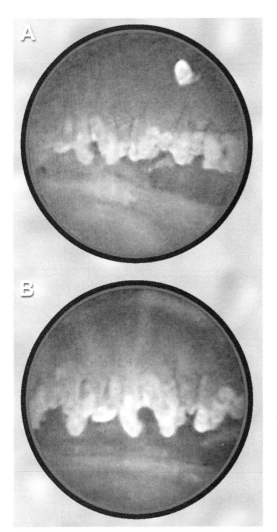

FIGURE 21-8. Eye with chronic uncontrolled open-angle glaucoma that developed after cataract surgery. **A:** Small piece of nucleus adherent to sulcus detected by endoscopy. **B:** Same area after aspiration of nuclear fragment.

patiently repeated as many times as necessary until all nuclear material has been removed from the eye.

The "divide and conquer" method used by many anterior segment phacoemulsification surgeons plays an important role for the posterior segment removal of the nucleus. Breaking this material into smaller pieces makes its removal through the needle more efficacious. Clearly, the larger the fragment is to begin with, the more important breaking it to smaller pieces becomes. It seems that nuclear fragments almost always fall onto the macula in the vitrectomized eye. Therefore, the surgeon should be careful, patiently and repeatedly shifting from the higher-magnification/close-up endoscopic image for engaging the fragment to the wide-field/distant placement of the endoscope when applying the fragmentation mode in the mid- or anterior vitreous cavity. Even greater care must be taken in the presence of retinal detachment.

All of these principles hold true when the entire crystalline lens has been dropped into the vitreous cavity. This situation can be somewhat time consuming because of the repetitions required for shifting endoscope field of view, aspirating lens material from the retinal surface, and fragmentation of the lens in the vitreous cavity away from the retinal surface. Nevertheless, a good outcome can usually be expected.

The ciliary sulcus and posterior iris region should be inspected endoscopically for nuclear fragments that may be "hiding." If missed, they can go on to create recurrent inflammation or glaucoma, yet they are simple enough to detect.

Once completed, it is important to inspect the retina for 360 degrees with the endoscope to detect any inadvertent retinal damage. Any breaks that are observed can be simultaneously photocoagulated.

ENDOSCOPIC VITRECTOMY FOR DISLOCATED INTRAOCULAR LENS IMPLANTS

The management of dislocated intraocular lens (IOL) implant is controversial, with some surgeons advocating repositioning of the IOL and others recommending exchange or removal; still others recommend no intervention at all. As in most of these situations, the decision must be made on a case-by-case basis. Complete removal of all anterior and posterior vitreous must be performed before one goes fishing for the errant IOL. If sufficient capsule seems to be present—and this can be easily and best assessed with endoscopy—the surgeon may elect to preserve it for repositioning or replacement of the IOL later in the procedure or during another surgery.

IMAGING AND MOBILIZING THE INTRAOCULAR LENS

First, a word about visualization. Some IOLs, particularly those with transparent haptics, can be difficult to find in the balanced saline solution–filled eye while imaging through the microscope. Furthermore, the implant may not have fallen posteriorly but rather may have become adherent to the retina more peripherally, making its identification even more difficult. The presence of hemorrhage or retinal detachment certainly compounds the situation. Endoscopy easily circumvents these issues. Perhaps because of the optics of imaging from within the eye, a transparent IOL in a clear liquid medium is still easily seen, whereas it may disappear when imaged from outside of the eye to the inside, as with the operating microscope.

Typically, the IOL will be lying on the retinal surface after vitrectomy. It must be grasped, usually by the haptic, with intraocular forceps (Fig. 22-1). Extreme care must be taken not to damage the underlying retina, and several variations on the method for accomplishing this task have been suggested. It is best to "float" the lens off of the retinal surface by injecting some material into the posterior segment. Many advocate perfluorocarbon liquid (PFCL) for this purpose. It is theoretically possible to float the IOL from the macula all the way to the sulcus by using this technique. Unfortunately, often the IOL is displaced laterally, toward the eye wall, where it will adhere, complicating removal. Furthermore, it may be difficult to remove all of the PFCL from the eye at the completion of surgery, thereby introducing another problem into the equation. An alternative approach is to inject viscoelastic over the optic nerve and macula in sufficient quantity to lift the IOL from the retinal surface. The haptic can then be grasped with an intraocular forceps and the implant maneuvered anteriorly. If these materials are not available or for some reason do not seem

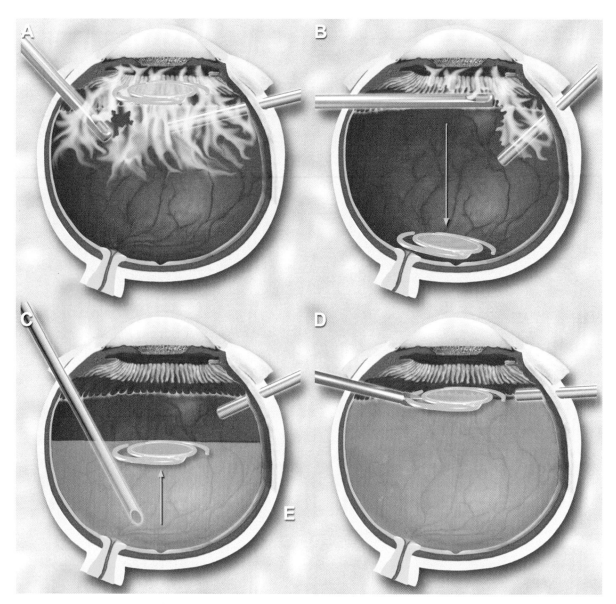

FIGURE 22-1. Dislocated lens implant. **A:** Vitrectomy frees the lens. **B:** The lens drops posteriorly. **C:** Perfluorocarbon liquid injection causes the lens to float off the retinal surface. **D:** Forceps are used to grab the lens for anterior placement.

to achieve the task at hand, the forceps can be used to grasp the IOL directly from the retinal surface, although great care must be taken not to traumatize the underlying tissue.

The next problem to consider is what exactly to do with the IOL once it has been lifted from the retina and moved toward the anterior segment.

INTRAOCULAR LENS EXPLANTATION

Often it is necessary to remove the IOL from the eye altogether. There are usually a few reasons this becomes necessary. The haptics of the IOL may be damaged and not amenable to repositioning; the style of the IOL may not lend itself to being sewn back into position; anatomic features may not permit lens replacement; or intraoperative conditions may become unsatisfactory for repositioning. In any event, surgery is initiated by removal of all vitreous from the anterior and posterior chambers. If a significant amount of lens capsule remains, it can be left intact for later IOL reimplantation.

Implants can be removed through a limbal or pars plana incision. In the long run, it probably does not make much difference which site is used, with anatomic and technical conditions determining the best course of action.

The first consideration relates to the IOL itself. Lens designs vary, making some more easily managed than others. IOL optic thickness, flexibility, and haptic design are all features that must be considered when deciding how to resolve the situation. If the goal is to limit the size of the incision used to remove the implant, some surgeons have advocated intraocular cutting of the IOL optic into segments as well as removal of the haptics, so that ultimately only a small incision is needed to remove all of the pieces.

This approach can indeed be useful with lenses that are flexible and thin. Endoscopic imaging provides a clear view of the pars plana so that a larger than usual incision can be created externally yet be monitored internally for the creation of retinal breaks or vitreous incarceration. The segments of the IOL can be closely scrutinized from the inside of the eye as they are passed through the incision to the external environment, ensuring that they do not traumatize the retina. After all of the pieces have been removed, a thin yellow line will be seen on the brown pars plana, denoting the incision site. Incidentally, this "yellow line sign" indicates surgical or traumatic laceration of the pars plana, which may prove to be of value when one is hunting for intraocular foreign bodies or evidence of perforation. At any rate, once this task has been completed, the enlarged sclerotomy can be sutured and the conjunctiva reapproximated. These same IOL fragments can also be removed from the limbus, again with the assistance of endoscopy to prevent trauma to adjacent tissue. Opinions vary but it seems that surgical trauma to the sclera would be less significant than to the cornea.

On the other hand, some IOL types defy this approach. For example, large-plate haptic silicone IOLs are impossible to refold within the eye and are quite thick. Attempts to cut them, even with large intraocular scissors, are usually unsuccessful. These types of implants are not amenable to repositioning because of their proclivity for falling posteriorly again. Finally, the geometry of the lens and its positioning holes makes the implant difficult to suture from within the eye. In effect, this style

of IOL must be removed through a large incision in one piece. Again, the surgeon has the option of explanting through a limbal or pars plana incision. The principles are the same for both approaches with one modification. Because it is known in advance that a large incision will be required and that it is less than optimal to create this incision once the forceps have grasped the IOL and brought it to the explantation site, the incision should be prepared before the lens is grasped.

Suppose that a 6-mm incision is needed and a pars plana exit has been selected (Figs. 22-2 and 22-3). The surgeon marks the extent of the site on the sclera 3.5 to 4.5 mm from the limbus, and the MVR blade is used to create the incision. One or two sutures are placed with a slip-knot to keep the edges of this relatively large wound approximated and water tight—all at the initiation of the vitrectomy. Once all of the vitreous has been removed, the IOL is grasped and brought toward the wound. Then the surgeon removes the endoscope from the eye, using this hand to untie the slip knots and move the sutures aside. At this point, the endoscope is reinserted to internally monitor removal of the IOL, which may now be easily completed through the large incision site. The opened slip-knot sutures are then tied, closing the wound. The vitrector is used to meticulously remove any residual vitreous or debris in this region, all of which may be well monitored endoscopically. More sutures can be used to close the sclerotomy as befits the situation and the surgeon's preference. Endoscopic photocoagulation of the pars plana incision site may relieve the surgeon's anxiety.

The other option is to explant the IOL through the limbus. The same basic principles apply. Following vitrectomy, the IOL is floated, then grasped and brought toward the wound. The limbal incision should be fashioned prior to grasping the IOL and closed with slip-knot sutures, as in the pars plana extraction. The endoscope is removed from the eye freeing the surgeon's second hand to open and displace the limbal sutures. The endoscope does not necessarily have to be introduced in this situation because the explantation can be monitored through the microscope. After removal of the IOL, the sutures are tied and, once again, any vitreous in the region must be meticulously excised.

It is at this point that endoscopy can again be useful in that any errant strands of vitreous that may be adherent to the wound or iris can be detected and removed. These adhesions are often missed by the microscope yet have the potential to create significant difficulties later on, particularly cystoid macular edema and retinal detachment. Therefore, their detection and excision is of great importance.

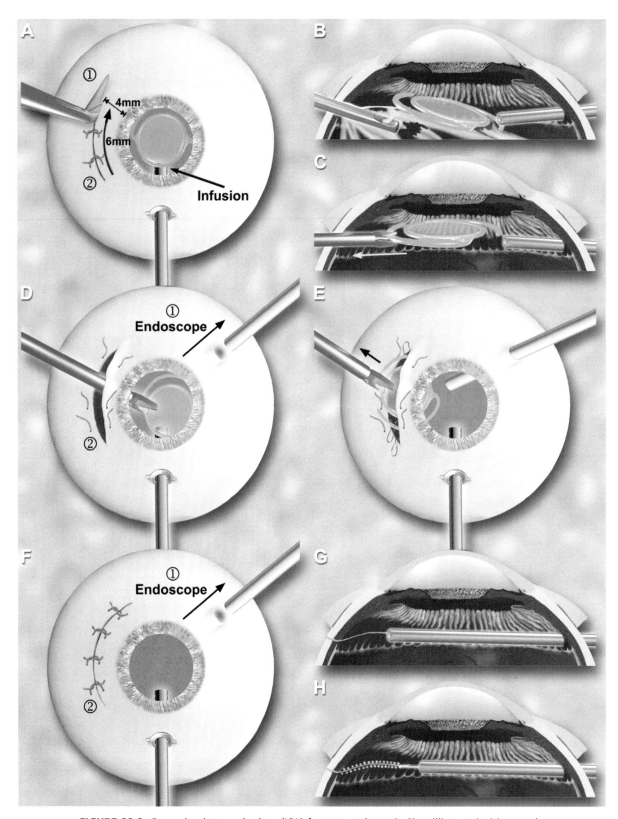

FIGURE 22-2. Removing intraocular lens (IOL) from pars plana. **A:** Six-millimeter incision made over pars plana temporally typically using corneoscleral scissors or some type of blade (1), and secured with several slipknots (2). **B:** Endoscopic vitrectomy with special attention to internal aspect of large pars plana incision site. **C:** When the IOL is freely mobile, it is floated from retinal surface, grasped with forceps, and brought to the large incision site. **D:** The surgeon removes the endoscope from the nasal sclerotomy (1) and uses this hand to untie the slipknots (2). **E:** The endoscope is reinserted to monitor explantation through the now-open large temporal sclerotomy site. **F:** Once the IOL is explanted, all instruments are removed from the eye (1) and slipknot sutures are permanently tied (2). **G:** The endoscope is reinserted nasally, and the ocular interior is inspected for breaks or residual vitreous. **H:** Endoscopic pars plana laser applications are made at the surgeon's discretion and the eye is closed.

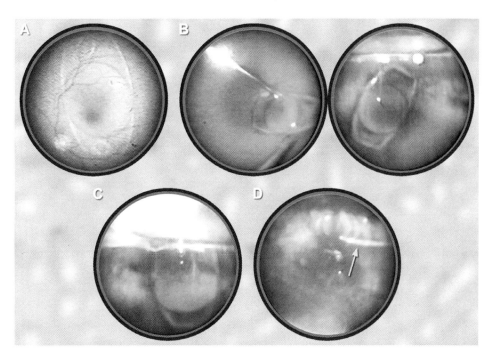

FIGURE 22-3. Explantation of dislocated intraocular lenses (IOLs). **A:** Plate haptic silicone IOL on retinal surface. Unlike other types of lens implants that dislocate posteriorly yet rarely become symptomatic or cause retinal damage, these lenses can be quite disturbing to the patient. If repositioned without fixation, they tend to fall posteriorly again. They are difficult or impossible to suture into position. These lenses require extraction. **B:** Plate haptic lens on posterior pole is grasped with forceps. **C:** The IOL is now partially removed from the pars plana. **D:** The IOL has been completely explanted, and the yellow line, indicating the internal aspect of the incision site, is photocoagulated.

REPOSITIONING OF A POSTERIORLY DISLOCATED INTRAOCULAR LENS

If the surgeon elects to lift the IOL from the retinal surface and reposition it in the sulcus, the same basic technique described in the previous explantation applies here. The lens is floated from the retinal surface, grasped with forceps, and then brought anteriorly. The next question is how exactly to position and secure the IOL in the sulcus. One option is to merely wedge the IOL into the sulcus without suturing, and this may indeed be satisfactory. This is especially true if there is a significant amount of capsule remaining. It is quite simple, under moderate- to wide-field endoscopic guidance, to place the IOL in the remains of the capsular bag and wedge it into the sulcus (Fig. 22-4). The precise location of each haptic can be fully assessed and the

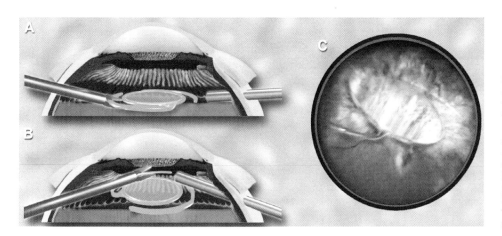

FIGURE 22-4. Repositioning intraocular lens (IOL) in sulcus. **A:** IOL floated from retina and grasped with forceps. **B:** Haptics wedged into sulcus under endoscopic guidance where stability can be assessed. **C:** Posterior chamber IOL on retinal surface. This style of lens implant is amenable to lifting from posterior segment and repositioning in sulcus without scleral fixation if there is adequate capsular support.

stability of the new arrangement can be appreciated far better than by microscope imaging.

Although it would seem to be a simple task to reposition a plate haptic lens in the sulcus compared with the difficulties of explantation, this approach cannot be considered. These lenses are so soft and flexible that they will surely fall posteriorly again. This is even true if there seems to be a substantial amount of capsular support. This style of lens, then, must be either sewn back into position, which is extremely difficult, or explanted.

SUTURING OF A POSTERIORLY DISLOCATED INTRAOCULAR LENS

Some surgeons believe that posteriorly dislocated IOLs should be sutured into position. Many variations of the technique required to do this have been reported; a simple one will be described here. In this particular approach, the three standard pars plana incision sites are created, along with a small paralimbal scleral incision and flap at the 3 o'clock and 9 o'clock positions (Fig. 22-5). After completion of the vitrectomy, the IOL is floated from the retinal surface. A suture of the surgeon's choice is prepared with the needle on one end and a small loop on the other. This loop can be tied and knotted or merely created by twisting the suture. While holding the endoscope in one hand, the surgeon inserts an intraocular forceps and the suture loop through the opposite paralimbal incision with the other hand. The loop is placed around one of the haptics and then the forceps is withdrawn. The endoscope is then switched to the opposite pars plana sclerotomy site while another suture loop and forceps are introduced through the second paralimbal incision. The process of placing the loop around the haptic is repeated.

At this point, all of the difficult work has been done. Each IOL haptic has a suture around it connected to a needle emanating from a paralimbal incision. The needle on each side is passed through one edge of the scleral wound and the suture is pulled on both sides, more or less simultaneously, raising the IOL into its proper position. The suture on each side is then tied to the sclera, and the flap is placed over the knot. The pars plana incisions are then closed in the surgeon's usual fashion.

PLACEMENT AND SUTURING OF AN INTRAOCULAR LENS FROM THE ANTERIOR SEGMENT

Many ophthalmologists prefer to manage the optical rehabilitation of the aphakic eye by securing an IOL in

the sulcus. Again, many techniques to accomplish this goal have been described, and a relatively simple method will be discussed here. A paralimbal scleral incision with flap is created at the 3 o'clock and 9 o'clock positions (Fig. 22-6). A 10-0 proline suture with a long straight (Keith) needle is passed through the superior edge of the incision while a 27-gauge needle is passed through the superior edge of the opposite incision. The suture needle is placed inside the barrel of the 27-gauge needle and then withdrawn from the eye so that an equal length of the suture exits from each sclerotomy. A similar process is performed through the inferior edge of each sclerotomy site. The purpose of a superior and inferior suture on each side is to limit the potential for creating a "propeller" effect that might arise if only a single suture were used. An appropriately sized clear corneal, tunnel, or other limbal incision is created superiorly to permit introduction of the IOL.

At this point, the endoscope can be inserted through this third incision to check the location of each suture internally, ensuring that their proper placement in the sulcus has been achieved. Each suture is then withdrawn through the superior incision with a hook or other instrument and is cut. The superior and inferior suture on each side can then be tied to the haptic or positioning hole of the IOL. The implant is maneuvered into position, and the sutures are tightened and tied on each side. At this point, the IOL should be securely and correctly positioned in the sulcus, achieving permanent stability.

HAPTIC EROSION OF TISSUE AND INTRAOCULAR HEMORRHAGE

Occasionally a patient presents with a new or recurrent hyphema or vitreous hemorrhage of undetermined cause. Some patients also demonstrate elements of red blood cell glaucoma. Initial conservative supportive measures may suffice, but in some eyes the problem becomes relentless. Endoscopy can be helpful in this situation because the internal aspect of previously fashioned incisions can be inspected for vascularization (Figs. 22-7 to 22-10). Perhaps more importantly, the points of IOL haptic content can be visually inspected from an anterior or posterior approach (or both). Sites representing haptic extrusion from the capsular bag, points of erosion, and bleeding may be detected that not only will serve to establish the cause of the patient's problem but can also be photocoagulated to prevent further occurrences. Sometimes, endoscopic inspection fails to reveal any underlying pathology.

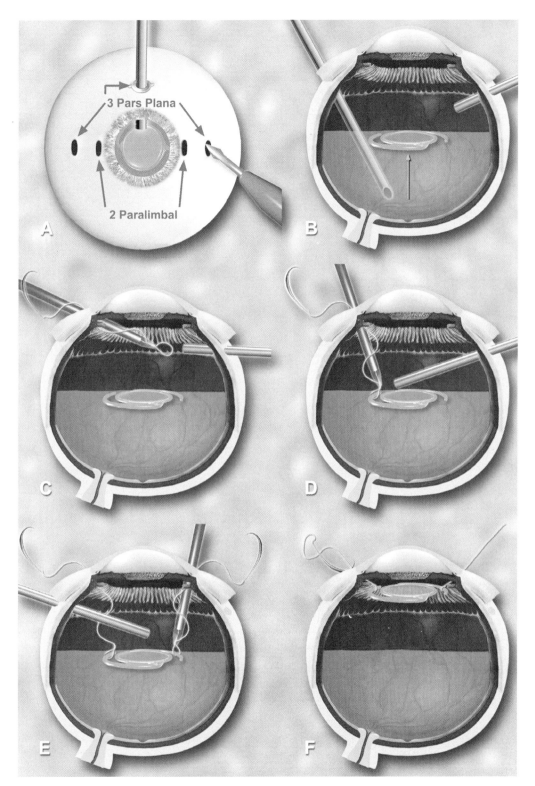

FIGURE 22-5. Intraocular suturing of dislocated posterior chamber intraocular lens (IOL) into position. **A:** Five incisions are made—three through the pars plana in their usual locations and two paralimbal, through the sulcus, at the 3 o'clock and 9 o'clock positions. **B:** A pars plana vitrectomy is performed and the lens floated from retinal surface with perfluorocarbon liquid or viscoelastic. **C:** A suture loop with needle on its other end placed around haptic with intraocular forceps through the limbal site. The needle end is still external to eye. **D:** The same step is repeated on opposite side. **E:** Both sutures are now pulled to raise the IOL into position and then the external needle on each side is secured to the paralimbal scleral incision edge and scleral flaps secured. **F:** The pars plana incisions are closed.

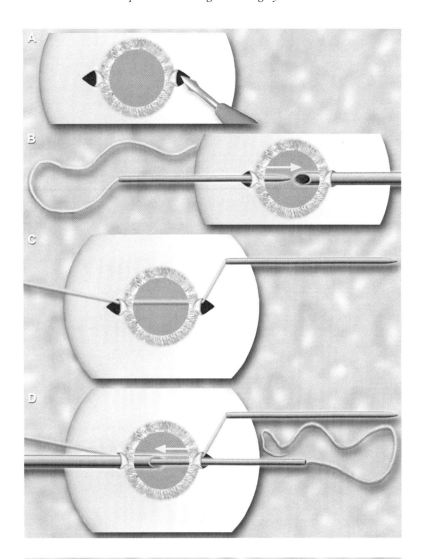

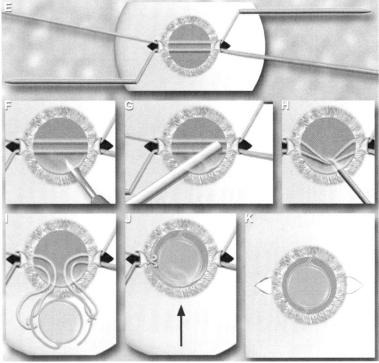

FIGURE 22-6. Securing a posterior chamber intraocular lens (IOL) in the sulcus of an aphakic eye. **A:** Paralimbal incisions with scleral flaps are fashioned at the 3 o'clock and 9 o'clock positions. **B:** A 10-0 proline suture on a long straight needle is passed through superior edge of one incision while a 27-gauge syringe needle is passed through the superior edge of the opposite incision. The long needle is placed in a 27-gauge needle lumen and then withdrawn from the eye. **C:** Now a suture stretches from the superior end of the incision to the superior edge of the other. **D:** This process is repeated for the inferior end of each incision. **E:** There are now two sutures that stretch from sulcus to sulcus. **F:** A superior limbal incision for IOL insertion is made. **G:** The endoscope is inserted through this incision to inspect for proper placement of the proline sutures in the sulcus. **H:** A hook is used to withdraw the sutures from the eye superiorly. **I:** They are cut and tied to the haptic or positioning holes of the IOL. **J:** The sutures are used to pull the IOL into proper position. **K:** Then they are tied and the scleral flap is closed over them. The IOL is now securely sutured in the sulcus.

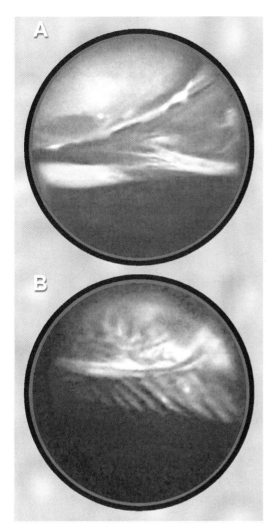

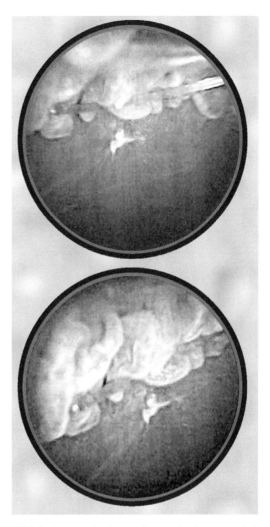

FIGURE 22-7. Suture of posterior chamber intraocular lens (IOL) in an aphakic eye. **A:** Inadequate capsular support necessitates securing IOL with suture. **B:** Image of same area after securing IOL. Note mild hemorrhage adjacent to suture site.

FIGURE 22-8. Intraocular hemorrhage of unknown etiology. At times, haptics can extrude through the capsular bag, piercing the ciliary body. This may be a cause of recurrent intraocular hemorrhage.

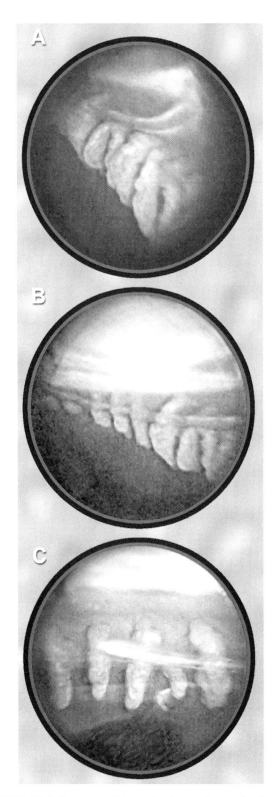

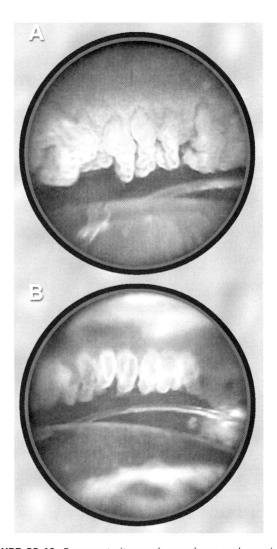

FIGURE 22-10. Recurrent vitreous hemorrhage and associated glaucoma of unknown etiology. **A:** Haptic extruding through capsular bag. **B:** Image after laser treatment of presumed erosion site.

FIGURE 22-9. Recurrent intraocular hemorrhage of unknown etiology. **A:** Haptic pierces through capsular bag at this point. **B:** The course of the "externalized" haptic is followed. **C:** Tip of haptic is now located along with presumed erosion site and area of hemorrhage.

23

ENDOSCOPIC VITRECTOMY FOR ENDOPHTHALMITIS

Infection within the eye, whether endogenous or exogenous, can be a devastating problem. Over the years, numerous treatment paradigms have evolved, and patients with this problem now have a significant opportunity for resolution. This discussion focuses on the role of endoscopic vitrectomy in the management of endophthalmitis and some of the advantages that this approach confers, rather than presenting an exhaustive examination of the causes, organisms, and medical therapy of endophthalmitis.

It would be fair to say that most cases of infectious endophthalmitis encountered in the United States represent a complication of cataract surgery. Gram-positive organisms are most commonly responsible. Nevertheless, the principles of vitrectomy in this situation are more or less the same, regardless of the cause or organism involved.

To begin, cultures may be taken from the ocular surface, anterior chamber, and vitreous aspirate in their usual manner. A standard three-port vitrectomy is then performed. Some surgeons consider it unnecessary to remove most of the vitreous but rather think it sufficient to remove just a core. Endoscopic imaging might dissuade one from this approach. Even in eyes with "early" infection, in which the vitreous appears to be clear on clinical examination, a significant vitritis is often apparent endoscopically. If one of the goals of surgery is to remove as much infectious material and inflammatory debris as possible, it follows that a complete vitrectomy is desirable.

When endophthalmitis is detected early in its course, particularly if it arises as a consequence of cataract surgery, most of the activity centers on the lens implant and anterior vitreous. Foci of infection may be detected in the region of the sulcus. Conventional imaging techniques do not permit much of a view of these areas, particularly if the cornea is edematous or the pupil miotic. Perhaps one of the reasons that even "successful" endophthalmitis vitrectomies often require considerable time to resolve after surgery is that a significant amount of infectious and inflammatory debris is left in the eye. Endoscopic vitrectomy at least offers the surgeon the opportunity to detect and remove most of this material. However, there may be a down side to this approach in that care must be taken not to destabilize the posterior chamber lens implant by aggressive removal of the

most anterior portion of the vitreous and its attachments to the lens capsule or zonules.

This is not to say that the anterior vitreous should be left intact. To the contrary, it is best to remove it in this situation. The surgeon should simply monitor the effect that this portion of the vitrectomy has on the intraocular lens so that if any pseudophacodenesis is detected it might be construed as a signal to move on.

Frequently, scattered deep and superficial retinal hemorrhages may be observed after removal of the vitreous debris. As long as the infection is eliminated and inflammation controlled postoperatively, such hemorrhages usually resolve spontaneously. While they are of little practical concern, it is important to search for retinal breaks at the conclusion of surgery. Endoscopic imaging is well suited for this purpose and is often superior to the indirect ophthalmoscope in this situation. Recall that many of these eyes have some element of corneal edema and miosis before surgery, and vitrectomy usually exacerbates the situation. Furthermore, because many of these eyes are in the immediate post-cataract surgery period with unhealed incisions, scleral depression may not be a great idea. Endoscopy can usually provide a high-magnification view with good resolution of the periphery without scleral depression, and any breaks that are detected may be simultaneously managed with photocoagulation. This is a very important feature of vitrectomy for this problem because the incidence of retinal detachment following treatment for endophthalmitis is about 15%. The endoscopic approach can substantially diminish the potential for this problem simply by providing the opportunity to clearly examine the retinal periphery at the conclusion of surgery (Fig. 23-1).

Eyes with endophthalmitis of several days' duration or more can develop inflammatory membranes on the retinal surface, the removal of which can usually be accomplished by aspiration through a soft-tipped extrusion cannula or brush. Perhaps high-dose corticosteroids applied at the appropriate time postoperatively would also make these membranes disappear, but then again, perhaps not. Removing as much inflammatory debris and membranes as possible at the time of surgery seems a more appropriate choice.

Although vitrectomy and intraocular antibiotic injection typically are sufficient to manage this problem, a small sub-

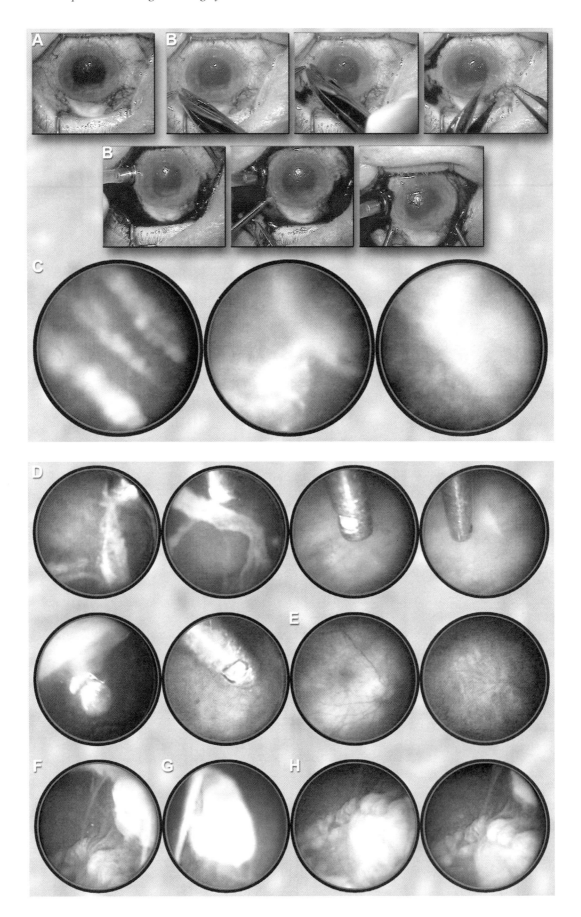

set of patients experience recurrent endophthalmitis despite best efforts by conventional techniques. In such eyes, one might wonder whether residual foci of infection remained and ultimately reactivated. Indeed, this seems to be true. In these uncommon situations in which recurrent infection occurs, one must seriously consider the possibility that residual foci exist that are not apparent upon examination using conventional techniques. Endoscopy can be quite valuable here because often these infectious sites are hidden on the posterior iris, inside the lens capsule peripherally, or adjacent to the ciliary body. Their endoscopic detection is straightforward, and combining this imaging technique with vitrectomy usually results in complete eradication of all hidden infectious foci. A published study (1) of vitrectomy for the treatment of *Propionibacterium acnes* endophthalmitis reported excellent outcomes in all but one patient, who experienced several recurrences of infection, each managed by vitrectomy. When confronted with yet another reactivation, the patient was referred for endoscopic vitrec-tomy, which resulted in apparent eradication of the problem (no recurrence in 2 years).

Endoscopic vitrectomy represents a significant advance in the management of endophthalmitis because it permits more complete removal of infectious and inflammatory debris, evaluation and elimination of some of the early intraocular complications of endophthalmitis (membrane formation, retinal breaks), and detection of more subtle foci of infection that can prove to be a problem later. In addition, endoscopic vitrectomy circumvents the intraocular imaging difficulties experienced with conventional techniques due to such anterior segment impediments as corneal edema or miosis.

REFERENCE

1. Aldave AJ, Srein JD, Deramo VA, et al. Treatment strategies for postoperative *Propionibacterium acnes* endophthalmitis. *Ophthalmology* 1999;106:2395–2401.

FIGURE 23-1. Endophthalmitis secondary to infected filtration bleb. **A:** External view. **B:** Creation of insertion sites. **C:** Appearance of infectious and inflammatory debris in the eye. **D:** Aspiration into vitrector. **E:** Vitreous cavity has been cleared of infectious and inflammatory debris. Note view of posterior pole and of peripheral retina. **F:** Internal view of infectious material oozing from trabeculectomy site into sulcus. **G:** Sclerostomy obstructed by infectious and inflammatory debris. **H:** Infectious material "dripping" down the face of the ciliary processes onto the intraocular lens.

ENDOSCOPIC VITRECTOMY FOR INTRAOCULAR FOREIGN BODY

There is some debate regarding the management of intraocular foreign body (IOFB), particularly as it relates to magnetic objects. Some surgeons believe that magnetic extraction is preferable, whereas others assert that vitrectomy is the best approach. Despite one's personal feelings on this issue, for the purposes of discussion only vitrectomy will be addressed.

Clinical management of IOFBs can be elusive because even the most thorough preoperative evaluation sometimes fails to uncover the presence of some intraocular fragments, particularly nonmetallic ones. To further confound the situation, many of these eyes have sustained significant anterior and posterior segment trauma. The value of conventional viewing techniques, such as the operating microscope or indirect ophthalmoscope, can be significantly diminished. Being able to image from within the eye can greatly assist efforts to identify and manage intraocular pathology in this situation.

First, all lacerations must be properly addressed. Then a three-port vitrectomy is initiated. If the correct placement of the infusion cannula cannot be verified by the usual means, inserting the endoscope through an opposing incision can be helpful in establishing its proper position before "opening" the infusion line. If subretinal placement is detected, the situation may be remedied by replacing the infusion cannula with a longer one, draining an adjacent choroidal effusion/hemorrhage (if responsible for the problem), or simply moving to another site. Vitrectomy is performed as completely as possible, with special care given to the removal of blood and any foreign debris that was introduced at the time of ocular penetration.

After the vitreous has been cleared, a careful search for one or more IOFBs should be made. Once located, the next step is to determine whether the IOFB is free or embedded in the eye wall. If embedded, it must be freed before extraction. This is usually a simple task. Such an IOFB can be manipulated with the IOFB forceps tip until it can be grasped and extracted. If it is even more stubborn, a pick or spatula can be used to dislodge it; then it can be grasped and removed with the forceps.

Next, the surgeon must estimate the size of the IOFB as compared with the size of the sclerotomy site through which the forceps is being introduced. If the IOFB is larger than the sclerotomy site, the site must be enlarged to accommodate it before extraction is attempted (Fig. 24-1). The sclera can be marked 3.5 to 4.5 mm from the limbus along the length of the desired incision, and then the sclerotomy can be safely enlarged in a limbus-parallel fashion using an MVR blade, scissors, or other instrument. The endoscope can verify proper placement of the incision in its internal aspect. Care should be taken not to make this opening too anteriorly because doing so would lacerate the ciliary processes, which have a tendency to bleed profusely, as well as hamper the subsequent extraction. Certainly, the surgeon does not want to make this incision too posteriorly; avoiding the retina is usually a good idea. Precisely measuring this site, rather than "guesstimating," is important.

The endoscopic image may also indicate that there is a surprising amount of residual vitreous in the eye, particularly adjacent to the area of the large sclerotomy. Under endoscopic guidance, this vitreous can be removed.

Once completed, the surgeon's preferred scleral suture is placed in an interrupted fashion and tied with slip-knots that can be easily opened.

The extraction wound is closed except for the portion through which the grasping instrument is passed. The IOFB, which has been previously freed of any attachments, is now grasped with forceps and brought to the extraction site. The endoscope can then be removed from the eye, freeing the surgeon's second hand to untie the slip-knots and open the wound. If all goes well, the IOFB will be easily removed from the eye. This procedure can be repeated as many times as necessary for multiple IOFBs. If the wound is too small to permit extraction, the surgeon can enlarge it at that time with the free second hand. Once completed, the sutures can be tied and the "enlarged" portion of the sclerotomy site closed.

It is important at this juncture to reinsert the endoscope to inspect the internal aspect of the extraction site and adjacent tissue. Any incarcerated vitreous must be removed with the vitrector. If all comes together well, a thin yellow line will be seen, representing the reapproximated edges of the extraction site set against the brown coloration of the pars plana. It seems like a good idea to photocoagulate around

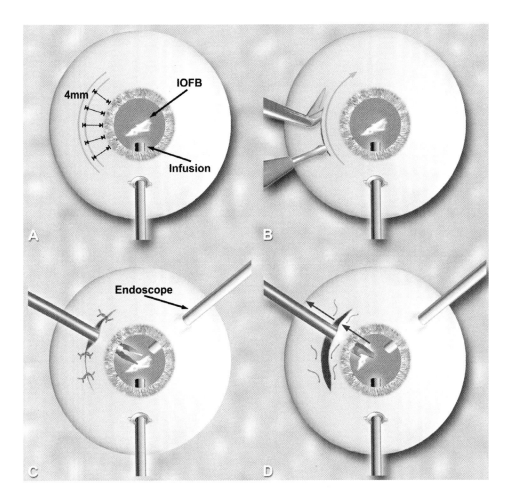

FIGURE 24-1. Enlargement of sclerotomy site to accommodate extraction of an intraocular foreign body (IOFB). **A:** The sclera is marked 3.5 to 4.5 mm from limbus along desired length of incision in a limbus-parallel manner. **B:** Sclerotomy is then enlarged to desired length with blade or scissors. **C:** Sutures are placed with slipknot to close the enlarged sclerotomy. **D:** The IOFB is grasped with forceps. The endoscope is removed from the eye, and this hand then unties the sutures, permitting extraction.

the yellow line as well as any other retinal pathology, although the value of this has not been assessed in a comparative manner. The ocular interior should then be reinspected for any residual pathology, particularly if multiple or difficult-to-visualize IOFBs (e.g., glass) were present (Fig. 24-2).

A few other details bear consideration. In many eyes with penetrating trauma, the residual vitreous is prone to contract, potentially creating a powerful focus of traction as well as a scaffold for future proliferation. With this in mind, all vitreous should be completely removed in the vicinity of perforation and extraction sites (Fig. 24-3). These areas should also be considered for photocoagulation.

As far as embedded IOFBs are concerned, once they are removed, by definition there is a retinal break. The vitreous in this area must be meticulously removed to prevent subsequent contraction and its consequences (Fig. 24-4). Laser retinopexy must also be applied. It has been my experience that placement of a segmental scleral buckle underlying the site of the embedded IOFB helps to prevent future retinal detachment, even though, theoretically, complete vitrectomy and laser retinopexy should be sufficient. Intraocular

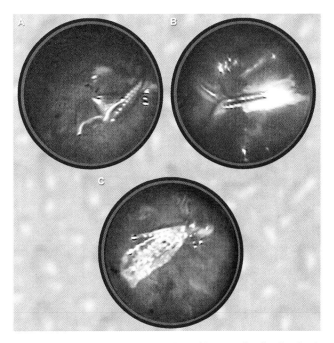

FIGURE 24-2. Endoscopic extraction of intraocular foreign bodies: **A:** metal, **B:** wood, **C:** glass.

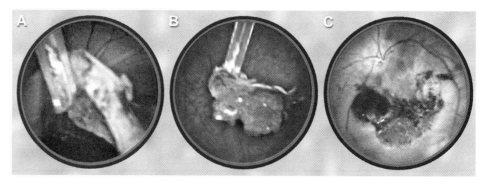

FIGURE 24-3. A metallic fragment perforates the eye. After vitrectomy, the fragment appears "rusty" and is lodged under the macula. **A:** A forceps is used to grasp the foreign body. **B:** Appearance of the foreign body as it is held in the midvitreous cavity. **C:** At the completion of surgery, the eye is filled with silicone oil.

antibiotics and steroids, long-acting gas or silicone oil injection, and lensectomy are administered at the surgeon's discretion.

Postoperatively, IOFB patients require close follow-up for the development of infection, inflammation, redetachment, proliferative vitreoretinopathy, and other problems. As in any iteration of penetrating ocular trauma, despite the surgeon's best efforts to meticulously manage these eyes, failure looms and patients should be forewarned so that they may have the appropriate expectations.

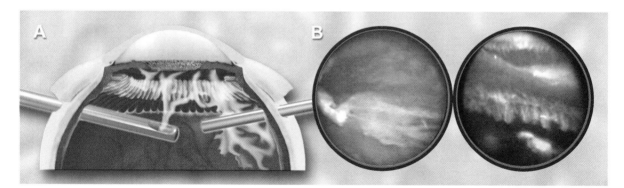

FIGURE 24-4. All vitreous should be excised from the vicinity of entry and extraction wounds to limit potential evolution of traction and proliferation. The yellow line identifies the extraction site.

ENDOSCOPIC VITRECTOMY FOR IRIS NEOVASCULARIZATION AND ITS CONSEQUENCES

Iris neovascularization (NVI) is the direct consequence of ocular schemia. The threshold for its development varies from eye to eye. Numerous etiologic factors culminate in a common pathway of neovascularization, intraocular hemorrhage, cataract formation, glaucoma, hypotony, blindness, and loss of the eye. Many of these patients present to the retinal surgeon at varying stages of this continuum, and their problems usually require some form of immediate intervention. The management of neovascular glaucoma has already been discussed, but the associated problems bear some scrutiny.

NVI usually first develops along the pupillary border or in the angle. It can be best detected when one almost "imagines" that it is present while viewing this portion of the iris with high magnification and illumination at the slit lamp (Fig. 25-1). The most subtle cases may not be readily apparent, but if the ophthalmologist stares at this region for a few seconds, the abnormal vessels might become visible. There are no "normal" vessels on the iris surface, so that if any vessels at all are detected, by definition they are neovascular in origin. Lightly pigmented or atrophic irides may present a diagnostic challenge in this regard. Fluorescein angiography of the iris can be helpful. While it should be clearly understood that many situations can cause iris vessels to leak this dye and that NVI does not necessarily involve leakage, if the iris in question is leaking fluorescein, especially while the fellow eye is not, it is a strong diagnostic point in favor of the pathologic nature of the iris vessels in question.

If a sufficient view of the retina is present, dense panretinal photocoagulation is required. This must be applied expeditiously because the progression from NVI with a partially open angle and normal intraocular pressure to a mostly obstructed drainage system with elevated intraocular pressure can occur within days or weeks. When ischemic central retinal vein occlusion is the underlying problem, rapid disease progression is of particular concern.

All of this is straightforward and does not usually present much of a diagnostic or therapeutic challenge. However, consider for a moment what should be done with the patient who has not only NVI but also one or more associated problems that make viewing, and therefore treating, the retina impossible. Hyphema, vitreous hemorrhage, miosis due to fibrovascular proliferation on the iris surface, and cataract are not uncommon features of ischemic ocular disorders. They also convert this situation to one that demands surgical intervention.

Although evacuation of a hyphema or vitreous hemorrhage is not the most complicated of procedures, it should be remembered that these are very compromised eyes that are already far along a downhill course and beginning to accelerate. It does not necessarily follow that promptly applied surgery with dense panretinal endophotocoagulation will result in disease stabilization. In fact, everyone involved should consider this to be a desperate situation.

In the past this state of affairs was managed by transscleral retinal cryoablation performed in a "blind" fashion. However, this did not prove to be an effective approach because titratable application is not possible. In addition, many of these eyes may still have good, or at least useful, vision. Extensive cryoablation, especially if heavy handed, often results in profound visual loss and is also painful.

Endoscopic vitrectomy and endophotocoagulation can be pivotal for a few reasons. If the pupil is miotic from fibrovascular proliferation on its surface, it will not dilate pharmacologically. Pupil-stretching maneuvers can induce more hemorrhage intraoperatively or postoperatively from rupture of these abnormal vessels. Furthermore, it is well known that the crystalline lens serves as a barrier between the anterior and posterior segments and has a beneficial effect on limiting the diffusion of "angiogenesis factor," the substance that theoretically promotes the development of NVI. If a cataract is present, even one that makes a posterior view impossible, it is best not to remove it while the proliferative process is accelerating.

Recalling that the goal of treatment is to access and ablate the ischemic retina in as atraumatic a manner as possible, the surgeon with the the use of endoscopy can adequately remove the vitreous and endophotocoagulate the retina in its entirety without disturbing the iris or lens. As

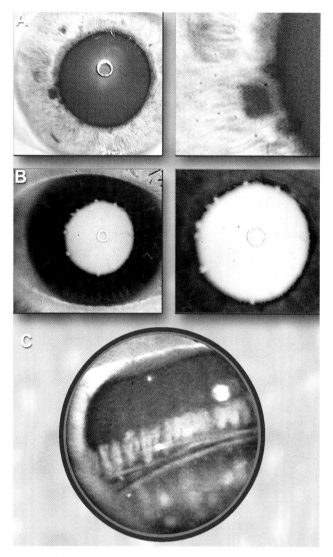

endoscopic vitrectomies go, this is a relatively easy procedure that patients can tolerate comfortably and that often proves effective in achieving the goal. If there were any question, the desired outcome here is to prevent the development of neovascular glaucoma (Fig. 25-2).

On the other hand, it is not uncommon to note persistent NVI despite dense and extensive panretinal photocoagulation. Nevertheless, this outcome is often satisfactory despite the fact that intermittent hyphema or vitreous hemorrhage may be noted periodically for years (Fig. 25-3). One might consider directly applying laser or wet-field ablation to NVI, but this method is ineffective. Once the eye has achieved a new steady state characterized by elimination or stabilization of NVI, the surgeon might address other issues, such as the presence of a significant cataract.

Finally, as observed with successfully managed neovascular glaucoma, progressive visual loss will develop in perhaps 20% of these eyes despite clear media and no other apparently active problems. This situation is undoubtedly due to ischemic compromise of the optic nerve and retina. Indeed, the optic nerve often demonstrates pallor and the retinal vasculature is markedly attenuated (Fig. 25-4). At this point, there is no intervention that would be of value.

FIGURE 25-1. Iris neovascularization (NVI). **A:** The earliest presentation of NVI can be quite subtle, requiring high magnification and illumination by slit examination. Small tufts at the pupillary border are barely evident here. **B:** Fluorescein angiography of the iris confirms their presence. **C:** Endoscopic appearance.

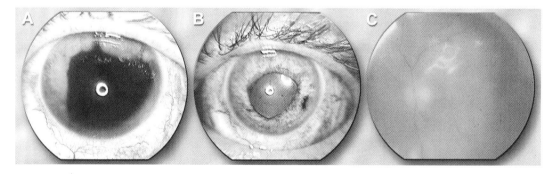

FIGURE 25-2. Management of iris neovascularization (NVI) in the absence of a posterior view. **A:** Iris neovascularization without glaucoma. **B:** Endoscopic vitrectomy and panretinal photocoagulation strictly avoiding lens. **C:** Management of recurrent vitreous hemorrhage and hyphema from NVI without glaucoma.

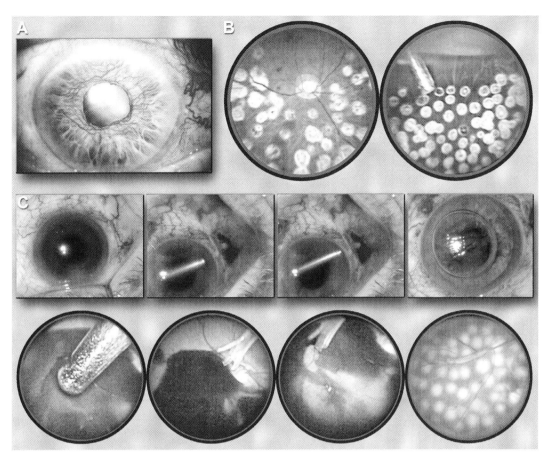

FIGURE 25-3. Recurrent hyphema and vitreous hemorrhage as a consequence of iris neovascularization (NVI). **A:** Patient with chronic NVI associated with ocular ischemic syndrome. The intraocular pressure is usually within normal limits. **B:** Vitrectomy clears hemorrhage. The patient experiences much improved visual aquity. **C:** Anterior and posterior segment hemorrhage with NVI blood is removed from anterior and posterior chambers permitting PRP, improved visual function, and regression of iris and retinal neovascularization.

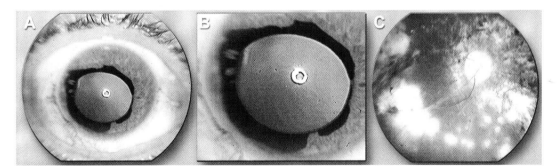

FIGURE 25-4. Regressed iris neovascularization (NVI) with poor residual visual function. **A:** Marked ectropion uveae following regression of NVI after dense panretinal photocoagulation. Note the presence of a good red reflex. **B:** Magnified view. **C:** Despite regression of severe iris and retinal proliferation, this patient's visual acuity is light perception. The media are clear, the IOP is within normal limits, and the retina is flat. Nevertheless, optic atrophy and poor retinal perfusion (characterized by attenuated vasculature) limit the visual potential of this eye.

26

ENDOSCOPIC VITRECTOMY FOR HYPOTONY

One may occasionally encounter a patient with a hypotonous eye and, for a variety of reasons, the patient and surgeon feel that some effort should be extended to reverse this essentially end-stage situation. The management of hypotony as a complication of glaucoma surgery has already been discussed, and the same principles universally apply.

Management will be discussed in the context of a progression from traction retinal detachment of proliferative vitreoretinopathy, proliferative diabetic retinopathy, or other posterior segment disease that results in fibrovascular proliferation to such a degree as to cause detachment of the ciliary body. There may also be an internal concentric tissue contraction of this gliotic tissue sufficient to cause the eye to "cave in" on itself. To be sure, many of these are lost eyes and do not warrant intervention of any kind. Even the most aggressive response usually results in failure.

On the other hand, desperate situations call for desperate measures. If the surgeon feels that anterior fibrovascular proliferation is at the root of the problem, the condition can be surgically addressed. This would be difficult or impossible by conventional means because the most significant pathology is lurking on the posterior aspect of the iris, ciliary body, and peripheral retina. These eyes usually present significant anatomic obstruction to a posterior segment view, such as cloudy cornea, miotic pupil, opacified and phimotic lens capsule, and opaque or hazy vitreous, all of which make microscope imaging of the region impossible. Furthermore, once surgery begins, there is often significant hemorrhage from these areas as the membranes are dissected away. While this feature may hinder the progress of endoscopic vitrectomy, it would render microscope-directed vitrectomy impossible.

There is a spectrum to the extent of vitreociliary traction that can be associated with hypotony (Fig. 26-1). At one extreme, the processes may appear to have a whitish discoloration to their surface yet exhibit no evident traction despite the presence of hypotony. A more severe manifestation is a fine translucent or white surface membrane with tractional elements characterized by elongation and distortion of the ciliary processes. In hypotony's most profound manifestation, dense white membranes cover the ciliary body, posterior iris, and pars plana and are associated with frank ciliary body detachment. In any event, the only therapeutic option would be to remove these membranes from the inner eye surface.

The dissection usually proceeds from anteriorly to posteriorly, starting with membranes adherent to the posterior surface of the iris (Figs. 26-2 to 26-7). It is often simplest to start with the MVR blade. The gliotic membrane is cut parallel to the iris (circumferentially), and the edge of the blade is rotated slightly so that it can be used for blunt dissection. It is then placed between the iris or ciliary body and the membrane. Once this is achieved, the blade can then be used to lift, rather than cut, this tissue from the surface to which it is adherent. In this way, vast areas of gliotic tissue can be rapidly removed. Often the ciliary body and other anatomy can be seen to "snap back" into a more normal-appearing configuration. Intraocular wet-field coagulation should be used to control any bleeding. Once this membrane has been removed from its most anterior connections, the remainder of its dissection, proceeding posteriorly, is often relatively simple. Endophotocoagulation, gas tamponade, or silicone oil injection can be applied at the surgeon's discretion.

Despite an outstanding surgery that, by its conclusion, had achieved the desired anatomic goal, many of these eyes will continue their downward course, with progressive decline in intraocular pressure and increasing media opacification. Probably less than half of the patients who have experienced "successful" endoscopic hypotony surgery seem to benefit from the intervention. Both the surgeon and the patient must be prepared for this eventuality.

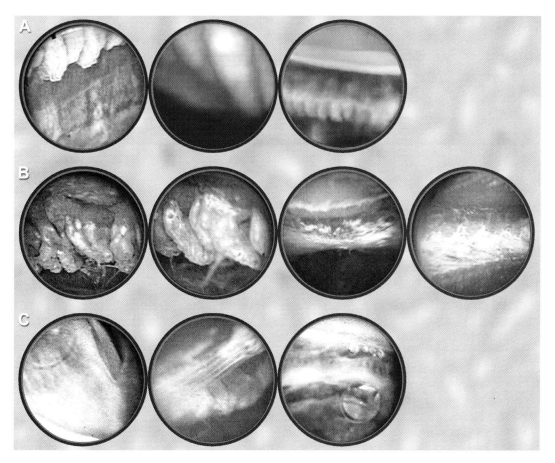

FIGURE 26-1. Spectrum of clinical appearance in hypotony of this type. **A:** White discoloration on ciliary process surface without apparent traction. **B:** Translucent, white, or pigmented membranes on ciliary process surface with distortion and elongation of ciliary process architecture. **C:** White membranes on posterior iris, lens, sulcus, or ciliary body, and peripheral retina with detachment of the ciliary body

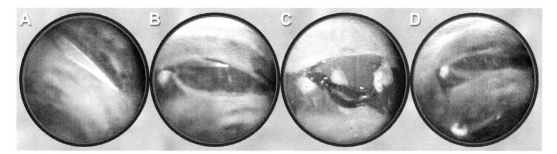

FIGURE 26-2. Endoscopic hypotony surgery. **A:** An MVR blade is inserted parallel to limbus between membrane and ciliary body or posterior iris. **B:** The blade is rotated and the flat edge used to lift or cut membrane from ocular structures. **C:** Forceps can also be used to grasp membrane and lift or pull it from the tissue surface. **D:** The process is continued until membrane traction releases and the ciliary body resumes a more normal position.

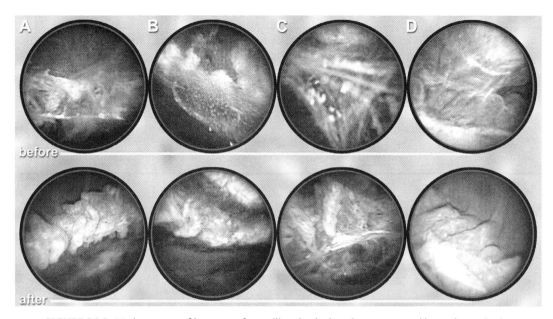

FIGURE 26-3. Various cases of hypotony from ciliary body detachment treated by endoscopic vitrectomy techniques. **A:** Ciliary processes are detached and distorted to the extent that they are unrecognizable. After membranectomy, the architecture is normalized. **B:** Membrane with pigment cells overlies and detaches ciliary body. After membranectomy, the anatomy becomes more recognizable, although there is still whitening of the ciliary process surface, flattening (atrophy?) of the tissue, and some residual distortion. **C:** Marked pretreatment traction and distortion. After endoscopic membranectomy, the appearance is much improved although a moderate degree of distortion remains. **D:** Anteriorly directed traction with ciliary body detachment created by membrane connecting posterior iris to the anterior portion of the ciliary processes. After surgery, the folded over edge of residual membrane can be seen. The ciliary body is now attached and demonstrates more normalized anatomy.

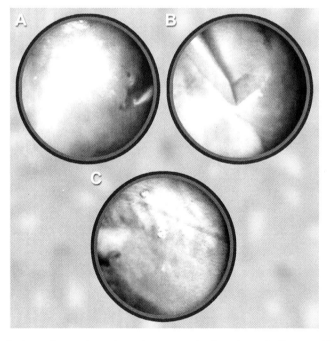

FIGURE 26-4. Endoscopic membranotomy in surgery for hypotony. **A:** Dense white membrane exerts traction from posterior iris, over the capsule–intraocular lens (IOL) complex to the ciliary body. **B:** MVR blade is used to incise and divide this membrane. **C:** In this situation, the cut membrane then contracts in a posterior direction allowing the architecture of the capsule-IOL and ciliary body to normalize.

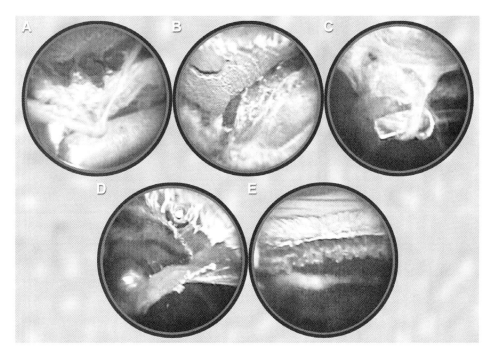

FIGURE 26-5. Endoscopic membranectomy using vitrector and forceps. **A:** Membrane is aspirated into the port of the vitrector to strip as much of it as possible. Cutting is used to remove the excised tissue from the eye. **B:** Ciliary body is now free of tractional elements and most of it spontaneously reattaches. Note that the superior edge of the processes on the left side of the photo remains detached from the eye wall. **C:** In the same eye, an extensive and dense area of membrane is grasped with the forceps and stripping is initiated. **D:** Membrane stripping continues, in this case in a circumferential direction. **E:** Normalized anatomy with reattachment of the ciliary body following extensive membrane removal.

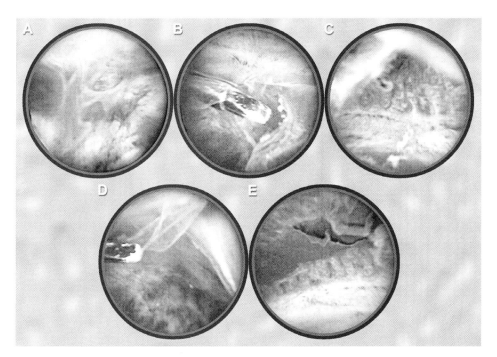

FIGURE 26-6. Forceps membranectomy in hypotony surgery. **A:** Marked anatomic disruption of the ciliary body with dense membranes extending from posterior iris to the peripheral retina, completely obscuring a view of the ciliary body. Membrane contraction results in collapse of the anterior–posterior diameter of the eye by retracting the iris toward the retina. **B:** Forceps are used to pull the membrane from the retina and ciliary body. **C:** A small area of ciliary process tissue has reattached following removal of tractional elements. **D:** Further stripping of the membrane along an extensive area of the ciliary ring is performed. **E:** The ciliary body is now attached although there is a tear in pigmented epithelium of the iris.

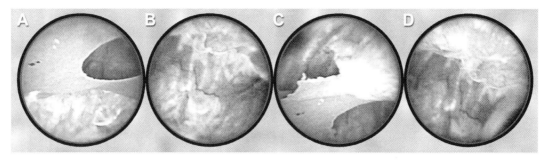

FIGURE 26-7. Severe tissue contraction in hypotony surgery. **A:** A tightly compacted area of adhesion exists between the ciliary process and the posterior iris to such an extent the virtually all of the iris pigmented epithelium is detached up to the pupil. This accounts for distinctive circular opening in the tissue. **B:** An MVR blade was used to incise and separate this connection. The cut membrane edge retracts anteriorly, relieving traction on the ciliary processes. Although they are still distorted, they are nevertheless attached. **C:** Dense adhesion and retraction of a portion of the iris epithelium to the ciliary processes despite relaxation of adjacent tissue. **D:** Same area after division of this membrane with reattachment of the ciliary body and anterior retraction of the cut edge of the membrane.

27

ENDOSCOPIC SURGICAL MANAGEMENT OF CHOROIDAL HEMORRHAGE AND EFFUSION

Although endoscopic management of choroidal hemorrhage and effusion has been discussed in the context of glaucoma surgery, massive hemorrhagic or serosanguinous effusion may evolve as a consequence of any type of intraocular surgery or on a spontaneous basis, most often associated with an eccentric focus of subretinal neovascularization. Risk factors for the development of this problem include anticoagulation, uncontrolled hypertension, aphakia, and previous vitrectomy.

Surgical management can be quite challenging. Sclerotomy sites should be fashioned in each of the quadrants involved, just as one would for pars plana vitrectomy (Fig. 27-1). Choroidal hemorrhage often begins to drain immediately (Fig. 27-2), although this maneuver alone is usually insufficient to address massive effusions. An anterior chamber maintainer can be placed at the limbus and the infusion begun. Presumably, increasing the pressure in the anterior segment and then in the posterior segment by this method will help to flatten the choroid and push the effusion out of the eye through the sclerotomies. The external surface of the eye can be massaged with a cotton-tipped applicator to help achieve this goal as well. If these maneuvers are successful in opening the funnel obscuring a posterior pole view, then no further intervention is required. On the other hand, if these measures fail to ameliorate the situation, vitrectomy is required.

Placement of a pars plana infusion cannula can be trying. The site must be chosen such that the tip of the cannula will not ultimately be positioned in the subretinal space. This can be a difficult task because the choroid is often bulging anteriorly and dense vitreous hemorrhage is not uncommon. If the infusion port cannot be verified to be within the vitreous cavity, a sclerotomy opposite its position can be created, followed by insertion and advancement of the endoscope. This approach often confirms the adequacy of infusion cannula positioning prior to initiating flow. If the infusion port were inadvertently misplaced, infusion would compound the difficulty that is already present.

Once all three vitrectomy sites have been created, the vitrectors and the endoscope can be inserted. The view will be terrible through the endoscope because of vitreous hemorrhage, but as the hemorrhage is cleared, better imaging will result. The goal of this portion of the surgery is to clear the vitreous cavity (Fig. 27-3). When this goal has been achieved, the surgeon must decide whether adequate choroidal drainage has taken place or if further intervention is required. When a substantial quantity of choroidals remains, especially those of the hemorrhagic type, and, even more importantly, when the submacular region is involved, further drainage is most likely necessary. Injection of perfluorocarbon liquid (PFCL) can be extremely useful at this juncture. Typically, a small amount of PFCL (0.5 to 1.0 mL) is injected over the optic nerve. Then the peripapillary choroid flattens by pushing the choroidal hemorrhage and fluid anteriorly and out through the sclerotomy sites. This process may take a few minutes, so that if at first not much seems to be changing, the surgeon should exercise patience. Once this brief equilibration period has elapsed, more PCFL can be injected until most of the choroidal hemorrhage has flattened. The periphery should be endoscopically examined for retinal breaks (iatrogenic or otherwise). These are especially likely to develop considering the constricted intraocular space within which the surgeon must work. If such pathology is detected, it is easily photocoagulated endoscopically. Air or balanced saline solution can then be exchanged for PCFL. Silicone oil can be injected at the surgeon's discretion.

Even though most of these eyes have high intraocular pressure, pain, and profound visual loss preoperatively, they often become comfortable and hypotonous immediately after surgery. Nevertheless, visual acuity is typically poor at this time and the prognosis for recovery is guarded. Still, the endoscopic approach may prove to be the only therapeutic method available to reverse choroidal hemorrhage and effusion.

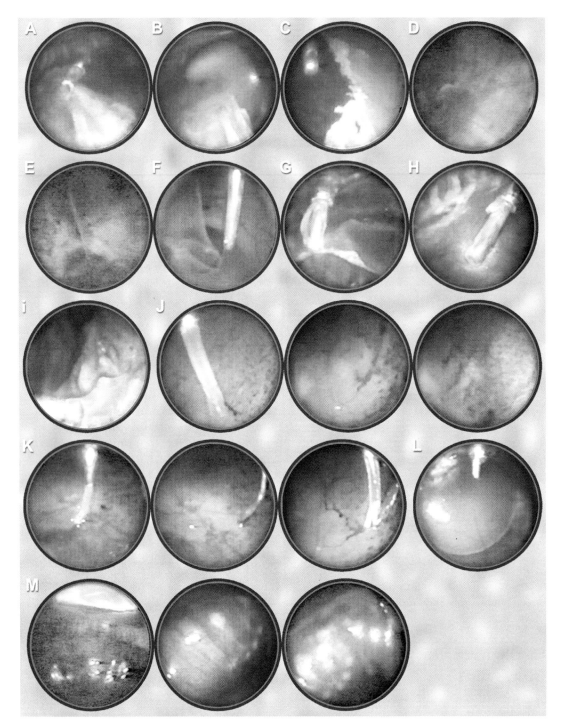

FIGURE 27-1. Management of massive choroidal and vitreous hemorrhage. **A:** Appearance of dense vitreous hemorrhage as it is being removed by the vitrector. **B:** "Plume" of chronic white vitreous hemorrhage. **C:** Is this a sheet of dehemoglobinized vitreous blood or is it blood covered retina? **D:** Viewing through this opening reveals an underlying choroidal hemorrhage. **E:** By manipulation of the endoscope through the opening, the posterior pole as well as vitreous and choroidal hemorrhage can be seen. **F:** The vitrector is then advanced to remove this material. **G:** Vitrectomy continues to remove the apron of blood. **H:** Hemorrhage is aspirated from the ciliary body surface. **I:** A retinal break is present and is flat on the surface of the underlying bulging choroid. **J:** A diffuse preretinal membrane with dots of brown hemorrhage can now be seen covering various portions of the retina. **K:** These are aspirated using a soft-tipped extrusion cannula. **L:** A small peripheral area of retinal detachment is found. **M:** At the completion of surgery, the vitreous cavity is clear, the retina is flat, laser has been applied to the retinal breaks, and most of the choroidal hemorrhage has been drained. There is still a peripheral ring of choroidal hemorrhage remaining.

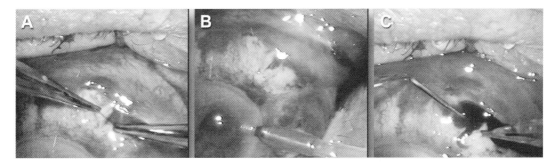

FIGURE 27-2. External view of draining a choroidal hemorrhage. **A:** A circumferentially oriented sclerotomy is fashioned 4 mm from the limbus. **B:** An anterior chamber maintainer is inserted through the peripheral clear cornea and infusion is begun. **C:** This maneuver was insufficient, so a cyclodialysis spatula was inserted, releasing some of the choroidal hemorrhage.

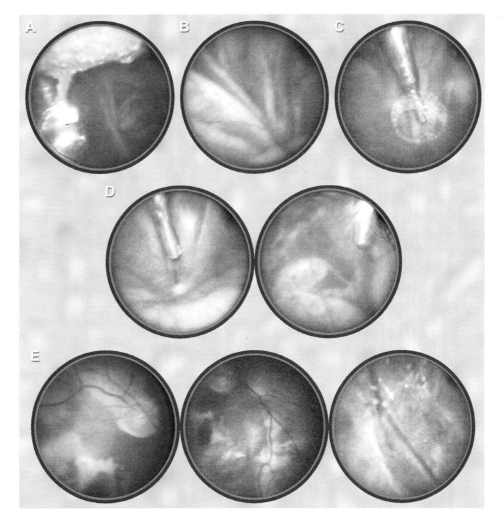

FIGURE 27-3. Endoscopic vitrectomy for draining a choroidal hemorrhage. **A:** The vitrector is introduced and can be seen removing blood from the posterior aspect of a shaggy-looking crystalline lens. **B:** Despite external maneuvers to drain the choroidal hemorrhage, vitrectomy was required and revealed a "closed funnel" appearance to the ocular interior. **C:** Perfluorocarbon liquid (PFCL) is introduced to force the choroidal hemorrhage out through the previously fashioned sclerotomies that were placed in each quadrant. **D:** Injection of PFCL continues until the retina and choroids flatten. Extensive and organizing choroidal hemorrhage can now be seen. **E:** Posterior and peripheral views of flattened retina and choroid with gliotic organization.

ENDOSCOPIC FLUORESCEIN ANGIOGRAPHY

Once the principles of endoscopic imaging were established, development of endoscopic fluorescein angiography was not much of a stretch. To achieve adequate resolution, certain technical requirements existed, among them sufficient illumination and video camera sensitivity as well as the proper filtration of light and image. The reward was high-resolution wide-field views of any interior region of the eye. An additional unique feature of this approach is that the angiographic imaging is initiated within the eye rather than from the standard external-to-internal configuration. Attainment of these images can create some novel opportunities in the management of glaucoma and vitreoretinal disease.

GLAUCOMA MANAGEMENT

Because the ciliary processes can be directly viewed and photocoagulated from a limbal wound in the phakic, aphakic, and pseudophakic eye in virtually any patient, the novel opportunity to angiographically study the ciliary processes before and after various forms of ablation arose.

To evaluate this technical adaptation in the context of imaging the ciliary body, four groups, each consisting of 20 patients undergoing endoscopic cyclophotocoagulation (ECP) for various mechanisms of uncontrolled glaucoma, were created (1). A clear corneal incision was used to access the ciliary processes in all cases. Neovascular glaucoma (NVG)

was present in 47 patients, aphakic/pseudophakic glaucoma in 29 patients, and congenital mechanisms in 4 patients.

■ Group 1 patients were injected with fluorescein and the ciliary process angiogram features noted. Then ECP was performed and the angiographic characteristics were once again delineated.
■ Group 2 eyes first underwent ECP, and then fluorescein angiography was performed.
■ Group 3 patients underwent ECP at least 2 months before the current study and failed to achieve adequate intraocular pressure (IOP) control. In this group, fluorescein was injected and ECP performed again.
■ Group 4 patients had failed previous transscleral cyclodestruction. Cyclocryotherapy (CCT) had been performed in 3 patients and laser transscleral cyclophotocoagulation (TSCPC) in 17 patients. Fluorescein was first injected and the processes angiographically imaged. ECP was then performed.
Results were as follows:
■ Group 1 patients demonstrated early and intense hyperfluorescence of the ciliary processes without leakage into the vitreous. As the study progressed to the recirculation phase, the processes remained intensely hyperfluorescent. When ECP was performed, the treated processes became slightly less hyperfluorescent and tended to remain in that state without leakage. It was difficult to distinguish between treated and untreated processes when fluorescein was injected before ECP (Fig. 28-1).

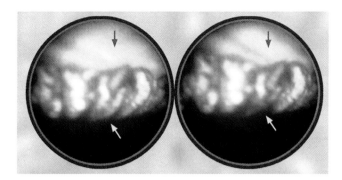

FIGURE 28-1. Group 1. Typically hyperfluorescent ciliary processes. Fluorescein injected prior to laser treatment. *(blue arrow)* Same ciliary process before and after endoscopic cyclophotocoagulation. Slightly less fluorescence is observed when comparing treated and untreated processes. Posterior iris hyperfluorescence *(red arrow)* indicative of iris neovascularization.

- Group 2 patients underwent ECP followed by fluorescein injection. The ciliary process tissue that was lasered appeared densely hypofluorescent initially and remained so throughout the study. Processes or portions of them that were not photocoagulated were markedly hyperfluorescent early in the study and remained in that state into the recirculation phase (Fig. 28-2).
- Group 3 patients were given injections before ECP. The processes or portions of them that were previously photocoagulated were densely hypofluorescent early in the study and continued to demonstrate hypofluorescence into the late phase. Previously untreated processes revealed initial marked hyperfluorescence and remained in that state throughout the angiogram (Fig. 28-3).
- Group 4 patients demonstrated identical findings to group 3, characterized by hypofluorescence of treated processes and hyperfluorescence of untreated ones (or portions of them). In addition, extensive regions of

hyperfluorescence and hypofluorescence were present in areas adjacent to the ciliary body. The former represents fluorescein staining of gliotic tissue, and the latter represents pigment deposition or vascular nonperfusion (Fig. 28-4). The records of all patients in this group indicated that 360 degrees of TSCPC had been previously applied. However, fluorescein angiography revealed that none of the patients experienced more than 120 degrees of ciliary process ablation, 9 of 20 patients had between 90 and 120 degrees of actual cyclodestruction, and 11 of 20 patients demonstrated an actual treatment zone of less than 90 degrees. (Table 28-1).

A number of interesting issues can be discerned from this small study. On the technical side, recall that the typical fundus camera engenders a study area of 30 to 60 degrees, most often confined to the posterior pole. The retinal periphery can be viewed by this technique in the hands of an experienced angiographer when the media are clear, the pupil is widely dilated, and the patient is cooperative. The ciliary body and posterior iris regions have not been previously elucidated by this technique. Intraoperative angiography, adapting the operating microscope as the imaging system, has been reported but suffers from the same limitations as the standard technique. Specifically, clear media and a widely dilated pupil are required to obtain a 30-degree field of view, and the retinal periphery, pars plana, ciliary body, and iris are not approachable. These limitations may be overcome by endoscopic fluorescein angiography.

The first two study groups were created to evaluate the angiographic effect of photocoagulation on the ciliary process before and after perfusion with fluorescein. Group 1 patients established the typical fluorescein angiographic characteristics of the ciliary body: early and intense hyperfluorescence that persists throughout the study. Once perfused with fluorescein and then photocoagulated, the ciliary

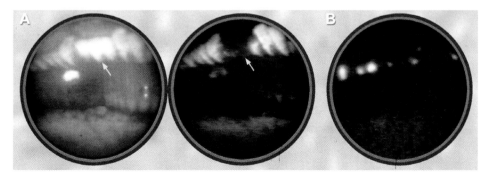

FIGURE 28-2. Group 2. **A:** Cluster of three photocoagulated ciliary processes. Fluorescein injected after endoscopic cyclophotocoagulation (ECP). (blue arrow) Densely hypofluorescent treated processes that contrast sharply with surrounding hyperfluorescent untreated ones. **B:** Fluorescein injection immediately after ECP demonstrates residual zones hyperfluorescence indicative of incomplete treatment to these individual processes. The surgeon now has the opportunity to achieve complete laser application to the ciliary process surface.

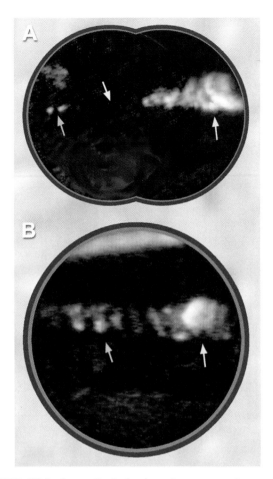

FIGURE 28-3. Group 3. A: Inadequate response to previous endoscopic cyclophotocoagulation (ECP). Fluorescein injection demonstrates area of scattered hyperfluorescence indicative of viable ciliary epithelium *(orange arrow)*. Adjacent zone of dense hypofluorescence *(yellow arrow)* has been adequately lasered. The region of hyperfluorescent processes *(blue arrow)* clearly distinguishes between site of previously treated and untreated tissue. If further ECP is indicated, it may be initiated at this point. **B:** Inadequate intraocular pressure response to previous ECP. Fluorescein injected prior to treatment. Note numerous small hyperfluorescent areas *(orange arrow)* revealing that portions of these processes are not completely lasered. One process appears to be entirely untreated *(blue arrow)*. Response to previous therapy and extent of further treatment must be judged considering this residual viable tissue.

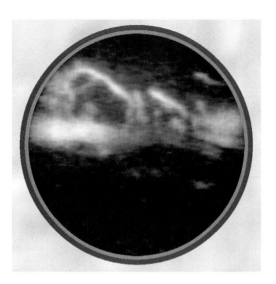

FIGURE 28-4. Group 4. Extensive mottled hyperfluorescence and hypofluorescence in eye with previous laser transscleral cyclophotocoagulation. The hypofluorescent zones indicate obliterated areas of iris and ciliary body. The hyperfluorescent region delineates a gliotic portion of the ciliary body.

angiogram was useful in delineating small areas of individual processes that were thought to have been adequately photocoagulated but had not been. Once these areas were identified, further ECP could be applied.

Groups 3 and 4 represented an outgrowth of the findings in group 2. When one is performing a second or subsequent ECP, it is sometimes clinically difficult to precisely identify previous treatment zones. To a lesser degree, this is also true in eyes that have undergone previous TSCPC. In these two groups, fluorescein was injected prior to ECP. Any ciliary process tissue that had been ablated did not perfuse with dye and was therefore hypofluorescent, whereas unaffected tissue demonstrated the typical fluorescent pattern of a "normal" ciliary process. In these two groups this technique was not only helpful in identifying tissue that could be used for treatment; it also clearly delineated the extent of previous applications that the eye actually sustained, rather than what the surgeon presumed to have taken place. With this information, treatment could be tailored using the patient's

processes became only slightly less fluorescent, possibly as a consequence of "blocked" fluorescence by the acutely whitened process surface.

Group 2 patients revealed a fluorescence pattern of significant utility. In this group, the treated processes were notably hypofluorescent while untreated processes, or untreated portions, were quite fluorescent. The treatment zone could be clearly delineated on an angiographic basis. Furthermore, segments of "treated" processes occasionally demonstrated persistent hyperfluorescence and when reevaluated endoscopically (but not angiographically) were observed to indeed have insufficient or no laser effect. The

TABLE 28-1. REPORTED VERSUS ACTUAL EXTENT OF CYCLODESTRUCTION IN 20 EYES WITH TRANSSCLERAL CYCLOPHOTOCOAGULATION

Extent of Cyclodestruction (degrees)		
Reported	Actual	*n*
360	120–360	0 (0%)
360	90–120	9 (45%)
360	<90	11 (55%)

IOP response to previous ciliary process applications and the known quantity of ciliary process tissue that was truly affected. For example, if a patient with congenital glaucoma and failed goniotomy, trabeculotomy, and 180 degrees of TSCPC was evaluated by endoscopic fluorescein angiography and found to have only 60 degrees of ciliary process hypofluorescence, the surgeon would know that insufficient cyclodestruction was previously effected and that additional significant treatment could be applied.

Another example would be a typical group 3 patient who underwent previous ECP yet failed to achieve adequate IOP control. Angiography would reveal that a number of processes that were previously photocoagulated demonstrated segments that were hyperfluorescent. This finding indicated that portions of these ciliary processes were not destroyed and continued to function. Treatment failure might then be attributed to missing these areas, and if they were to be photocoagulated the extent of a new treatment zone might be minimized.

Endoscopic fluorescein angiography elucidated a curious finding in group 4 patients. All of these eyes were reported to have complete cyclophotocoagulation yet ultimately demonstrated an unacceptable level of IOP control. This diagnostic technique clearly indicated that these patients in no way experienced the degree of cyclodestruction that was presumed to have occurred. The inability of TSCPC to effect a titratable tissue response, and therefore be effective in the management of glaucoma in a given eye, is apparent in this group of patients, as judged by the tissue effect. It is also clear that the untoward reactions associated with the transscleral route of cyclodestruction are related to, among other factors, damage to adjacent nonciliary process tissue. This was particularly striking in patients with congenital glaucoma in whom the ciliary processes were situated more anteriorly than expected. In these patients, a pigmentary and gliotic response was observed to involve the pars plana, whereas the ciliary processes were not incorporated into the treatment zone.

It should be noted that what ultimately brought group 4 patients to this trial was failure to attain adequate IOP control. In this group, the surgeon overestimated the extent of true cycloablation. Unfortunately, and to be fair, angiographic evaluation of patients who experienced good IOP control following TSCPC or CCT has not been performed. Nevertheless, one might surmise that these eyes would demonstrate a closer correlation between the extent of estimated and actual cyclodestruction.

To conclude, endoscopic fluorescein angiography can distinguish treated from untreated ciliary processes or portions of them, on surgeon demand, in a given eye, regardless of lens status. The value of this technique lies in its ability to assess the adequacy of ECP immediately after treatment so that the therapeutic goal anticipated by the surgeon is, in fact, achieved. Alternatively, it can precisely delineate the true extent of previous cyclodestruction,

whether applied transsclerally or by ECP. The surgeon may then correlate this information with the observed IOP response so that a decision regarding the amount of further ciliary process photocoagulation can be made.

DIAGNOSIS AND MANAGEMENT OF RETINAL DISORDERS

Fluorescein angiography is an essential tool in the diagnosis and management of retinal and choroidal disorders. This diagnostic modality generally provides a 30- to 60-degree field of view and is largely directed to the posterior pole. Peripheral fundus imaging is dependent on the presence of a widely dilated pupil, clear media, and a cooperative patient. Even under these circumstances, it is difficult to study the retinal/choroidal periphery.

Although the operating microscope has been adapted by several investigators to permit intraoperative study of the retina, the limitations of this technology are similar to those of the standard fundus camera—specifically, the limited field of view and need for a widely dilated pupil in an eye with clear media.

This unique technology allows fluorescein studies to be performed of the retina, subretinal space, pars plana, ciliary body, and posterior iris region during the course of intraocular surgery. The immediate interpretation of these findings may assist in the management of the patient's surgical problem. Anterior segment opacification, pupillary miosis, lens status, and presence of intraocular gas or vitreous substitute do not diminish the surgeon's ability to survey the ocular interior angiographically.

One hundred patients undergoing vitrectomy for various retinal/choroidal disorders were evaluated (2). Standard three-port vitrectomy was performed, thus clearing the vitreous cavity of hemorrhage or debris. Reattachment of the retina was performed as required. The ophthalmic endoscope provided illumination and "photography" in these procedures. Because of to the sensitivity of the imaging system, a bright flash was not necessary. Rather, filtered light from the system's standard source was employed. When the eye was either fluid or gas filled, 5 mL of sterile 10% sodium fluorescein was intravenously injected. Typically, the laser endoscope was held in mid-vitreous cavity and directed to the posterior pole. The retinal and choroidal vasculature could be seen to fill whereupon the endoscope could be directed to a particular area of interest as the study continued; or it could be used to pan the ocular interior. By moving the tip of the endoscope around the interior of the eye, just as one would manipulate an endoilluminator, an angiographic sweep of the ocular interior, from posterior pole to peripheral retina, to ciliary body and posterior iris; could be made (Fig. 28-5).

The relative merits of angiography in fluid- versus air-filled eyes were examined. If a panoramic view were desired,

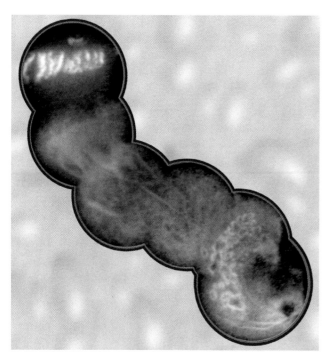

FIGURE 28-5. Fluorescein perfusing retinal and choroidal vasculature imaged through the endoscope. Montage of scan incorporating disc, macula, retinal periphery, pars plana, ciliary body, and posterior iris.

the endoscope would be held at a distance from the target tissue, increasing the field of view but minimizing the image size. A gas-filled eye would enhance this effect.

On the other hand, by advancing the tip of the endoscope toward the target tissue, the field of view would become smaller but the magnification would be increased. Fluid or gas fill made little difference in this situation.

Any observations made with this technology can be simultaneously recorded on a variety of image capture devices, most commonly the videocassette recorder, truly bridging the gap between angioscopy and angiography.

The patients evaluated by this methodology presented with an array of retinal disorders, including complications of diabetic retinopathy, retinal venous obstruction, retinal vasculitis associated with cytomegalovirus, and subretinal neovascularization associated with the age-related form of macular degeneration.

General Characteristics

General Image Quality

The angiographic image quality produced by this technology was comparable to that obtained by standard fundus photography/angiography instrumentation. The major retinal vessels could be easily delineated as could the arterial, laminar venous, venous, and recirculation phases of perfusion. The capillary bed of the retina was well defined, as was choroidal perfusion. Pathologic states of the retina—including microa-

neurysms, zones of capillary nonperfusion, neovascular membranes, vessel wall staining, and frank occlusions—could be easily observed.

Capillary Perfusion

After initial fluorescein perfusion of the major retinal vessels and capillaries, a survey of the mid- and far periphery was performed for 360 degrees. In eyes undergoing surgery for the effects of diabetic proliferative disease, varying states of capillary nonperfusion were evident. Typically, intense nonperfusion was observed in the far retinal periphery. Usually, there were no capillaries evident between the vortex veins and the retinal insertion. This effect seemed to be more profound nasally than temporally. As the level of schemia increased, the nonperfusion appeared to extend more posteriorly. Macular and paramacular nonperfusion seemed to be advanced manifestations of a process that was initiated peripherally.

Disc and Retinal Neovascularization

The pathologic process underlying disc and retinal neovascularization created the typical, increasingly hyperfluorescent pattern of a focal nature, with extravasation of fluorescein into the vitreous cavity as the study progressed into its recirculation phase. If there were extensive or numerous zones of neovascularization, it was more efficacious to record these findings when the eye was air filled rather than fluid filled because the progressive leakage of fluorescein into the fluid-filled vitreous cavity would ultimately obscure the view. In the air-filled eye, this progressive hyperfluorescence tended to remain localized. Although retinal neovascularization can typically be identified using the operating microscope, occasionally what appeared to be a small hemorrhage on the retinal surface was angiographically revealed to be a small tuft of active neovascularization.

Iris Neovascularization

There are numerous pathologic states that might result in fluorescein leakage from the iris. In the setting of vitrectomy for complications of ocular proliferation, iris neovascularization would be the most likely cause of this angiographic finding. Progressive hyperfluorescence from the posterior iris surface was observed in many patients who demonstrated iris neovascularization when examined preoperatively by slit-lamp biomicroscopy. Occasionally, the diabetic patient with recurrent vitreous hemorrhage of unknown etiology and without preoperative angiographic or clinical evidence of iris neovascularization may demonstrate progressive hyperfluorescence from the posterior iris at the time of endoscopic vitrectomy. Recurrent hemorrhage was presumed to result from posterior iris neovascularization. This situation might perhaps represent the earliest manifestations of anterior hyaloidal fibrovascular proliferation. Mostly, patients with retinal or disc neovasculariza-

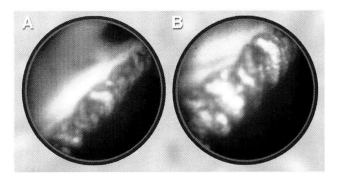 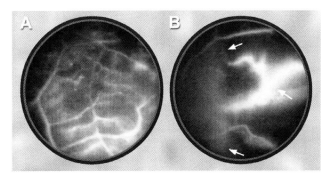

FIGURE 28-6. Posterior iris neovascularization. **A:** Demonstrates endoscopic angiogram of posterior iris to edge of pupil with marked hyperfluorescence, typical of posterior iris neovascularization. Progressive hyperfluorescence of the posterior iris is often indicative of neovascularization. Ciliary body demonstrates normal fluorescence pattern. **B:** Is higher magnification view of this same area achieved by advancing the endoscope tip closer to the target. Posterior neovascularization of the iris can be a cause of recurrent vitreous hemorrhage but need not be associated with active disc or retinal neovascularization.

FIGURE 28-7. Vessel wall staining. **A:** Angiographic manifestation of damage to the vessel wall itself. This is often found in zones of capillary nonperfusion. This vessel is in the far periphery of an eye with diabetic retinopathy. **B:** Vessel wall staining in retinal vasculitis associated with cytomegalovirus infection. The border of perfused and nonperfused retina is indicated by *white arrows*.

tion but without iris involvement were not observed to have iris fluorescein leakage, instead displaying hypofluorescence of the posterior iris surface (Fig. 28-6).

Vessel Wall Staining

Vessel wall staining is a characteristic of blood vessel wall damage, and in diabetic patients was typically observed in regions of capillary nonperfusion (Fig. 28-7). In patients with cytomegalovirus retinitis and retinal detachment, prominent areas of vessel wall staining, perhaps signifying active inflammation, were present. Adjacent capillary nonperfusion was typically observed.

Subretinal Neovascularization

Three patients in this study underwent submacular surgery for the management of extensive hemorrhage associated with the exudative phase of age-related macular degeneration. After creation of a retinotomy, removal of hemorrhage, and intravenous fluorescein injection, the choroid could be easily viewed as diffusely and homogeneously hyperfluorescent. The perfusion of the overlying retina did not interfere with choroidal angiography. In all three patients, the mound of subretinal neovascularization was densely hypofluorescent, with only a thin rim of mottled hyperfluorescence at its base. As the study progressed into the recirculation phase, all of the structures in this region diminished in their fluorescent pattern (Fig. 28-8).

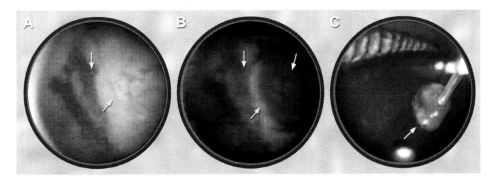

FIGURE 28-8. Subretinal neovascularization. Surprisingly, when imaged subretinally, neovascular membranes were densely hypofluorescent with only a rim of mottled hyperfluorescence that diminished into the recirculation phase. **A:** Endoscopic image of subretinal space. White arrow indicates edge of elevated neurosensory retina. Note hemorrhage of surface of RPE at base of subretinal neovascular complex *(yellow arrow)*. Subretinal neovascular complex viewed without overlying neurosensory retina *(purple arrow)*. **B:** Endoscopic angiogram of same area. Yellow arrow indicates hypofluorescence of hemorrhage on RPE surface while the subretinal neovascular complex is hypofluorescent *(white arrow)*. Note rim of mottled hyperfluorescence at neovascular complex base *(blue arrow)*. **C:** Endoscopic view of subretinal neovascular complex *(white arrow)* held in anterior vitreous cavity. Note ciliary processes in background of anterior chamber pseudophakic eye.

CONCLUSION

Fluorescein angiography is a standard diagnostic tool that has been invaluable in the management of many ophthalmic disorders. However, its intraoperative application is uncommon, with only a few reports of operating microscope adaptation for this purpose. While such technology may be useful, its value may be diminished by limitations inherent in operating microscope imaging of the ocular interior. Specifically, the cornea, state of the pupil, lens, and posterior media may serve as an impediment to viewing. Even under ideal circumstances, viewing of the peripheral retina, pars plana, ciliary processes, and posterior iris is difficult or impossible. Scleral depression of these regions, while possibly allowing the surgeon to view them, also alters their appearance and relationship to surrounding structures in comparison with endoscopic visualization without scleral depression. The ophthalmic laser endoscope permits high-resolution imaging of these structures despite anterior segment conditions that preclude a posterior view. Adaptation of the laser endoscopy system to perform fluorescein angiography has enabled angiographic study of regions that are typically difficult to image intraoperatively.

For example, in the diabetic eye undergoing vitrectomy for opaque media, nonperfusion was evident more peripherally. This information is not often obtainable preoperatively. However, during the course of vitrectomy, when the media have been cleared and the retina attached, endophotocoagulation may be selectively applied to those areas that appear to be the most ischemic angiographically. The areas of retina with poorest perfusion that presumably facilitated the development of ocular proliferation may be specifically addressed at the time of surgery. This highly selective approach to intraoperative retinal ablation defined the regions most requiring intervention, permitting the remainder to be photocoagulated postoperatively. The value of selective intraoperative retinal ablation requires substantiation.

Alternating between angiographic and routine endoscopic imaging was helpful in the characterization of specific lesions. An example of this would be the endoscopic detection of what appeared to be a retinal hemorrhage but proved to be a small tuft of retinal neovascularization. Converting to the angiographic image would reveal a lesion that was markedly hyperfluorescent with progressive fluorescein leakage, typical of active neovascularization, rather than a hypofluorescent area, which would be expected with hemorrhage. Focal laser ablation would then be effected in the former, whereas no treatment would be required in the latter.

Marked abnormality of the macular capillary bed with extensive fluorescein leakage was observed in a number of patients undergoing vitrectomy for complications of diabetic retinopathy. Even with macular reattachment, a satisfying event for the surgeon, this intraoperative finding predicted a poor functional outcome for the patient.

The angiographic findings during subretinal surgery were surprising. A well-demarcated area of lacy hyperfluorescence with progression of this phenomenon into the latter phases of the study was the expectation. Issues of "occult" subretinal neovascularization would be moot because angiographic imaging was performed beneath the neurosensory retina. Nevertheless, these lesions proved to be densely hypofluorescent throughout the study, with only a small rim of mottled hyperfluorescence at the lesion's base. It may be concluded that few, if any, vessels existed in these lesions. In addition, angiographic characteristics may be explained by the presence of neovascularization in the sub-RPE space in patients with the age-related form of macular degeneration. Under these circumstances, hyperfluorescence from vessel leakage might be obscured by overlying RPE. Patients with subretinal neovascularization associated with the presumed ocular histoplasmosis syndrome, wherein neovascularization arising from the choroid proliferates in the subneurosensory retinal space rather than under the RPE, have not been evaluated. On a practical level, the angiogram obtained from patients with subretinal neovascularization associated with the age-related form of macular degeneration was not helpful in their management.

Filling the eye with gas enhanced the clarity of angiographic images in the presence of active neovascularization because it prevented diffusion of fluorescein into the vitreous cavity. No complications related to the use of fluorescein were observed in this study. The safety of this diagnostic agent has been well established. Furthermore, there was no evidence of retinal phototoxicity in these patients. Because a flash technique was not employed during fluorescein imaging, retinal irradiance was minimized.

Presumed posterior iris neovascularization was observed in a number of patients and was characterized by progressive hyperfluorescence from the posterior iris surface. This finding was quite striking because typically, the posterior iris surface was observed to be hypofluorescent. Vitreous hemorrhage, in the absence of disc or retinal neovascularization, might be considered to arise from this previously unreported pathologic state.

Endoscopic fluorescein angiography is a unique method for studying the ocular interior. However, its indication in the management of various retinal or choroidal disorders requires further study. Still, it is a unique intraoperative tool that permits evaluation of essentially any intraocular area with a field of view up to 110 degrees. The purpose of this approach is to elucidate the anatomy of a specific region, delineate pathology, and allow more directed intraoperative photocoagulation so as to gain information regarding prognosis, and to perhaps uncover unexpected pathology at the time of surgery that can then be immediately addressed. It has proved to be a safe and simple technique in this group of patients undergoing vitrectomy for a variety of vitreo-retinal disorders. The indication for endoscopic fluorescein angiography in the management of specific disease processes has yet to be determined.

REFERENCES

1. Uram M. Endoscopic fluorescein angiography of the ciliary body in glaucoma management. *Ophthalmic Surg Lasers* 1996;27:174–178.
2. Uram M. Endoscopic fluorescein angiography. *Ophthalmic Surg Lasers* 1996;27:849–855.

ENDOSCOPIC TRANSCANALICULAR LASER DACRYOCYSTORHINOSTOMY

TECHNOLOGY 228   TECHNIQUE 229

TECHNOLOGY

It would be fair to say that nowadays dacryocystorhinostomy (DCR) is not often performed by most ophthalmologists, even though there are many patients who would benefit from this surgery. There are a number of reasons why this situation has evolved, including difficulty of the classic surgical procedure, unfamiliar instrumentation, and intraoperative bleeding, to name a few. To many ophthalmologists, DCR may seem a heavy-handed approach to a less than threatening problem that is often restricted to the elderly. Conservative—that is, nonsurgical—management seems to be the option most often elected.

The development of endoscopy has created an alternate method of examining the region of the middle turbinate that previously could be accessed only by an external-to-internal route. Placing an endoscope in the nasal cavity and viewing "upward," toward the orbit, afforded an excellent opportunity to develop a different approach to this surgery.

The ultimate goal of intervention is to create a large osteotomy that connects the remains of the lachrymal drainage system to the nose. Whether this is achieved with hammer and osteotome, with a drill, or by some other means may not make much of a difference in the long run; however, in terms of patient morbidity, there can be a substantial benefit to one technique over the other.

To digress for a moment, ophthalmologists are well acquainted with laser delivery systems through air (slit lamp or indirect ophthalmoscope) or liquid media (endophotocoagulation). This noncontact methodology has been the universal mode in the management of ophthalmic diseases. There is, however, another means of directing the laser to the target tissue, so-called contact laser delivery. The intent of this approach is to pass laser energy through a quartz fiber with a sharply honed orbital or elliptical tip and actually touch the tissue. Instead of shooting out from the fiber, the laser concentrates in the tip, with little laser energy escaping to a distant site. The tip itself becomes quite hot. At lower energy levels, it can be used for cauterization (Table 29-1). At higher levels, the tip becomes hotter and can be used for cutting, incision, or excision. At even higher levels, the tip can become sufficiently hot so as to vaporize any tissue it contacts, including blood vessels, mucosa, soft tissue, tumors, and bone. What this phenomenon of vaporization is actually achieving is turning the contacted tissue into a plume of smoke.

Unlike the relatively lower-powered lasers (1 to 2 W) typically used in ophthalmology, tissue vaporization, especially of bone, requires the use of substantially higher levels. The development of high-power solid-state lasers, such as neodymium:yttrium-argon-garnet (Nd:YAG) or holmium:YAG, has created an opportunity for their application in DCR. For some time, the transnasal approach to the middle meatus, combined with transnasal high-powered contact laser application, has been used for the creation of a large osteotomy without the need for skin dissection or other components of the classical technique. To be sure, the efficacy of this approach has been debated, as it seems to be somewhat less reliable than the more typical methodology. This appears to be particularly true of the holmium laser, the impression being that the osteotomies close more frequently, resulting in treatment failure.

As an alternative, a higher powered (15-W) semiconductor diode laser tuned to the 810-nm wavelength has been used as a substitute for these other lasers in this application (Fig. 29-1). From a scientific or medical viewpoint, there is little advantage to this technology. On the other hand, there are two distinct benefits to such lasers over the holmium

TABLE 29-1. CONTACT LASER TISSUE POWER DENSITY AND TISSUE EFFECT

Relative Power	Tissue Effect
Low	Cauterization
Moderate	Incision
	Cutting
	Excision
High	Vaporization

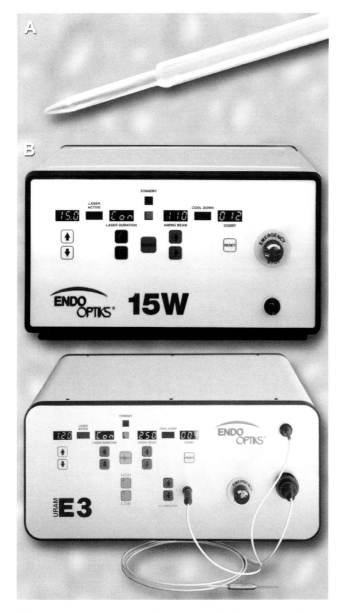

FIGURE 29-1. Instrumentation required for transcanalicular laser dacryocystorhinostomy. **A:** Contact laser fiber. **B:** High-power 810-nm diode laser as separate unit or incorporated into the endoscopy system.

and Nd:YAG lasers. First, they are about 80% less expensive; second, they are relatively small and lightweight. Such a device is about the size of a briefcase and can be easily carried. These lasers can also be integrated with an endoscopy system.

In certain respects, the tissue effect experienced with the contact laser mode is independent of the wavelength. At first, this might seem like a ridiculous assertion because, as ophthalmologists, we are well acquainted with the variability of tissue response to even relatively small changes in wavelength. As an example, one can clearly perceive the difference between a green laser applied to the retina and a red laser. Shouldn't it follow that at geometrically higher power levels these wavelength differences would become even more evident? The answer to this question is simply that the tissue effect does not result from the application of a particular wavelength but rather (and perhaps oversimplistically) that the laser merely serves to heat the tip of the contact fiber. Thus, it is this "hot" tip that induces the tissue response. In this instance, the laser power level is more significant than the wavelength.

TECHNIQUE

Because these contact laser fibers have a small outer diameter (about 1 mm or less), they can be passed down the inferior canaliculus into what remains of the lachrymal sac and drainage system. This characteristic creates a unique opportunity. Instead of endoscopically viewing and applying high-power contact laser transnasally, an alternative approach is to divide these functions. In this technique, general, local, or even topical anesthesia can be used.

First, and this is a key step, the middle turbinate must be pushed medially. This can be easily accomplished with any spatulated surgical instrument, such as a bone elevator. It is critical to move the turbinate to view the laser fiber entering the nasal antrum in the region of the middle meatus. If left in place, the osteotomy could theoretically still be performed but the surgeon would have no way of visualizing the process.

Next, the endoscope is placed into the nasal antrum, viewing "upward" toward the orbit (Fig. 29-2). Because this is a relatively large space, it is not necessary to use a microendoscope; indeed, almost any endoscope will work. A larger gauge ear–nose–throat endoscope (3 to 5 mm in diameter) can subserve the visualization function quite well.

A contact laser fiber can then be directed through the inferior canaliculus in a "downward" direction. A fiber with a sharp conical tip is usually best. It is passed inferiorly and nasally as far as it can go and then is gently

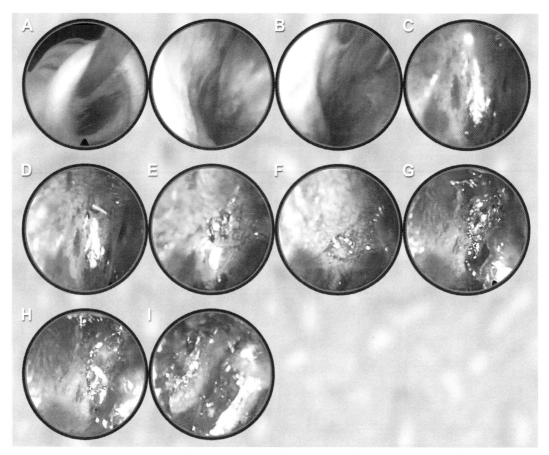

FIGURE 29-2. The procedure. **A:** Endoscopic view "upward" in nasal antrum. **B:** The surgeon medializes the middle turbinate, in this instance with a large forceps. **C:** "Downward"-directed tip of contact laser fiber begins to appear as it vaporizes lachrymal bone and mucosa. **D:** Tip of contact laser fiber clearly enters nasal antrum. **E:** Manipulation of laser fiber continues while continuously fired laser enlarges osteotomy without hemorrhage. **F:** Vaporization of bone and mucosa. **G:** Enlargement of osteotomy continues. Note char at edges of the antrosotomy. **H:** Tissue vaporization and enlargement of antrostomy continues. **I:** View into osteotomy obtained by advancing endoscope into site.

embedded in the bone. Visualization of the canalicular system is not necessary, nor is the creation of a false passageway en route to the lachrymal bone a significant issue because the goal of the treatment is to essentially vaporize this region. There is a substantial added advantage in directing the laser into the nose rather than toward the orbit. A severe complication of transnasal DCR is blindness, presumably arising from inadvertent orbital optic nerve damage. By directing the laser in the opposite direction, the potential for this devastating outcome is eliminated.

If using the high-powered semiconductor 810-nm diode laser, the typical initial settings are 7 W of power with pulse duration set at continuous wave. At the outset, the tip cannot be seen by the endoscope because it is on

the other side of the lachrymal bone and nasal mucosa. As the laser is fired it begins to vaporize a small opening into the nasal antrum. The fiber tip then becomes visible. At this point, all the surgeon must do is manipulate the laser fiber in such a manner as to enlarge the osteotomy to the desired size, perhaps 10 to 15 mm. Unlike the holmium laser, which makes a finer edge to the osteotomy, almost like an incision with a blade, the diode laser creates a thick perimeter of black charring. Perhaps it is this feature that accounts for poor wound healing by increasing the probability that the osteotomy will remain patent.

Typically, there is no bleeding because the blood vessels are being vaporized along with the bone and mucosa. Because laser hemostasis occurs at lower power levels than vaporization, if any untoward hemorrhage were to

TABLE 29-2. SUMMARY OF TRANSCANALLICULAR LASER DACRYOCYSTORHINOSTOMY TECHNIQUE

1. Medialize middle turbinate.
2. Pass contact laser fiber "downward" through inferior canaliculus.
3. Enbed fiber tip in bone.
4. Insert endoscope into nasal antrum viewing "upward."
5. Fire laser on continuous-wave mode until tip enters nasal antrum.
6. Manipulate fiber while firing laser to enlarge osteotomy.
7. Place silicone tubes.

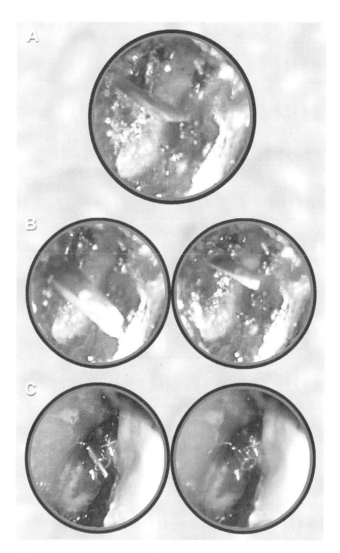

FIGURE 29-3. Conjunctival dacryocystorhinostomy (C-DCR) following completion of the above-described maneuvers. **A:**Entry of needle for tube insertion in C-DCR. **B:** Enlargement of entry site with hemostat. **C:** Insertion of tube.

develop, applying the fiber tip to the area and treating with the same or lower power would suffice in controlling the situation.

Once this large osteotomy is created, the laser fiber and endoscope are removed. Silicone tubes should then be placed. Although the surgery may be successful without them, the potential for success is increased by tube placement. The nose can then be packed with gauze.

It should be apparent that there is no skin incision using this approach, nor is the approach as traumatic as the classical hammer and osteotome or drill method of osteotomy creation. Once the surgeon is adept at this technique, it can be performed quite rapidly (Table 29.2 and Fig. 29-3).

Complications with this approach have been few. Pain, hemorrhage, and facial swelling are uncommon. Infection has not yet been encountered. However, it is important to ensure that the tip of the contact laser fiber is lightly embedded in the bone. If it is only in a subcutaneous location, firing of the laser may result in burning through skin. In the only patient who experienced this event, spontaneous tissue granulation occurred, with an excellent cosmetic and functional outcome. Nevertheless, the lesson was well taken.

A particular advantage to this approach can be appreciated when reoperation from previously failed DCR is required (Fig. 29-4). While the classic method can be challenging because of the need for more extensive dissection in a previously operated field, transcanalicular laser DCR is simpler. Recall that there is no dissection per se in this approach, and so issues of hemorrhage and the sometimes lengthy establishment of tissue planes are moot. Indeed, even less laser power is required in this technique because there is no bone to penetrate. Fibrovascular tissue closes the osteotomy, and often only 3 to 5 W of laser power is required for vaporization. Furthermore, by the surgeon's

knowing that the individual involved has a propensity for closure, the osteotomy size can be adjusted to address this potential.

It can certainly be said that the classic methods for DCR can be effective. The impetus for changing to the transcanalicular laser approach centers not only on its apparent efficacy but also on its simplicity, reduced anesthesia requirement, absence of skin incision, and ease of repetition. Perhaps this combination of attributes will increase the attractiveness of this technique as a solution.

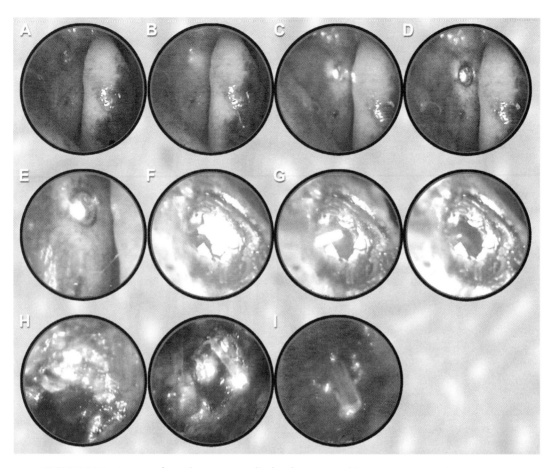

FIGURE 29-4. Images of another transcanalicular dacryocystorhinostomy case. **A:** Pretreatment view after medialization of the middle turbinate. **B:** Submucosal infrared laser emission detected by video camera as white "flash." **C:** White area enlarges and charring of mucosa begins. **D:** A well-defined small area of mucosal charring has evolved in this case. **E:** Further laser application is initiated. **F:** Antrostomy is enlarged. **G:** Further laser is applied, finally opening antrostomy site. **H:** Small gas bubbles form as vaporization continues. **I:** Tube is placed.

SUGGESTED READING

Aaberg TM. Management of anterior and posterior proliferative vitreoretinopathy. 45th Edward Jackson Memorial Lecture. *Am J Ophthalmol* 1988;106:519–532.

Agarwal A, Brummer TA, Tawansy KA, et al. Endoscopic assisted pars plana vitrectomy and glaucoma shunt placement. *Invest Ophthalmol Vis Sci* 2001;42:2349.

Aiello AL, Tran UT, Rao NA. Post natal development of the ciliary body and pars plana. *Arch Ophthalmol* 1992;110:802–805.

Akimoto M, Tanihara H, Negri A, et al. Surgical results of trabeculotomy ab externo for developmental glaucoma. *Arch Ophthalmol* 1994;112:1540–1549.

Akova Y, Bulut S, Duman S. Late bleb-related endophthalmitis after trabeculectomy with mitomycin C. *Ophthalmic Surg Lasers* 1990;30:146–151.

Aldave AJ, Srein JD, Deramo VA, et al. Treatment strategies for postoperative *Proprionobacterium acnes* endophthalmitis. *Ophthalmology* 1999;106:2395–2401.

al Faran MF, Tomey KF, al Mutlaq FA. Cyclocryotherapy in selected cases of congenital glaucoma. *Ophthalmic Surg* 1990;21:794–798.

Allen RC, Bellows AR, Hutchinson BT, Murphy SD. Filtration surgery in the treatment of neovascular glaucoma. *Ophthalmology* 1982;89:1181–1187.

Alpar JJ. Glaucoma after intraocular lens implantation: surgery and recommendations. *Glaucoma* 1985;7:241–250.

Aminlari A. Cyclocryotherapy in congenital glaucoma. *Glaucoma* 1981;3:331–332.

Ando F, Kawai T. Transscleral contact cyclophotocoagulation for refractory glaucoma: a comparison of the results of pars plicata and pars plana irradiation. *Lasers Light Ophthalmol* 1993;5:143.

Ashkenazi I, Melamed S, Avni I, et al. Risk factors associated with late infections of filtering blebs and endophthalmitis. *Ophthalmic Surg* 1991;22:570–582.

Assia EI, Apple DJ. Side-view analysis of the lens. I. The crystalline lens and the evacuated bag. *Arch Ophthalmol* 1992;110:89–97.

Avery RL, Hickenbotham D, deJuan E. Intraoperative fluorescein angioscopy in subretinal surgery [letter]. *Arch Ophthalmol* 1992;110:1518–1519.

Balazsi G. Noncontact thermal mode Nd:YAG laser transscleral cyclophotocoagulation in the treatment of glaucoma: intermediate follow-up. *Ophthalmology* 1991;98:1858–1863.

Barkan O. Technique of goniotomy. *Arch Ophthalmol* 1938;19:217–221.

Barkana Y, Morad Y, Ben-nun J. Endoscopic photocoagulation of the ciliary body after repeated failure of transscleral diode laser cyclophotocoagulation. *Am J Ophthalmol* 2002;133:405–407.

Beauchamp GR, Parks MM. Filtering surgery in children: barriers to success. *Ophthalmology* 1979;86:170–180.

Beckman H, Kinoshita A, Rota AN, Sugar HS. Transscleral ruby laser irradiation of the ciliary body in the treatment of intractable glaucoma. *Trans Am Acad Ophthalmol Otolaryngol* 1972;76:423–436.

Beckman H, Sugar HS. Neodymium laser cyclocoagulation. *Arch Ophthalmol* 1973;90:27–28.

Beckman H, Waelterman J. Transscleral ruby laser cyclophotocoagulation. *Am J Ophthalmol* 1984;98:788–795.

Bellows AR. Cyclocryotherapy for glaucoma. *Int Ophthalmol Clin* 1981;21:99–111.

Bellows AR, Grant WM. Cyclocryotherapy of chronic open-angle glaucoma in aphakic eyes. *Am J Ophthalmol* 1978;85:615–621.

Ben-nun J. Cornea sparing by endoscopically guided vitreoretinal surgery. *Ophthalmomlogy* 2001;108:1465–1470.

Berke SJ, Cohen AJ, Sturm RT. Endoscopic cyclophotocoagulation and phacoemulsification in the treatment of medically controlled primary angle glaucoma. *J Glaucoma* 2000;9:129.

Bietti G. Surgical intervention on the ciliary body: new trends for the relief of glaucoma. *JAMA* 1950;142:889–897.

Blomquist PH, Gross RL, Koch DD. Effect of transscleral neodymium:YAG cyclophotocoagulation on intraocular lenses. *Ophthalmic Surg* 1990;21:223–226.

Bloom M, Weber PA. Probe orientation in contact Nd:YAG laser cyclophotocoagulation. *Ophthalmic Surg* 1992;23:364–366.

Bock CJ, Freedman SF, Buckley EG, Shields MB. Transscleral diode laser cyclophotocoagulation for refractory pediatric glaucomas. *J Pediatr Ophthalmol Strabismus* 1977;34:235–238.

Brancato R, Giovanni L, Trabucchi G, Pietroni C. Contact transscleral cyclocoagulation with YAG laser in uncontrolled glaucoma. *Ophthalmic Surg* 1989;20:547–551.

Brancato R, Leoni G, Trabucchi G. Transscleral contact cyclophotocoagulation with Nd:YAG laser CW: experimental study on rabbit eyes. *Int J Tissue React* 1987;9:493–498.

Brancato R, Trabucchi G, Verdi M, et al. Diode and Nd:YAG laser contact transscleral cyclophotocoagulation in a human eye: a comparative histopathologic study of the lesions produced using a new fiberoptic probe. *Ophthalmic Surg* 1994;25:607–611.

Branch Retinal Vein Occlusion Study Group. Argon laser scatter photocoagulation for prevention of neovascularization and vitreous hemorrhage in branch vein occlusion. *Arch Ophthalmol* 1986;104:34–41.

Cairns JE. Trabeculectomy: preliminary report of a new method. *Am J Ophthalmol* 1968;66:673–679.

Caronia RM, Sturm RT, Marmor MA, Berke SJ. Treatment of a cyclodialysis cleft by means of ophthalmic laser endoscope endophotocoagulation. *Am J Ophthalmol* 1999;128:760–761.

Charles S. Endophotocoagulation. *Retina* 1981;1:117–120.

Chen J, Cohn RA, Lin SC, et al. Endoscopic photocoagulation of the ciliary body for treatment of refractory glaucomas. *Ophthalmology* 1997;124:787–796.

Chen TC, Wilensky JT, Viana MAG. Long-term follow-up of initially successful trabeculectomy. *Ophthalmology* 1997;104:1120–1125.

Christman LM, Wilson ME. Motility disturbances after Molteno implants. *J Pediatr Ophthalmol Strabismus* 1992;29:44–48.

Ciardella AP, Fisher YL, Carvalho C, et al. Endoscopic vitreoretinal surgery for complicated proliferative diabetic retinopathy. *Retina* 2001;21:20–27.

Cohen EJ, Schwartz LW, Luskind RD, et al. Neodymium:YAG laser transscleral cyclophotocoagulation for glaucoma after penetrating keratoplasty. *Ophthalmic Surg* 1989;20:713–716.

Coleman AL, Smyth RJ, Wilson MR, Tam M. Initial clinical experience with the Ahmed Glaucoma Valve implant in pediatric patients. *Arch Ophthalmol* 1997;115:186–191.

Costa VP, Moster MR, Wilson RP, et al. Effects of topical mitomycin-C on primary trabeculectomies and combined procedures. *Br J Ophthalmol* 1993;77:693–697.

Crymes BM, Gross RL. Laser placement in noncontact Nd:YAG cyclophotocoagulation. *Am J Ophthalmol* 1990;110:670–673.

Danis RP, Ciulla TA, Pratt LM, Anliker W. Intravitreal triamcinolone acetonide in exudative age-related macular degeneration. *Retina* 2000;20:244–250.

Davidson PC, Sternberg P Jr. Potential retinal phototoxicity. *Am J Ophthalmol* 1993;116:497–500.

deLuise VP, Anderson DR. Primary infantile glaucoma (congenital glaucoma). *Surv Ophthalmol* 1983;28:1–23.

Derbolav A, Vass C, Menapace R, et al. Long-term effect of phacoemulsification on intraocular pressure after trabeculectomy. *J Cataract Refract Surg* 2002;28:425–430.

De Roeth A Jr. Ciliary body temperatures in cryosurgery. *Arch Ophthalmol* 1971;85:204.

De Roeth A Jr. Cryosurgery for the treatment of glaucoma. *Trans Am Ophthalmol Soc* 1965;63:189.

De Smet MD. Retinal transscleral photocoagulation under endoscopic control. *Retina* 2000;20:3:316–317.

Devenyi RG, Trope GE, Hunter WH, Badeeb O. Neodymium:YAG transscleral cyclocoagulation in human eyes. *Ophthalmology* 1987;94:1519–1522.

Diabetic Retinopathy Vitrectomy Study Research Group. Early vitrectomy for severe vitreous hemorrhage in diabetic retinopathy. Diabetic Retinopathy Vitrectomy Study Report 2. *Arch Ophthalmology* 1985;103:1644–51

Diabetic Retinopathy Vitrectomy Study Research Group. Two year course of visual acuity in severe proliferative diabetic retinopathy with conventional management. Diabetic Retinopathy Vitrectomy Study Report 1. *Ophthalmology* 1985;92:492–501

Diabetic Retinopathy Vitrectomy Study Research Group. Early vitrectomy for severe proliferative diabetic retinopathy in eyes with useful vision. Diabetic Retinopathy Vitrectomy Study Report 3. *Ophthalmology* 1988;1307–1320.

Diabetic Retinopathy Vitrectomy Study Research Group. Early vitrectomy for severe proliferative diabetic retinopathy in eyes with useful vision: Clinical applications of results of a randomized trial. Diabetic Retinopathy Vitrectomy Study Report 4. *Ophthalmology* 1988; 1321–1334.

Diabetic Retinopathy Vitrectomy Study Research Group. Early vitrectomy for severe vitreous hemorrhage in diabetic retinopathy. Four years results of a randomized trial. Diabetic Retinopathy Vitrectomy Study Report 5. *Arch Ophthalmology* 1990;108:958–964.

Dickens CJ, Nguyen N, Mora JS, et al. Long-term results of noncontact transscleral neodymium:YAG cyclophotocoagulation. *Ophthalmology* 1995;102:1777–1781.

Egbert PR, Fiadoyor S, Budenz DL, et al. Diode laser transscleral cyclophotocoagulation as a primary surgical treatment for primary open angle glaucoma. *Arch Ophthalmol* 2001;119:345–355.

Eguchi S, Araie M. A new ophthalmic electronic video endoscope system for intraocular surgery. *Arch Ophthalmol* 1990;108:1778–1781.

Eid TE, Katz JL, Spaeth GL, Augsburger JJ. Long-term effects of tube-shunt procedures on management of refractory childhood glaucomas. *Ophthalmology* 1997; 104:1101–1106.

Endophthalmitis Vitrectomy Study Group. Results of the Endophthalmitis Vitrectomy Study: a randomized trial of immediate vitrectomy and of intravenous antibiotics for the treatment of postoperative bacterial endophthalmitis. *Arch Ophthalmol* 1995;113:1479–1496.

Fankhauser F. Contact Nd:YAG laser cyclophotocoagulation. *Ophthalmic Surg* 1992;23:299–300.

Fankhauser F, Kwasniewska S, England C, Durr U. Diode versus Nd:YAG laser for cyclodestructive procedures. *Ophthalmic Surg* 1993;24:566–567.

Fankhauser F, van der Zypen E, Kwasniewska S, et al. Transscleral cyclophotocoagulation using a neodymium:YAG laser. *Ophthalmic Surg* 1986;17:94–100.

Fellenbaum PS, Almeida AR, Minckler DS, et al. Krupin disc implantation for complicated glaucomas. *Ophthalmology* 1994;101:1178–1182.

Ferry AP. Histopathologic observations on human eyes following cyclocryotherapy for glaucoma. *Trans Am Acad Ophthalmol Otol* 1977;83:90–101.

Fisher YL, Slakter JS. A disposable ophthalmic endoscopic system. *Arch Ophthalmol* 1994;112:984–986.

Fisher Y, Turtz A, Gold M, et al. Use of sodium hyaluronate in reformation and reconstruction of the persistent flat anterior chamber in the presence of severe hypotony. *Ophthalmic Surg* 1982;13:819–821.

Fluorouracil Filtering Surgery Study Group. Three-year follow-up of the Fluorouracil Filtering Surgery Study. *Am J Ophthalmol* 1993;115:82–92.

Foulks GN. Glaucoma associated with penetrating keratoplasty. *Ophthalmology* 1987;94:871–874.

Freedman J. Clinical experience with the Molteno dual-chamber single-plate implant. *Ophthalmic Surg* 1992;23:238–241.

Freedman SF, McCormick M, Cox TA. Mitomycin-C augmented trabeculectomy in postoperative wound modulation in pediatric glaucoma. *Journal American Academy of Pediatric Ophthalmology & Strabisimus* 1999;3:117–124.

Furia M, Hamard H, Puech M, et al. Cloutage retinien avec film video-endoscopique U-MATIC ["Retinal nailing" with U-MATIC video-endoscopy film]. *Bull Soc Ophtalmol Fr* 1987;87:1395–1403.

Furia M, Hamard H, Puech M. Endoscopie oculaire. I. Modele experimental d'étude de l'implantation en chambre posterieure apres extraction extra-capsulaire du cristallin [Ocular endoscopy. I. Experimental model for studying implantation into the posterior chamber after extracapsular extraction of the crystalline lens]. *Bull Soc Ophtalmol Fr* 1987;87:759–760.

Gass JDM. Biomicroscopic and histopathologic considerations regarding the feasibility of surgical excision of subfoveal neovascular membranes. *Am J Ophthalmol* 1994;118:285–298.

Gayton J. Combined surgery with an endoscopic laser. In: *Maximizing results: strategies in refractive, corneal, cataract and glaucoma surgery.* Thorofare, NJ: Slack, 1996:224–234.

Gayton JL. Combined cataract and glaucoma surgery: trabeculectomy vs. endoscopic laser cyclophotocoagulation. *Journal American Society of Cataract & Refractive Surgery* 1999;25:1212–1219.

Gayton JL. Traumatic aniridia during endoscopic laser cycloablation. *J Cataract Refract Surg* 1998;24:134–135.

Gayton JL, Van Der Karr M, Sanders V. Combined cataract and glaucoma surgery: trabeculectomy vs. endoscopic laser cyclophotocoagulation. *Journal American Society of Cataract & Refractive Surgery* 1999;25:1212–1219.

Gimbel HV, Meyer D, DeBroff BM, et al. Intraocular pressure response to combined phacoemulsification and trabeculectomy ab externo versus phacoemulsification alone in primary open angle glaucoma. *J Cataract Refract Surg* 1995;21:653–660.

Googe JM, Bessler M, Hoskins JC, Miller JH. Intraoperative fluorescein angiography. *Ophthalmology* 1993;100:1167–1170.

Gressel MG, Heuer DK, Parrish RK II. Trabeculectomy in young patients. *Ophthalmology* 1984;91:1242–1246.

Gross RL, Feldman RM, Spaeth GL, et al. Surgical therapy of chronic glaucoma in aphakia and pseudophakia. *Ophthalmology* 1988;95:1195–1201.

Haller JA Transvitreal endocyclophotocoagulation. *Trans Am Ophthmol Soc* 1996;94:589–676.

Hampton C, Shields MB. Transscleral neodymium-YAG cyclophotocoagulation: a histopathologic study of human autopsy eyes. *Arch Ophthalmol* 1988;106:1121.

Hampton C, Shields MB, Miller KN, Blasini M. Evaluation of a protocol for transscleral neodymium:YAG cyclophotocoagulation in one hundred patients. *Ophthalmology* 1990;97:910–917.

Hardten DR, Brown JD. Malignant glaucoma after Nd:YAG cyclophotocoagulation [letter]. *Am J Ophthalmol* 1990;111:245–247.

Hardten DR, Brown JD. Transscleral Nd:YAG cyclodestruction: comparison of 180-degree and 360-degree initial treatments. *Ophthalmic Surg* 1993;24:181–184.

Hayashi M, Yablonski ME, Boxrud C, et al. Decreased formation of aqueous humor in insulin-dependent diabetic patients. *Br J Ophthalmol* 1989;73:621–623.

Hennis HL, Affia E, Stewart WC, et al. Transscleral cyclophotocoagulation using a semiconductor diode laser in cadaver eyes. *Ophthalmic Surg* 1992;22:374–378.

Hennis JL, Stewart WC. Semiconductor diode laser transscleral cyclophotocoagulation in patients with glaucoma. *Am J Ophthalmol* 1992;113:81–85.

Hennis HL, Stewart WC. The use of 5-fluorouracil in patients with combined trabeculectomy and cataract extraction. *Ophthalmic Surg* 1991;22:451–463.

Henry JC, Krupin T, Schmitt M, et al. Long-term follow-up of pseudoexfoliation and the development of elevated intraocular pressure. *Ophthalmology* 1987;94:545–552.

Heuck M, Sonnsjoe B, Krakan CET. Measurement of progressive disc change in glaucoma. *Ophthalmic Surg* 1992;23:672–679.

Hill Ra, Nguyen QH, Baerveldt G, et al. Trabeculectomy and Molteno implantation for glaucomas associated with uveitis. *Ophthalmology* 1993;100:903–909.

Immonen I, Puska P, Raitta C. Transscleral contact krypton laser cyclophotocoagulation for treatment of glaucoma. *Ophthalmology* 1994;101:876–882.

Ip MS, Kumar KS. Intravitreous triamcinolone acetonide as treatment for macular edema from central retinal vein occlusion. *Arch Ophthalmol* 2002;120:1217–1219.

Iwach AG, Drake MV, Hoskins HD Jr, et al. A new contact neodymium:YAG laser for cyclophotocoagulation. *Ophthalmic Surg* 1991;22:345–248.

Jacobi PC, Dietlein TS, Krieglstein GK. Microendoscopic trabecular surgery in glaucoma management. *Ophthalmology* 1999;106:538–544.

Jaffe TW, Barak A, Melamed S, Glovinski Y. Intraocular pressure increments after cataract extraction in glaucomatous eyes with functioning filtering blebs. *Ophthalmic Surg Lasers* 1997;28:657–661.

Jahne MG. [25 years of Cardona keratoprosthesis after severe chemical eye burns: long-term outcome of 4 eyes]. *Klin Monatsbl Augenheilkd* 2000;216:191–196.

Jonas JB, Sofker A. Intraocular injection of crystalline cortisone as adjunctive treatment of diabetic macular edema. *Am J Ophthalmol* 2001;132:425–427.

Joos KM, Alward WL, Folberg R. Experimental endoscopic goniotomy: a potential treatment for primary infantile glaucoma. *Ophthalmology* 1993;100:1066–1070.

Joos KM, Bueche MJ, Palmberg PF, et al. One-year follow-up results of combined mitomycin C trabeculectomy and extracapsular cataract extraction. *Ophthalmology* 1995;102:76–83.

Joos KM, Shen JH. An ocular endoscope enables a goniotomy despite a cloudy cornea. *Arch Ophthalmol* 2001;119:134–135.

Joos KM, Shen J-H, Parel J-M, Rol P. In vitro examination of the anterior chamber angle with a gradient-index (GRIN) lens endoscope. *Lasers Ophthalmol* 1994;2:2330.

Kalenak JW, Parkinson JM, Kass MA, Kolker AE. Transscleral neodymium:YAG laser cyclocoagulation for uncontrolled glaucoma. *Ophthalmic Surg* 1990;21:346–351.

Kangas TA, Greenfield DS, Flynn HW Jr, et al. Delayed-onset endophthalmitis associated with conjunctival filtering blebs. *Ophthalmology* 1997;104:746–752.

Kattan HM, Flynn HW, Pflugfelder SC, et al. Nosocomial endophthalmitis survey: current incidence of infection after intraocular surgery. *Ophthalmology* 1991;98:227–238.

Katz LJ, Cantor LB, Spaeth GL. Complications of surgery in glaucoma: early and late bacterial endophthalmitis following glaucoma filtering surgery. *Ophthalmology* 1985;92:959–963.

Klapper RM, Wandel T, Donnenfeld E, Perry HD. Transscleral neodymium YAG thermal cyclophotocoagulation in refractory glaucoma: a preliminary report. *Ophthalmology* 1988;95:719–722.

Koch FH, Luloh KP, Augustin AJ, et al. Subretinal surgery with gradient index endoscopes. *Ophthalmologica* 1997;211:283–287.

Koch FH, Schmidt HP, Monks T, et al. The retinal irradiance and spectral properties of the multiport illumination system for vitreous surgery. *Am J Ophthalmol* 1993;116:489–496.

Kong YT, Kim TI, Kong BW. A report of 131 cases of endoscopic laser lacrimal surgery. *Ophthalmology* 1994;101:1793–1800.

Konstas AG, Jay JL, Marshall GE, Lee WR. Prevalence, diagnostic features, and response to trabeculectomy in exfoliation syndrome. *Ophthalmology* 1993;100:619–625.

Kora Y, Yaguchi S. Sutured secondary posterior chamber lens with endoscopic control. *Ocular Surg News* 1990.

Koryllos K. Trabeculectomy: a new glaucoma operation. *Bull Soc Hellen Ophthalmol* 1967;35:147–157.

Kosoko O, Gaasterland DE, Pollack IP, Enger CL. Long-term outcome of initial ciliary ablation with contact diode laser transscleral cyclophotocoagulation for severe glaucoma. The Diode Laser Ciliary Ablation Study Group. *Ophthalmology* 1996;103:1294–1300.

Kozarsky AM, Knight SH, Waring GO III. Clinical results with a ceramic keratoprosthesis placed through the eyelid. *Ophthalmology* 1987;94:904–911.

Krebs DB, Liebmann JM, Ritch R, Speaker M. Late infectious endophthalmitis from exposed glaucoma setons. *Arch Ophthalmol* 1992;110:174–175.

Krupin T, Johnson MF, Becker B. Anterior segment schemia after cyclocryotherapy. *Am J Ophthalmol* 1977;84:426–433.

Krupin TH, Juzych MS, Shin DH. Adjunctive mitomycin-C in primary trabeculectomy in phakic eyes. *Am J Ophthalmol* 1994;119:30–39.

Krupin T, Mitchell K, Becker B. Cyclocryotherapy in neovascular glaucoma. *Am J Ophthalmol* 1978;86:24–26.

Kwiterovich KA, Maguire MG, Murphy RP, et al. Frequency of adverse systemic reactions after fluorescein angiography: results of a prospective study. *Ophthalmology* 1991;98:1139–1142.

Lam S, Tessler HH, Lam BL, Wilensky JT. High incidence of sympathetic ophthalmia after contact and noncontact neodymium:YAG laser cyclotherapy. *Ophthalmology* 1992;99:1818–1822.

Landers MB III, Trese MT, Stefansson E, Bessler E. Argon laser intraocular photocoagulation. *Ophthalmology* 1982;89:785–788.

Larrson LI, Pach JM, Brubaker RF. Aqueous humor dynamics in patients with diabetes mellitus. *Am J Ophthalmol* 1995;120:362–367.

Lavin MJ, Franks WA, Wormald RPL, Hitchings RA. Clinical risk factors for failure in glaucoma tube surgery: a comparison of three tube designs. *Arch Ophthalmol* 1992;110:480–485.

Leagis JM, Rol P, Briat B, et al. Endoscope rigide à lentilles de GRIN. *J Fr Ophthalmol* 1997;20:439–443.

Lecoq PJ, Billotte C, Combe JC. Interet de la videoendoscopie vitreo-retinienne [Value of vitreoretinal videoendoscopy]. *J Fr Ophthalmol* 1986;9:427–429.

Lecoq PJ, Billotte C, Combe JC, Hamel C. Plaidoyer en

favour de l'endoscopie pour certaines interventions retinovitreennes [A plea for endoscopy in various retino-vitreous operations]. *Bull Oc Ophtalmol Fr* 1987;87: 575–576.

Lee PF. Argon laser photocoagulation of the ciliary processes in cases of aphakic glaucoma. *Arch Ophthalmol* 1979;97:2135–2138.

Lee PF, Pomerantzeff O. Transpupillary cyclophotocoagulation of rabbit eyes: an experimental approach to glaucoma surgery. *Am J Ophthalmol* 1971;71:911–920.

Legeais JM, Renard G, Parel JM, et al. Keratoprosthesis with biocolonizable microporous fluorocarbon haptic: preliminary results in a 24-patient study. *Arch Ophthalmol* 1995;113:757–763.

Leon CS, Leon JA. *Endoscopie chirurgicale oculaire.* Paris: Medsi/McGraw-Hill, 1990.

Leon CS, Leon JA. Microendoscopic ocular surgery. I. Endoscopic equipment/methodology applied to cataract surgery with intraocular lens implantation. *J Cataract Refract Surg* 1991;17:568–572.

Leon CS, Leon JA. Microendoscopic ocular surgery. II. Preliminary results from the study of glaucomatous eyes. *J Cataract Refract Surg* 1991;5:573–576.

Levin PS, StormoGipson J. Endocanalicular laser-assisted dacryocystorhinostomy: an anatomic study. *Arch Ophthalmol* 1992;110:1488–1490.

Lewis A, Aaberg TM. Anterior proliferative vitreoretinopathy. *Am J Ophthalmol* 1988;105:227–284.

Lloyd MA, Baerveldt G, Fellenbaum PS, et al. Intermediate-term results of randomized clinical trial of the 350- vs 500-mm^2 Baerveldt implant. *Ophthalmology* 1994; 101:1456–1464.

Lloyd MA, Heuer DK, Baerveldt G, et al. Combined Molteno implantation and pars plana vitrectomy for neovascular glaucomas. *Ophthalmology* 1991;98:14–15.

Lumme P, Laatikainen L. Exfoliation syndrome and cataract extraction. *Am J Ophthalmol* 1993;116:51–55.

Lund OE. Limits and possibilities of optical keratoprosthesis: a clinical and histopathological report. *Klin Monatsbl Augenheilkd* 1982;180:3–12.

Mandal AK, Walton DS, John T, Jayagandan A. Mitomycin-C augmented trabeculectomy in refractory congenital glaucoma. *Ophthalmology* 1997;104;996–1001.

Mandelbaum S, Forster RK, Gelender H, Culbertson W. Late-onset endophthalmitis associated with filtering blebs. *Ophthalmology* 1985;92:964–972.

Mao LK, Stewart WC, Shields MB. Correlation between intraocular pressure control and progressive glaucomatous damage and primary open-angle glaucoma. *Am J Ophthalmol* 1991;111:51–55.

Marsh P, Wilson DJ, Samples JR, Morrison JC. A clinicopathologic correlative study of noncontact transscleral Nd:YAG cyclophotocoagulation. *Am J Ophthalmol* 1993;115:597–602.

Martidis A, Duker JS, Greenberg PB, et al. Intravitreal triamcinolone for refractory diabetic macular edema. *Ophthalmology* 2002;109:920–927.

Maus M, Katz LJ. Choroidal detachment, flat anterior chamber, and hypotony as complications of neodymium:YAG laser cyclophotocoagulation. *Ophthalmology* 1990;97:69–72.

McCartney DL, Memmen JE, Stark WJ, et al. The efficacy and safety of combined trabeculectomy, cataract extraction, and intraocular lens implantation. *Ophthalmology* 1988;95:754–757.

McDonnell PJ, Robin JB, Schanzlin DJ, et al. Molteno implant for control of glaucoma in eyes with penetrating keratoplasty. *Ophthalmology* 1988;95:364–369.

McGuigan LJ, Gottsch J, Stark WJ, et al. Extracapsular cataract extraction and posterior chamber intraocular lens implantation in eyes with pre-existing glaucoma. *Arch Ophthalmol* 1986;104:1301–1313.

McPherson SD Jr. Results of external trabeculotomy. *Am J Ophthalmol* 1973;76:918–922.

Medow N, Haley J, Lima F. Initial ciliary ablation with TSPC [letter]. *Ophthalmology* 1997;104:171–172.

Medow NB, Sauer HL. Endoscopic goniotomy for congenital glaucoma. *J Pediatr Ophthalmol Strabismus* 1997;34: 258–259.

Meisler DM, Palestine AG, Vastine DW, et al. Chronic *Propionibacterium* endophthalmitis after extracapsular cataract extraction and intraocular lens implantation. *Am J Ophthalmol* 1986;92:964–972.

Menikoff JA, Speaker MG, Marmor M, Raskin EM. A case-control study of risk factors for postoperative endophthalmitis. *Ophthalmology* 1991;98:1761–1768.

Mermoud A, Salmon JF, Alexander P, et al. Molteno tube implantation for neovascular glaucoma: long-term results and factors influencing outcome. *Ophthalmology* 1993;100:897–902.

Merritt JC. Transpupillary photocoagulation of the ciliary processes. *Ann Ophthalmol* 1976;8:325–328.

Michels M, Lewis H, Abrams CW, et al. Macular phototoxicity caused by fiberoptic endoillumination during pars plana vitrectomy. *Am J Ophthalmol* 1992;114: 287–296.

Michels R. *Vitreous surgery.* St Louis: CV Mosby, 1981.

Mietz H, Krieglstein GK. Three-year follow-up of trabeculectomies performed with different concentrations of mitomycin-C. *Ophthalmic Surg Lasers* 1998;29:628–634.

Migdal C, Gregory W, Hitchings GW. Long-term functional outcome after early surgery compared with laser and medicine in open-angle glaucoma. *Ophthalmology* 1994;101:1651–1657.

Mizota A, Takaso M, Asangi K, et al. Internal contact sclerostomy with an erbium laser and intraocular fiberscope. *Laser Light Ophthalmol* 1995;7:57–64.

Mochizuki M. Transpupillary cyclophotocoagulation in hemorrhagic glaucoma: a case report. *Jpn J Ophthalmol* 1975;19:191–198.

Molteno AC. New implant for drainage in glaucoma: clinical trial. *Br J Ophthalmol* 1969;53:606–615.

Mora JS, Iwach AG, Gaffney MM, et al. Endoscopic diode laser cyclophotocoagulation with a limbal approach. *Ophthalmic Surg Lasers* 1997;28:118–123.

Munden PM, Alward WLM. Combined phacoemulsification, posterior chamber intraocular lens implantation, and trabeculectomy with mitomycin-C. *Am J Ophthalmol* 1994;119:20–29.

Murchison JF Jr, Shields MB. An evaluation of three surgical approaches for coexisting cataract and glaucoma. *Ophthalmic Surg* 1989;20:393–402.

Murray TG, Boldt C, Lewis H, et al. A technique for facilitative visualization and dissection of the vitreous base, pars plana and pars plicata. *Arch Ophthalmol* 1991; 109:1458–1459.

Naveh N, Kotass R, Golvinsky J, et al. The long-term effect on intraocular pressure of a procedure combining trabeculectomy and cataract surgery, as compared to trabeculectomy alone. *Ophthalmic Surg* 1990;21:339–351.

Neeley DE, Plager DA. Endocyclophotocoagulation for the management of difficult pediatric glaucomas. *Journal American Academy of Pediatric Ophthalmology & Strabisimus* 2001;5:221–229.

Netland PA, Terada H, Dohlman CH. Glaucoma associated with keratoprosthesis. *Ophthalmology* 1998;105: 751–757.

Netland PA, Walton DS. Glaucoma drainage implants in pediatric patients. *Ophthalmic Surg* 1993;24:723–729.

Norris JL. Vitreous surgery viewed through an endoscope. *Dev Ophthalmol* 1981;2:15–16.

Norris JL, Cleasby GW. An endoscope for ophthalmology. *Am J Ophthalmol* 1978;85:420–422.

Norris JL, Cleasby GW. Intraocular foreign body removal by endoscopy. *Ann Ophthalmol* 1982;14:371–372.

Norris JL, Cleasby GW, Nakanishi AS, Martin LJ. Intraocular endoscopic surgery. *Am J Ophthalmol* 1981;91: 603–606.

Noureddin BN, Wilson-Holt N, Lavin M, et al. Advanced uncontrolled glaucoma: Nd:YAG cyclophotocoagulation or tube surgery. *Ophthalmology* 1992;99:430–437.

Nouri-Mahdavi K, Brigatti L, Weitzman M, Caprioli J. Outcomes of trabeculectomy for primary open angle glaucoma. *Ophthalmology* 1995;102:1760–1769.

Parc CE, Johnson DH, Oliver JE, et al. The long-term outcome of glaucoma filtration surgery. *Am J Ophthalmol* 2001;132:27–35.

Park HJ, Weitzman M, Caprioli J. Temporal corneal phacoemulsification combined with superior trabeculectomy. *Arch Ophthalmol* 1997;115:318–323.

Parrish CM, O'Day DM. Traumatic endophthalmitis. *Int Ophthalmol Clin* 1987;27:112–119.

Patel A, Thompson JT, Michels RG, Quigley HA. Endolaser treatment of the ciliary body for uncontrolled glaucoma. *Ophthalmology* 1986;93:825–830.

Pavlin CJ, Harasiewicz K, Foster FS. Ultrasound biomicroscopy of anterior segment structures in normal and glaucomatous eyes. *Am J Ophthalmol* 1992;113:381–389.

Peyman GA, Conway MD, Raichand M, Lin J. Histopathologic studies of transscleral argon-krypton photocoagulation with an exolaser probe. *Ophthalmic Surg* 1984;15:496–501.

Peyman GA, Lee KJ. Multifunction endolaser probe. *Am J Ophthalmol* 1992;114:103–104.

Peyman G, Shulman J. *Intravitreal surgery: principles and practice*. Norwalk, CT: Appleton-Century-Crofts, 1986.

Phelan MJ, Higginbotham EJ. Contact transscleral Nd:YAG laser cyclophotocoagulation for the treatment of refractive pediatric glaucoma. *Ophthalmic Surg Lasers* 1995;26:401–403.

Phillips WB II, Wong TP, Bergren RL, et al. Late-onset endophthalmitis associated with filtering blebs. *Ophthalmology* 1994;25:88–91.

Plager DA, Neeley DE. Intermediate-term results of endoscopic diode laser cyclophotocoagulation for pediatric glaucoma. *Journal American Academy of Pediatric Ophthalmology & Strabisimus* 1999;3:131–137.

Polack F, De Roeth A. Effect of freezing on the ciliary body. *Invest Ophthalmol* 1964;3:164.

Prum BE Jr, Shields SR, Simmons RB, et al. The influence of exposure duration in transscleral Nd:YAG laser cyclophotocoagulation. *Am J Ophthalmol* 1992;114: 560–567.

Quigley HA. Histological and physiological studies of cyclocryotherapy in primate and human eyes. *Am J Ophthalmol* 1976;82:722–727.

Quigley HA. Open-angle glaucoma. *N Engl J Med* 1993; 328:1097–1106.

Rao GN, Blatt HL, Aquavella JV. Results of keratoprosthesis. *Am J Ophthalmol* 1979;88:190–196.

Ritch R. 5-Fluorouracil filtering surgery and neovascular glaucoma. [Discussion] *Ophthalmology* 1995;106:892–893.

Roth M, Epstein DL. Exfoliation syndrome. *Am J Ophthalmol* 1980;89:477–481.

Ryan S. *Retina*. St Louis: CV Mosby, 1989.

Sato Y, Berkowitz BA, Wilson CA, de Juan E Jr. Blood–retinal barrier breakdown caused by diode vs argon laser endophotocoagulation. *Arch Ophthalmol* 1992;110: 277–281.

Savage JA, Thomas JV, Belcher C III, Simmons RJ. Extracapsular cataract extraction and posterior chamber lens implantation in glaucomatous eyes. *Ophthalmology* 1985;92:1506–1516.

Schubert HD, Federman JL. A comparison of CW Nd:YAG contact transscleral cyclophotocoagulation with cyclocryopexy. *Invest Ophthalmol Vis Sci* 1989;30: 536–542.

Schuman JS, Bellows AR, Shingleton BJ, et al. Contact transscleral Nd:YAG laser cyclophotocoagulation: midterm results. *Ophthalmology* 1992;99:1089–1094.

Schuman JS, Noecker RJ, Puliafito CA, et al. Energy levels and probe placement in contact transscleral semiconductor diode laser cyclophotocoagulation in human cadaver eyes. *Arch Ophthalmol* 1992;109:1534–1538.

Schuman JS, Puliafito CA, Allingham RR, et al. Contact transscleral continuous wave neodymium:YAG laser cyclophotocoagulation. *Ophthalmology* 1990;97:571–580.

Shields MB. Combined cataract extraction and glaucoma surgery. *Ophthalmology* 1982;89:231–239.

Shields MB. Cyclodestructive surgery for glaucoma: past, present, and future. *Trans Am Ophthalmol Soc* 1985;83:285–303.

Shields MB. Intraocular cyclophotocoagulation. *Trans Ophthalmol Soc UK* 1986;105:237–241.

Shields MB. Intraocular cyclophotocoagulation: histopathologic evaluation in primates. *Arch Ophthalmol* 1985;103:1731–1735.

Shields MB, Chandler DB, Hickingbotham D, Klintworth GK. Intraocular cyclophotocoagulation: histopathologic evaluation in primates. *Arch Ophthalmol* 1985;103:1731–1735.

Shields MB, Shields SE. Non-contact transscleral Nd:YAG cyclophotocoagulation: a long-term follow-up of 500 patients. *Trans Am Ophthalmol Soc* 1994;92:271–278.

Shields SM, Stevens JL, Kass MA, et al. Histopathologic findings after Nd:YAG transscleral cyclophotocoagulation. *Am J Ophthalmol* 1988;106:100–110.

Sherwood MB, Smith MF. Prevention of early hypotony associated with Molteno implants by a new occluding stent technique. *Ophthalmology* 1993;100:85–90.

Sherwood MB, Smith MF, Driebe WT Jr, et al. Drainage tube implants in the treatment of glaucoma following penetrating keratoplasty. *Ophthalmic Surg* 1993;24:185–189.

Shin DH, Simone PA, Song MS, et al. Adjunctive subconjunctival mitomycin-C in glaucoma triple procedure. *Ophthalmology* 1995;102:550–1558.

Shingleton BJ, Gamell LS, O'Donoghue MW, et al. Long-term changes in intraocular pressure after clear corneal phacoemulsification: normal patients versus glaucoma suspect and glaucoma patients. *J Cataract Refract Surg* 1999;25:885–890.

Shingleton BJ, Jacobson LM, Kuperwaser MC. Comparison of combined cataract and glaucoma surgery using planned extracapsular and phacoemulsification techniques. *Ophthalmic Surg Lasers* 1995;26:414–419.

Sidoti PA, Baerveldt G. Glaucoma drainage implants. *Curr Opin Ophthalmol* 1994;11:85–98.

Sidoti PA, Dunphy TR, Baerveldt G, et al. Experience with the Baerveldt glaucoma implant in treating neovascular glaucoma. *Ophthalmology* 1995;102:1107–1118.

Siegner SW, Netland PA, Urban RC Jr, et al. Clinical experience with the Baerveldt glaucoma drainage implant. *Ophthalmology* 1995;102:1298–1307.

Silicone Oil Study Group. Vitrectomy with silicone oil or sulfahexafluoride in eyes with severe proliferative vitreoretinopathy: results of a randomized clinical trial. Silicone Study Report No. 1. *Arch Ophthalmol* 1992;110:770–779.

Silicone Oil Study Group. Vitrectomy with silicone oil or sulfahexafluoride in eyes with severe proliferative vitreoretinopathy: results of a randomized clinical trial. Silicone Study Report No. 2. *Arch Ophthalmol* 1992;110:780–792.

Simmons RB, Shields MB, Blasini M, et al. Transscleral Nd:YAG cyclophotocoagulation with a contact lens. *Am J Ophthalmol* 1991;112:671–677.

Simmons RB, Stern RA, Teekhasaenee C, Kenyon KR. Elevated intraocular pressure following penetrating keratoplasty. *Trans Am Ophthalmol Soc* 1989;87:79–91.

Singh AD, Singh A, Whitmore I, Taylor E. Endoscopic visualisation of the human nasolacrimal system: an experimental study. *Br J Ophthalmol* 1992;76:663–667.

Smiddy WE, Michels RG, Green WR. Lens and peripheral retinal relationships during vitrectomy. *Retina* 1991;11:199–203.

Smith R. A new technique for opening the canal of Schlemm. *Br J Ophthalmol* 1960;44:370–375.

Smith RS, Boyle E, Rudt LA. Cyclocryotherapy: a light and electron microscopic study. *Arch Ophthalmol* 1977;95:285–288.

Stewart WC, Crinkley CM, Carlson AN. Results of trabeculectomy combined with phacoemulsification versus trabeculectomy combined with extracapsular cataract extraction in patients with advanced glaucoma. *Ophthalmic Surg* 1994;25:621–627.

Stocker FW. Response of chronic simple glaucoma to treatment with cyclodiathermy puncture. *Arch Ophthalmol* 1945;34:181–186.

Stolzenburg S, Kresse S, Muller-Stolzenburg W. Thermal side reactions during in vitro contact cyclophotocoagulation with the continuous wave Nd:YAG laser. *Ophthalmic Surg* 1990;21:356–368.

Sturmer J, Broadway DC, Hitchings RA. Young patient trabeculectomy: assessment of risk factors for failure. *Ophthalmology* 1993;10:928–939.

Susanna R, Oltrogge EW, Carani JCE, et al. Mitomycin as adjunct chemotherapy with trabeculectomy in congenital and developmental glaucomas. *J Glaucoma* 1995;4:15–17.

Tello C, Walsh J, Rosen R, et al. High resolution endoscopic evaluation of anterior segment structures. *Invest Ophthalmol Vis Sci* 2001;42:767.

Thorpe HE. Ocular endoscope. *Trans Am Acad Ophthalmol Otolaryngol* 1934;39:422–424.

Ticho U, Ophir A. Late complications after glaucoma filtration surgery with adjunctive 5-fluorouracil. *Am J Ophthalmol* 1993;115:506–510.

Tomey KF, Traverso CE. The glaucomas in aphakia and pseudophakia. *Surv Ophthalmol* 1991;36:79–112.

Torii H, Takahashi K, Yoshitomi F, et al. Mechanical detachment of the anterior hyaloid membrane from the posterior lens capsule. *Ophthalmology* 2001;108:2182–2185.

Trevisani MG, Allingham RR, Shields MB. Histologic comparison of contact transscleral diode cyclophotocoagulation and endoscopic diode cyclophotocoagulation. *Invest Ophthalmol Vis Sci* 1995;36:4.

Trope GE, Ma S. Mid-term effects of neodynium:YAG transscleral cyclocoagulation in glaucoma. *Ophthalmology* 1990;97:73–75.

Tsai JC, Feuer WJ, Parrish RK III, Grajewski AL. 5-Fluorouracil filtering glaucoma surgery and neovascular glaucoma: long-term follow-up of the original pilot study. *Ophthalmology* 1995;102:887–893.

Uram M. Combined phacoemulsification, endoscopic cyclophotocoagulation, and intraocular lens insertion in glaucoma management. *Ophthalmic Surg* 1995;26: 346–352.

Uram M. Diode laser endocyclodestruction. *Ophthalmic Surg* 1994;25:268–269.

Uram M. Endoscopic cyclophotocoagulation in glaucoma management. *Curr Opin Ophthalmol* 1995;11:19–29.

Uram M. Endoscopic cyclophotocoagulation in glaucoma management: indications, results, and complications. *Ophthalmic Pract* 1995;13:173–185.

Uram M. Endoscopic cyclophotocoagulation in the management of aphakic and pseudophakic glaucoma. ARVO abstract, 1996.

Uram M. Endoscopic cyclophotocoagulation in the management of keratoprosthesis glaucoma *(in press)*.

Uram M. Endoscopic fluorescein angiography. *Ophthalmic Surg Lasers* 1996;27:849–855.

Uram M. Endoscopic fluorescein angiography of the ciliary body in glaucoma management. *Ophthalmic Surg Lasers* 1996;27:174–178.

Uram M. Laser endoscope in the management of proliferative vitreoretinopathy. *Ophthalmology* 1994;101:1404–1408.

Uram M. Ophthalmic laser microendoscope ciliary process ablation in the management of neovascular glaucoma. *Ophthalmology* 1992;99:1823–1828.

Uram M. Ophthalmic laser microendoscope endophotocoagulation. *Ophthalmology* 1992;99:1829–1832.

Uram M. Transcanalicular diode laser dacryocystorhinostomy. Presented at the meeting of the American Society of Cataract and Refractive Surgery, Seattle, WA, June 1–4, 1996.

Uram M. Transscleral Nd:YAG laser cyclodestruction. *Ophthalmic Surg* 1993;24:133.

van der Zypen E, England C, Fankhauser F, et al. The effect of transscleral cyclophotocoagulation on rabbit ciliary body vascularisation. *Graefes Arch Clin Exp Ophthalmol* 1989;227:172–179.

Volkov VV, Danilov AV, Vassin LN, Frolov YA. Flexible endoscope for intraocular surgery. *Arch Ophthalmol* 1990;108:1037–1038.

Volkov VV, Danilov AV, Vassin LN, Frolov YA. Flexible endoscopes: ophthalmoendoscopic techniques and case reports. *Arch Ophthalmol* 1990;108:956–957.

Wallace DK, Plager DA, Snyder SK, et al. Surgical results of secondary glaucomas in childhood. *Ophthalmology* 1998;105:101–111.

Walton DS, Grant WM. Penetrating cyclodiathermy for filtration. *Arch Ophthalmol* 1970;83:47–48.

Weekers R. Effects of photocoagulation of the ciliary body upon ocular tension. *Am J Ophthalmol* 1961;52: 156–163.

Weve H. Die Zyklodiatermie das Corpus ciliare bei Glaukom. *Zentralbl Ophthalmol* 1933;29:562–569.

Wheatcroft S, Singh A, Casey T, McAllister J. Treatment of glaucoma following penetrating keratoplasty with transscleral YAG cyclophotocoagulation. *Int Ophthalmol* 1992;16:397–400.

Wilensky JT, Welch D, Mirolovich M. Transscleral cyclocoagulation using a neodymium:YAG laser. *Ophthalmic Surg* 1985;16:95–99.

Wolner B, Liebmann JM, Sassani JW, et al. Late bleb-related endophthalmitis after trabeculectomy with adjunctive 5-fluorouracil. *Ophthalmology* 1991;98: 1053–1060.

Wong PC, Ruderman JM, Krupin T, et al. 5-Fluorouracil after primary combined filtration surgery. *Am J Ophthalmol* 1994;117:149–154.

Wright MM, Grajewski AL, Feuer WJ. Nd:YAG cyclophotocoagulation: outcome of treatment for uncontrolled glaucoma. *Ophthalmic Surg* 1991;22:279–283.

Yannuzzi LA, Gitter KA, Schatz H. *The macula: a comprehensive text and atlas.* Baltimore: Williams & Wilkins, 1979.

Zarbin MA, Michels RG, de Bustros S, et al. Endolaser treatment of the ciliary body for severe glaucoma. *Ophthalmology* 1988;95:1639–1648.

Zeimer RC, Wilensky JT, Gieser DK, Vianna MA. Association between intraocular pressure peaks and progression of visual field loss. *Ophthalmology* 1991;98:64–69.

Zivojnovic R. *Silicone oil in vitreoretinal surgery.* Dordrecht: Martinus Nijhoff/Dr. W. Junk Publishers, 1987.

SUBJECT INDEX

Page numbers followed by f refer to figures; page numbers followed by t refer to tables.